T0264216

Recent Advances in Management of Heart Failure

Editors

RAGAVENDRA R. BALIGA
UMESH C. SAMAL

HEART FAILURE CLINICS

www.heartfailure.theclinics.com

Consulting Editor
EDUARDO BOSSONE

Founding Editor
JAGAT NARULA

October 2018 • Volume 14 • Number 4

ELSEVIER

1600 John F. Kennedy Boulevard • Suite 1800 • Philadelphia, Pennsylvania, 19103-2899

http://www.theclinics.com

HEART FAILURE CLINICS Volume 14, Number 4
October 2018 ISSN 1551-7136, ISBN-13: 978-0-323-64125-8

Editor: Stacy Eastman
Developmental Editor: Laura Fisher

© **2018 Elsevier Inc. All rights reserved.**

This periodical and the individual contributions contained in it are protected under copyright by Elsevier, and the following terms and conditions apply to their use:

Photocopying
Single photocopies of single articles may be made for personal use as allowed by national copyright laws. Permission of the Publisher and payment of a fee is required for all other photocopying, including multiple or systematic copying, copying for advertising or promotional purposes, resale, and all forms of document delivery. Special rates are available for educational institutions that wish to make photocopies for non-profit educational classroom use. For information on how to seek permission visit www.elsevier.com/permissions or call: (+44) 1865 843830 (UK)/(+1) 215 239 3804 (USA).

Derivative Works
Subscribers may reproduce tables of contents or prepare lists of articles including abstracts for internal circulation within their institutions. Permission of the Publisher is required for resale or distribution outside the institution. Permission of the Publisher is required for all other derivative works, including compilations and translations (please consult www.elsevier.com/permissions).

Electronic Storage or Usage
Permission of the Publisher is required to store or use electronically any material contained in this periodical, including any article or part of an article (please consult www.elsevier.com/permissions). Except as outlined above, no part of this publication may be reproduced, stored in a retrieval system or transmitted in any form or by any means, electronic, mechanical, photocopying, recording or otherwise, without prior written permission of the Publisher.

Notice
No responsibility is assumed by the Publisher for any injury and/or damage to persons or property as a matter of products liability, negligence or otherwise, or from any use or operation of any methods, products, instructions or ideas contained in the material herein. Because of rapid advances in the medical sciences, in particular, independent verification of diagnoses and drug dosages should be made.

Although all advertising material is expected to conform to ethical (medical) standards, inclusion in this publication does not constitute a guarantee or endorsement of the quality or value of such product or of the claims made of it by its manufacturer.

Heart Failure Clinics (ISSN 1551-7136) is published quarterly by Elsevier Inc., 360 Park Avenue South, New York, NY 10010-1710. Months of publication are January, April, July, and October. Business and editorial offices: 1600 John F. Kennedy Boulevard, Suite 1800, Philadelphia, PA 19103-2899. Periodicals postage paid at New York, NY, and additional mailing offices. Subscription prices are USD 252.00 per year for US individuals, USD 471.00 per year for US institutions, USD 100.00 per year for US students and residents, USD 294.00 per year for Canadian individuals, USD 545.00 per year for Canadian institutions, USD 309.00 per year for international individuals, USD 545.00 per year for international institutions, and USD 100.00 per year for Canadian and foreign students/residents. To receive student and resident rate, orders must be accompanied by name of affiliated institution, date of term, and the *signature* of program/residency coordinator on institution letterhead. Orders will be billed at individual rate until proof of status is received. Foreign air speed delivery is included in all *Clinics* subscription prices. All prices are subject to change without notice. **POSTMASTER:** Send address changes to *Heart Failure Clinics*, Elsevier Health Sciences Division, Subscription Customer Service, 3251 Riverport Lane, Maryland Heights, MO 63043. **Customer Service: 1-800-654-2452 (US and Canada). From outside of the US and Canada, call 314-447-8871. Fax: 314-447-8029. For print support, E-mail: JournalsCustomerService-usa@elsevier.com. For online support, E-mail: JournalsOnlineSupport-usa@elsevier.com.**

Reprints. For copies of 100 or more of articles in this publication, please contact the Commercial Reprints Department, Elsevier Inc., 360 Park Avenue South, New York, NY 10010-1710. Tel.: 212-633-3874; Fax: 212-633-3820; E-mail: reprints@elsevier.com.

Heart Failure Clinics is covered in *MEDLINE/PubMed (Index Medicus).*

Contributors

CONSULTING EDITOR

EDUARDO BOSSONE, MD, PhD, FCCP, FESC, FACC
Director, "Cava de' Tirreni and Amalfi Coast,"
Division of Cardiology, Heart Department,
University Hospital, Cardiology Division,
University of Salerno, Salerno, Italy

EDITORS

RAGAVENDRA R. BALIGA, MD, MBA, FACP, FRCP, FACC
Inaugural Director, Cardio-Oncology Center of
Excellence, Associate Director, Division of
Cardiovascular Medicine, Professor of Internal
Medicine, The Ohio State University Wexner
Medical Center, Columbus, Ohio, USA

UMESH C. SAMAL, MD, FACC, FISE, FIAE, FIACM
Ex-Professor of Cardiology and Professor of
Internal Medicine, PMCH, Patna, India;
National Convener, Heart Failure Council
(Subspecialty), Cardiological Society of India,
India

AUTHORS

UMAIR AHMAD, MD
Department of Cardiology, The Ohio State
University Wexner Medical Center, Columbus,
Ohio, USA

NATASHA L. ALTMAN, MD
Section of Advanced Heart Failure and
Transplant, Division of Cardiology, Assistant
Professor, Department of Medicine, University
of Colorado Denver, Aurora, Colorado, USA

MICHELE ARCOPINTO, MD
Department of Translational Medical Sciences,
Federico II University, Naples, Italy

RAGAVENDRA R. BALIGA, MD, MBA, FACP, FRCP, FACC
Inaugural Director, Cardio-Oncology Center of
Excellence, Associate Director, Division of
Cardiovascular Medicine, Professor of Internal
Medicine, The Ohio State University Wexner
Medical Center, Columbus, Ohio, USA

EDUARDO BOSSONE, MD, PhD, FCCP, FESC, FACC
Director, "Cava de' Tirreni and Amalfi Coast,"
Division of Cardiology, Heart Department,
University Hospital, Cardiology Division,
University of Salerno, Salerno,
Italy

ELISA BRADLEY, MD
Assistant Professor of Internal Medicine,
Department of Physiology and Cell Biology,
The Ohio State University, Nationwide
Children's Hospital, Davis Heart and
Lung Research Institute, Columbus, Ohio,
USA

OMER CAVUS, MD
Research Assistant, Department of Physiology
and Cell Biology, Davis Heart and Lung
Research Institute, The Ohio State University,
Columbus, Ohio, USA

ANTONIO CITTADINI, MD
Interdisciplinary Research Centre in
Biomedical Materials, Department of
Translational Medical Sciences, Federico II
University, School of Medicine, Naples,
Italy

JUAN A. CRESTANELLO, MD
Senior Associate Consultant, Department of
Cardiovascular Surgery, Mayo Clinic,
Rochester, Minnesota, USA

ROBERTA D'ASSANTE, PhD
IRCCS SDN, Naples, Italy

ANITA DESWAL, MD, MPH
Professor of Medicine, Baylor College of
Medicine, Chief, Cardiology, Michael E. DeBakey
VA Medical Center, Houston, Texas, USA

KATHERINE DODD, DO, MPH
Cardiovascular Fellow, Division of
Cardiovascular Medicine, The Ohio State
University, Columbus, Ohio, USA

SITARAMESH EMANI, MD
Section of Advanced Heart Failure and Cardiac
Transplant, The Ohio State University Wexner
Medical Center, Columbus, Ohio, USA

VERONICA FRANCO, MD, MSPH
Associate Professor of Clinical Medicine,
Division of Cardiovascular Disease;
Co-Director Pulmonary Hypertension
Program, Advanced Heart Failure, LVAD
and Transplantation Program, The Ohio
State University, Columbus, Ohio,
USA

MAHAZARIN GINWALLA, MD, MS, FACC
Assistant Professor, Division of Cardiovascular
Medicine, Harrington Heart & Vascular
Institute, University Hospitals Cleveland
Medical Center, Cleveland, Ohio,
USA

CHRISTOPHER M. HRITZ, MD
Assistant Professor-Clinical, The Ohio State
University Wexner Medical Center, Columbus,
Ohio, USA

AHMET KILIC, MD
Division of Cardiac Surgery, Department of
Surgery, The Johns Hopkins Hospital,
Baltimore, Maryland, USA

ARMAN KILIC, MD
Division of Cardiac Surgery, Department of
Cardiothoracic Surgery, UPMC Heart and
Vascular Institute, University of Pittsburgh
Medical Center, Pittsburgh, Pennsylvania,
USA

BHAVANA KONDA, MD, MPH
Division of Medical Oncology, Assistant
Professor, Department of Internal Medicine,
The Ohio State University, Columbus, Ohio,
USA

BRENT C. LAMPERT, DO, FACC
Associate Professor of Clinical Medicine,
Division of Cardiovascular Medicine, The
Ohio State University, Heart Failure and
Transplantation, The Ohio State University
Wexner Medical Center, Columbus, Ohio,
USA

DANIEL J. LENIHAN, MD, FACC
Division of Cardiovascular Diseases,
Professor, Department of Internal Medicine,
Washington University in St. Louis, St Louis,
Missouri, USA

SCOTT M. LILLY, MD, PhD
Associate Professor, Department of
Cardiology, The Ohio State University Wexner
Medical Center, Interventional Cardiology,
Columbus, Ohio, USA

ALBERTO M. MARRA, MD
IRCCS SDN, Naples, Italy

AJITH NAIR, MD
Assistant Professor, Department of Medicine,
Section of Cardiology, Baylor College of
Medicine, Houston, Texas, USA

AMIT PATEL, MD
Advanced Heart Failure and Cardiac
Transplantation, St. Vincent Medical Group,
Indianapolis, Indiana, USA

AARTHI SABANAYAGAM, MD
Assistant Professor of Internal Medicine,
The Ohio State University, Nationwide
Children's Hospital, Davis Heart and Lung
Research Institute, Columbus, Ohio,
USA

ANDREA SALZANO, MD
Department of Translational Medical Sciences, Federico II University, Naples, Italy; Department of Cardiovascular Sciences, University of Leicester, Glenfield Hospital, Leicester, United Kingdom

IBRAHIM SULTAN, MD
Division of Cardiac Surgery, Department of Cardiothoracic Surgery, UPMC Heart and Vascular Institute, University of Pittsburgh Medical Center, Pittsburgh, Pennsylvania, USA

VARUN SUNDARAM, MD, FRCP
Assistant Professor, Department of Cardiology, Royal Brompton Hospital, Royal Brompton and Harefield NHS Foundation Trust, Royal Brompton Hospital and National Heart and Lung Institute, Imperial College London, London, United Kingdom; Case Western Reserve University School of Medicine, Cleveland, Ohio, USA

TORU SUZUKI, MD, PhD
Department of Translational Medical Sciences, Federico II University, Naples, Italy

DAVID S. TOFOVIC, MD
Department of Medicine, University Hospitals Cleveland Medical Center, Cleveland, Ohio, USA

AJAY VALLAKATI, MD, MPH
Division of Cardiovascular Diseases, Assistant Professor, Department of Internal Medicine, The Ohio State University, Columbus, Ohio, USA

ALI VAZIR, MBBS, PhD, FESC, FRCP
Consultant Cardiologist and Honorary Clinical Senior Lecturer, Department of Cardiology, Royal Brompton Hospital, Royal Brompton and Harefield NHS Foundation Trust, Consultant Cardiologist, Honorary Clinical Senior Lecturer, Royal Brompton Hospital and National Heart and Lung Institute, Imperial College London, London, United Kingdom

JORDAN WILLIAMS, BS
Research Assistant, Department of Physiology and Cell Biology, Davis Heart and Lung Research Institute, The Ohio State University, Columbus, Ohio, USA

Contents

> The burden of heart failure is projected to increase over the next decade; it is predicted that 1 in every 33 Americans will be affected by heart failure. Given that heart failure currently results in more than 1 million hospitalizations every year and the estimated 5-year mortality is approximately 50%, therapies that will improve survival and the economic burden are urgently needed. It is anticipated that the cost of managing heart failure is going to be approximately $70 billion in 2030. Therefore, the recent addition of the combination of sacubitril/valsartan (LCZ696) to guideline-directed medical therapies should ameliorate this burden.

> Heart failure affects more than 6 million people in the United States each year, and the prognosis is poor. The elevated heart rate in patients with heart failure is problematic, because it increases myocardial oxygen demand, decreases myocardial perfusion, and has been associated with increased rates of hospitalization and mortality. For these reasons, heart rate reduction has long been a therapeutic target in heart failure. Ivabradine is a selective inhibitor of the sinoatrial pacemaker modulating "f-current" (I_f) and provides heart rate reduction that can be beneficial in patients with heart failure with reduced ejection fraction.

> Several studies have shown that growth hormone (GH) deficiency is common in chronic heart failure and is associated with impaired functional capacity and poor outcomes. Data derived from animal models showed beneficial effects of GH treatment on peripheral vascular resistance, cardiac function, and survival. Despite this solid background, when translated onto the clinical field, these results did not lead to unequivocal results. This article focuses on the assessment of GH deficiency in chronic heart failure, the underlying molecular background, the impact on disease progression and outcomes, the effects of GH therapy, and the novel and more encouraging approach of GH-replacement therapy.

> Ultrafiltration (UF) mechanically removes excess fluid volume through an extracorporeal circuit and has been applied to clinical situations in which volume removal is the mainstay of therapy. Because of this ability, UF serves as an enticing method to treat acute heart failure (AHF) in which most symptoms are driven by

congestion due to excess volume. Additional physiologic properties of UF and the biochemical composition of the extracted fluid confer additional theoretic benefits in the treatment of AHF. Herein the concepts underlying UF, clinical evidence evaluating its efficacy, and ongoing challenges understanding the role of UF are reviewed.

More than 50% of patients with clinical heart failure have a preserved ejection fraction. Despite mortality that is similar to or slightly lower than heart failure with reduced ejection fraction, trials to date have not shown a therapy that imparts a mortality benefit in heart failure with preserved ejection fraction (HFpEF). HFpEF represents a heterogeneous disorder with a complex pathophysiologic basis, and this may contribute to the negative results in clinical trials. Geographic variations in both patient selection and adherence to study medications confound the interpretation of the trial results. Mineralocorticoid receptor antagonists may be useful in selected patients.

Iron deficiency anemia is both a comorbid condition and an indicator of poor prognosis in heart failure. The mechanisms by which this occurs are multiple and complex. Recent robust randomized clinical trials have shown significant improvements in quality of life and rates of hospitalization with intravenous repletion of iron. In this article, the authors review the mechanisms by which iron deficiency affects heart failure and the evidence behind repletion. There remains a good deal to learn about long-term effects of intravenous iron repletion, and clinical trials are ongoing in this regard.

Pulmonary hypertension (PH) due to left heart disease, or WHO group 2 PH, is the most frequent cause of PH. It affects approximately 50% to 60% of patients with heart failure with preserved ejection fraction as well as 60% of those with heart failure with reduced ejection fraction and contributes significantly to disease progression and unfavorable outcomes. The diagnosis of PH is associated with poor prognosis and significant morbidity and mortality.

Improvements in detection and treatment of cancer have resulted in a significant increase in cancer survivors. However, cancer survivorship comes with long-term risk of adverse effects of cancer therapies, including cardiomyopathy, heart failure, arrhythmias, ischemic heart disease, atherosclerosis, thrombosis, and hypertension. There is a renewed interest in understanding the pathophysiology of cancer therapeutics–related cardiac dysfunction. In recent years, efforts have been directed to the management of cancer therapeutics–related cardiac dysfunction. This article discusses the pathophysiology and molecular mechanisms that contribute to cancer therapeutics–related cardiac dysfunction and presents an approach to the evaluation and treatment of these patients.

There are more than 1 million adults with congenital heart disease (ACHD) in the United States. Heart failure (HF) is the most common late cardiovascular complication. These patients are challenging to manage given their diverse presentation, anatomy, and complex hemodynamics. Examination of the underlying anatomy is crucial because many require late transcatheter and surgical interventions after developing HF. Management of arrhythmia is equally important because this can modify HF symptoms. A multidisciplinary team with expertise in the care of ACHD-HF is critical.

Severe right ventricular (RV) failure is a significant cause of morbidity and mortality, with an in-hospital mortality rate up to 70% to 75%. Medical management is employed and is successful for most of these patients. However, a small percentage of patients will continue to have persistent RV failure, for which mechanical support is used for management.

Mitral valve diseases are common causes of congestive heart failure. Chronic primary and secondary (functional) mitral valve regurgitation are the most common reasons. Valve repair for primary mitral regurgitation cures mitral valve disease, whereas in functional regurgitation, mitral valve repair is associated with high failure rates secondary to persistent/progressive ventricular dysfunction and remodeling. Most patients are managed with strict adherence to the valve guidelines. Mitral valve replacement has an increased role in the management of functional mitral regurgitation. Surgery for mitral valve disease is indicated in symptomatic patients with severe valve disease and in asymptotic patients before irreversible ventricular damage occurs.

Inotropes are medications that improve the contractility of the heart and are used in patients with low cardiac output or evidence of end-organ dysfunction. Since their initial discovery, inotropes have held promise in alleviating symptoms and potentially increasing longevity in such patients. Decades of intensive study have further elucidated the benefits and risks of using inotropes. In this article, the authors discuss the history of inotropes, their indications, mechanism of action, and current guidelines pertaining to their use in heart failure. The authors provide insight into their appropriate use and related shortcomings and the practical aspects of inotrope use.

Cardiac palliative care is a multidisciplinary approach provided alongside standard heart failure management to improve a patient's quality of life. In this article the authors review the role of palliative care in heart failure management, including recent studies exploring the benefits of palliative care consultation in the inpatient and outpatient setting. They also discuss approaches to goals-of-care discussions and challenges providing end-of-life care in this patient population.

Convergence of the fields of heart failure (HF) and interventional cardiology has led to the formation of a discipline referred to as interventional HF. Although the term may be applied to essentially any invasive procedure performed in patients with HF (eg, coronary angiography, percutaneous coronary intervention, invasive assessment of hemodynamics), it is more commonly reserved for the application of invasive diagnostic or therapeutic procedures to improve the clinical decision-making, functional status, and outcomes of patients with HF. This article reviews developing modalities.

Sleep-disordered breathing (SDB) is highly prevalent in heart failure (HF). The presence of SDB in patients with HF appears to be associated with an increased risk of cardiovascular morbidity and mortality. In this article, the authors describe the types, pathophysiology, and consequences of SDB and discuss ways in which SDB can be diagnosed. They also lay emphasis on the recent randomized controlled trials that have had a major impact on how SDB is managed and highlight the complex relationship between SDB and outcomes.

HEART FAILURE CLINICS

SERIES OF RELATED INTEREST

Cardiology Clinics
http://www.cardiology.theclinics.com/

THE CLINICS ARE AVAILABLE ONLINE!
Access your subscription at:
www.theclinics.com

Preface

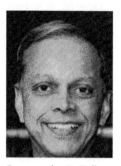

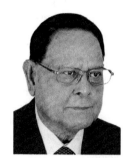

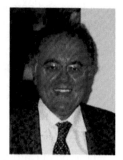

Ragavendra R. Baliga,
MD, MBA, FACP, FRCP, FACC

Umesh C. Samal, MD, FACC, FISE,
FIAE, FIACM

Eduardo Bossone, MD, PhD,
FCCP, FESC, FACC

Editors

The burden of heart failure is projected to increase over the next decade, and it is predicted that 1 in every 33 Americans will be affected by heart failure.[1] Given that heart failure currently results in over 1 million hospitalizations every year and the estimated 5-year mortality is approximately 50%, therapies that will improve survival and economic burden are urgently needed.[2] It is anticipated that the cost of managing heart failure will be approximately $70 billion in 2030.[3]

Keeping this in mind, we have put together this issue of *Heart Failure Clinics* with a focus on recent advances in the management of heart failure. The topics have focused on management of the patient with clinical heart failure, and the contributors are international experts in the field. The management of heart failure spans multiple dimensions,[4] including newer pharmacologic agents, utilization of a wide variety of devices, including ultrafiltration,[5] ventricular assist devices, and extracorporeal membrane oxygenation, newer noninvasive methods of hemodynamic monitoring,[6] surgical management of heart valves deficits, management of accompanying comorbidities, such as sleep apnea, and utilization of palliative care options, including continuous ambulatory inotropic therapy. These topics have been discussed by experts in the field with day-to-day experience in utilizing these options, and therefore, this issue should be a valuable resource to those who are actively involved in the management of heart failure.

However, we do realize that management of heart failure includes management of subclinical disease (including asymptomatic left ventricular dysfunction, management of endothelial dysfunction, autonomic dysfunction, myocardial ischemia, including vulnerable plaque and cardiac arrhythmia) and primordial prevention. The latter includes management of both traditional risk factors (including age, gender, family history, smoking, hypertension, dyslipidemia, diabetes, sedentary lifestyle, and obesity) and nontraditional risk factors (including air pollution, psychosocial stressors, and so forth).

It is well recognized that even passive exposure to tobacco or air pollution has persistent vascular consequences, including mobilization of dysfunctional endothelial progenitor cells that have impaired nitric oxide production.[7] Therefore, some of the future advances in the management of heart failure will require continued efforts to tobacco control and containment of air pollution. Considerable data strongly support the role of lifestyle interventions to improve glucose and insulin homeostasis—both increased physical activity and decreased calorie intake, particularly carbohydrate intake, should reduce the burden of diabetes mellitus, which in turn translates into reduction of major coronary events and consequent heart failure. An escalating body of evidence suggests that psychosocial risk factors, such as depression,[8] may exacerbate the development of heart failure, and together with associated unhealthy behaviors, may result in worsening myocardial ischemia and life-threatening ventricular arrhythmias. Therefore, management of psychosocial factors, behavioral interventions, and complementary preventive strategies should delay the onset or prevent overt heart failure.

Heart Failure Clin 14 (2018) xiii–xiv
https://doi.org/10.1016/j.hfc.2018.08.014
1551-7136/18/© 2018 Published by Elsevier Inc.

We hope that this issue of *Heart Failure Clinics* will serve as a stimulus for the reader to pursue changing paradigms and perceptions in the management of heart failure in their day-to-day clinical practice. And the topics in this issue should also provide a nidus for leaders in the field of heart failure to reflect on current concepts and knowledge and propose new clinical and preclinical studies to reduce dismal mortality in heart failure.

Ragavendra R. Baliga, MD, MBA, FACP,
FRCP, FACC
Division of Cardiovascular Medicine
The Ohio State University
Wexner Medical Center
200 Davis Heart and Lung Research Institute
473 West 12th Avenue
Columbus, OH 43210-1252, USA

Umesh C. Samal, MD, FACC, FISE, FIAE, FIACM
Internal Medicine
PMCH, Patna, India

Eduardo Bossone, MD, PhD, FCCP, FESC, FACC
Cardiology Division
"Cava de' Tirreni and Amalfi Coast" Hospital
Cardiothoracic and Vascular Department-
University Hospital, Salerno, Italy

Via Pr. Amedeo, 36
Lauro, Avellino 83023, Italy

E-mail addresses:
rrbaliga@gmail.com (R.R. Baliga)
drsamal.hffi@gmail.com (U.C. Samal)
ebossone@hotmail.com (E. Bossone)

REFERENCES

1. Benjamin EJ, Blaha MJ, Chiuve SE, et al. Heart disease and stroke statistics—2017 update: a report from the American Heart Association. Circulation 2017;135(10):e146–603.
2. Ponikowski P, Voors AA, Anker SD, et al. 2016 ESC guidelines for the diagnosis and treatment of acute and chronic heart failure: the task force for the diagnosis and treatment of acute and chronic heart failure of the European Society of Cardiology (ESC) developed with the special contribution of the Heart Failure Association (HFA) of the ESC. Eur Heart J 2016; 37(27):2129–200.
3. Heidenreich PA, Albert NM, Allen LA, et al. Forecasting the impact of heart failure in the United States: a policy statement from the American Heart Association. Circ Heart Fail 2013;6(3):606–19.
4. Baliga RR, Young JB. Clinical trials to "real-world" heart failure: applying risk stratification to deliver personalized care. Heart Fail Clin 2011;7(4):xi–xiv.
5. Haas GJ, Pestritto VM, Abraham WT. Ultrafiltration for volume control in decompensated heart failure. Heart Fail Clin 2008;4(4):519–34.
6. Baliga RR, Young JB. Editorial: bench to bedside to home: homing-in on therapy that begins at home. Heart Fail Clin 2009;5(2):xiii–xiv.
7. Heiss C, Amabile N, Lee AC, et al. Brief secondhand smoke exposure depresses endothelial progenitor cells activity and endothelial function: sustained vascular injury and blunted nitric oxide production. J Am Coll Cardiol 2008;51(18):1760–71.
8. Baliga RR, Young JB. Editorial: depression in heart failure is double trouble: warding off the blues requires early screening. Heart Fail Clin 2011;7(1):xiii–xvii.

Sacubitril/Valsartan
The Newest Neurohormonal Blocker for Guideline-Directed Medical Therapy for Heart Failure

Ragavendra R. Baliga, MD, MBA, FRCP, FACC

KEYWORDS

- Sacubitril • Valsartan • Neurohormonal blocker • Heart failure

KEY POINTS

- The burden of heart failure is projected to increase over the next decade, and it is predicted that 1 in every 33 Americans will be affected by heart failure.
- The recent addition of the combination of sacubitril/valsartan (LCZ696) to guideline-directed medical therapies should ameliorate this burden.
- Neprilysin inhibition is associated with significant improvements in survival.
- Despite substantial reductions in mortality with neprilysin inhibition, the mortality rate among patients with heart failure remains high around 20% over 2 years in the intervention arm of Prospective comparison of ARNi with ACEi to Determine Impact on Global Mortaility and morbidity in Heart Failure (PARADIGM_HF) suggesting that opportunities to reduce mortality in heart failure remain.

INTRODUCTION

The burden of heart failure is projected to increase over the next decade, and it is predicted that 1 in every 33 Americans will be affected by heart failure.[1] Given that heart failure currently results in more than 1 million hospitalizations every year and the estimated 5-year mortality is approximately 50%, therapies that will improve survival and the economic burden are urgently needed. It is anticipated that the cost of managing heart failure is going to be approximately $70 billion in 2030.[2] Therefore, the recent addition of the combination of sacubitril/valsartan (LCZ696) to guideline-directed medical therapies should ameliorate this burden.

PHARMACOLOGY

Sacubitril, a prodrug, is an inhibitor of neprilysin, a neutral endopeptidase, that is responsible for degradation of biologically active vasoactive peptides, including natriuretic peptides (brain natriuretic peptide [BNP] and N-terminal [NT]-proBNP) and bradykinin (**Figs. 1** and **2**). ProBNPs convert into NT-proBNP and BNP. BNP acts by natriuresis, diuresis, vasodilatation, antiproliferative vascular effects, and decreased sympathetic tone. Degradation of BNP into breakdown products is inhibited neprilysin resulting in an increase in natriuretic peptides, including BNP, which have vasodilator properties, facilitate sodium excretion, and most likely have effects on cardiac remodeling. Therefore, when patients are on neprilysin inhibitors, BNP cannot be used to monitor therapy; in fact, NT-proBNP is a biomarker of choice in patients on neprilysin inhibition.

NEUROHORMONAL BLOCKADE

The Metoprolol CR/XL Randomised Intervention Trial in Congestive Heart Failure (MERIT-HF[3])

Disclosure: The author has nothing to disclose.

Division of Cardiovascular Medicine, The Ohio State University Wexner Medical Center, 200 Davis Heart and Lung Research Institute (HLRI), 473 West 12th Avenue, Columbus, OH 43210-1252, USA
E-mail address: rrbaliga@gmail.com

Heart Failure Clin 14 (2018) 479–491
https://doi.org/10.1016/j.hfc.2018.06.012
1551-7136/18/© 2018 Elsevier Inc. All rights reserved.

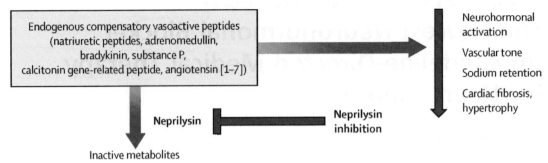

Fig. 1. The actions of vasoactive peptides in heart failure. Many endogenous compensatory vasoactive peptides act to antagonize the maladaptive mechanisms of heart failure (neurohormonal activation, vascular tone, sodium retention, and cardiac hypertrophy and fibrosis). Because these peptides are degraded by a common enzyme (neprilysin), their favorable actions are enhanced when a neprilysin inhibitor is included as part of the neurohormonal inhibitory strategy used to treat chronic heart failure. (*From* Packer M, McMurray JJV. Importance of endogenous compensatory vasoactive peptides in broadening the effects of inhibitors of the renin-angiotensin system for the treatment of heart failure. Lancet 2017;389:1832; with permission.)

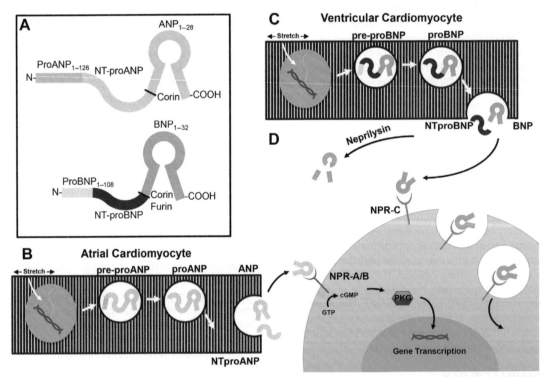

Fig. 2. Atrial natriuretic peptide (ANP) and BNP physiology. (*A*) Molecular structure of ANP (*top*) and BNP (*bottom*) showing enzymatic cleavage sites and end-product fragments. (*B*) Production and processing of ANP by atrial cardiac myocyte in response to mechanical stretch stimulus. (*C*) Production and processing of BNP by ventricular cardiac myocyte in response to mechanical stimulus. (*D*) Effects of ANP and BNP on target tissues. Both ANP and BNP bind natriuretic peptide receptor (NPR)A and NPR-B on target cells, inducing cleavage of guanosine triphosphate (GTP) to cyclic guanosine monophosphate (cGMP) by cytoplasmic G proteins, initiating an intracellular cGMP signaling cascade involving protein kinase G (PKG), ultimately leading to downstream transcription of genes involving smooth muscle cell relaxation, diuresis, and natriuresis (depending on target tissue). Both ANP and BNP are broken down in serum by circulating endogenous peptidases, including neprilysin. ANP and BNP are also degraded (to a lesser extent) by cellular uptake through binding NPR-C, undergoing receptor-mediated endocytosis and intracellular breakdown by lysosomes. (*From* Maisel AS, Duran JM, Wettersten N. Natriuretic peptides in heart failure. Heart Fail Clin 2018;14:15; with permission.)

showed that more patients in New York Heart Association (NYHA) class 2 and class 3 die of sudden death (**Fig. 3**). In NYHA class 2, 64% died of sudden death; in NYHA class 3, 59% died of sudden death; in class 2 only 12% died of systolic heart failure; in class 3 only 26% died of pump function or heart failure. In NYHA class 4, 56% died of loss of pump function or heart failure; only 33% died of sudden death in NYHA class 4 heart failure. Traditional inhibitors of the renin-angiotensin system, even under optimal conditions, lead only to a small relative reduction that is 5% to 18% (**Table 1**), compared with placebo, in reducing the risk of cardiovascular death in patients with chronic heart failure and heart failure with reduced ejection fraction[4–8]; clinical trials have struggled to identify a favorable effect of these drugs on the symptoms or quality of life.[9–12] So the survival benefit of angiotensin-converting enzyme (ACE) inhibitors and angiotensin receptor blockers (ARBs) is relatively small, and there is a tremendous opportunity to improve survival in patients with heart failure with reduced ejection fraction.

There were 4 early clinical trials investigating the role of neprilysin inhibition in hypertension and/or heart failure. Ruilope and colleagues[13] studied 1328 patients with hypertension in a randomized controlled dose ranging study. The primary end point was reduction in blood pressure between groups at 8 weeks. The main findings of this study (**Fig. 4**) were a significant reduction in systolic and diastolic blood pressure with neprilysin inhibitor 200 mg versus valsartan 160 mg, and there was a significant reduction in ambulatory blood pressure with neprilysin compared with valsartan.[13] In a randomized controlled dose ranging trial reported by Kario and colleagues,[14] which was studied in 389 Asians with hypertension, neprilysin inhibition showed significant reduction in systolic and diastolic blood pressures. The Prospective comparison of ARNI [angiotensin receptor neprilysin inhibitor] with ARB on Management Of heart failUre with preserved ejectioN fraction trial (PARAMOUNT)[15] studied 301 patients with heart failure with preserved ejection fraction; Solomon and colleagues[15] compared neprilysin inhibitor LCZ696 200 mg twice a day with valsartan 160 mg twice a day. This trial was a randomized controlled trial whereby the primary end point was a reduction in NT-proBNP at 12 weeks. The main findings were a significant reduction in NT-proBNP at 12 weeks with neprilysin inhibitor LCZ696 as well as a reduction in the left atrial volume at 36 weeks. There was an improvement in NYHA class in patients receiving LCZ696 when compared to the placebo.

These findings prompted the investigators to conduct the PARADIGM-HF[16] heart failure trial reported by McMurray and colleagues,[16] which studied 8442 patients with systolic heart failure. This randomized controlled trial compared LCZ696 200 mg twice a day with enalapril 10 mg twice a day. The primary outcome was cardiovascular mortality or heart failure hospitalization. Although the primary end point was cardiovascular death or hospitalization for heart failure, the study was designed as a cardiovascular mortality trial. The sample size of the trial, therefore, was determined by the effect on cardiovascular mortality and not the primary end point. In the PARADIGM-HF study, the inclusion criteria included chronic heart failure NYHA class 2 to 4

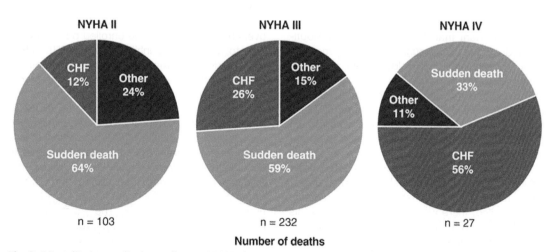

Fig. 3. Mortality in systolic depending on NYHA class. CHF, congestive heart failure. (*From* MERIT-HF Study Group. Effect of metoprolol CR/XL in chronic heart failure: Metoprolol CR/XL Randomised Intervention Trial in Congestive Heart Failure (MERIT-HF). Lancet 1999;353(9169):2005; with permission.)

Table 1
Number need to treat for mortality

Guideline Recommended Therapy	Relative Risk Reduction in Mortality (%)	Number Needed to Treat for Mortality	Number Needed to Treat for Mortality (Standardized to 36 mo)	Relative Risk Reduction in HF Hospitalizations (%)
ACEI/ARB	17	22 over 42 mo	26	31
Beta-blocker	34	28 over 12 mo	9	41
Aldosterone antagonist	30	9 over 24 mo	6	35
Hydralazine/nitrate	43	25 over 10 mo	7	33
CRT	36	12 over 24 mo	8	52
ICD	23	14 over 60 mo	23	NA
ARNI	16	36 over 27 mo	27	21

Benefit of angiotensin receptor neprilysin inhibitor therapy incremental to that achieved with ACE inhibitor therapy. For the other medications shown, the benefits are based on comparisons with placebo control.

Abbreviations: ACEI, angiotensin-converting enzyme inhibitor; ARB, angiotensin receptor blocker; ARNI, angiotensin receptor neprilysin inhibitor; CRT, cardiac resynchronization therapy; ICD, implantable cardioverter-defibrillator; NNT, number needed to treat.

Modified from Baliga RR, Dec GW, Narula J. Practice guidelines for the diagnosis and management of systolic heart failure in low- and middle-income countries. Glob Heart 2013;8(2):159; and Fonarow GC, Yancy CW, Hernandez AF, et al. Potential impact of optimal implementation of evidence-based heart failure therapies on mortality. Am Heart J 2011;161(6):1026; with permission.

with a left ventricular ejection fraction of 40% or less (see **Table 1**). It was then amended to less than 35% 1 year after the study was started. In addition to a reduction in ejection fraction, patients had to have a serum BNP of 150 pg/mL or greater or an NT-proBNP of 600 or greater or they had to have a BNP of 100 pg/mL or greater or an NT-proBNP of 400 or greater with heart failure hospitalization in the last 12 months. The patients needed to be stable on an ACE inhibitor or an ARB with the dose greater than or equal to 10 mg/dL of enalapril for at least 4 weeks. The patients were expected to be on beta-blocker therapy for 4 weeks unless it was not tolerated; it was important that the patients were on optimized dosing of background heart failure medications, particularly mineralocorticoid receptor antagonists. The key exclusion criteria were a history of angioedema, an estimated glomerular filtration rate (eGFR) less than 30 mL/min per 1.73 m^2 body surface area, a serum potassium greater than 5.2 mmol/L, symptomatic hypotension with a systolic blood pressure less than 100 mm Hg, and acutely decompensated heart failure. The study design first involved a single-blind run-in period wherein 10,000 patients were enrolled; there was a 19.7% attrition of this cohort, and more than 8000 were randomized. For the first 2 weeks, all patients were started on enalapril 10 mg twice a day, and then they were randomized to 2 arms; in the first arm the patients were on LCZ696, and in the second arm they

continued on enalapril. If they tolerated the enalapril or the LCZ696, they were then randomized to a double-blind period. During the single-blind run-in period, the dosage of LCZ696 was 100 mg twice a day for the first 2 weeks and then was increased to 200 mg twice a day after 2 weeks. In the double-blind period of the study, 8399 patients were enrolled. They were randomized 1:1 to sacubitril and valsartan 97 and 103 mg twice a day, respectively, or they were randomized to enalapril 10 mg twice a day. The median follow-up was 27 months for the study because the Data Safety Monitoring Board recommended that the trial be stopped early because of the overwhelming benefit. The enrolled patients were able to tolerate ACE inhibitors and ARBs before they randomized these patients to the double-blind period. When they enrolled in the study, they found that the predictors for noncompletion were a lower eGFR, a higher NT-proBNP, lower systolic blood pressure, and ischemic causes of heart failure.[17] The proportion of patients who withdrew from the study because of adverse events were actually higher during the enalapril run-in period than during the LCZ696 run-in period after adjustment for the longer duration of LCZ696 exposure. The most common causes for withdrawal from the study during the run-in period were hypotension, cough, hyperkalemia, and renal dysfunction. During the run-in period, 8 patients did not take enalapril and took only LCZ696.

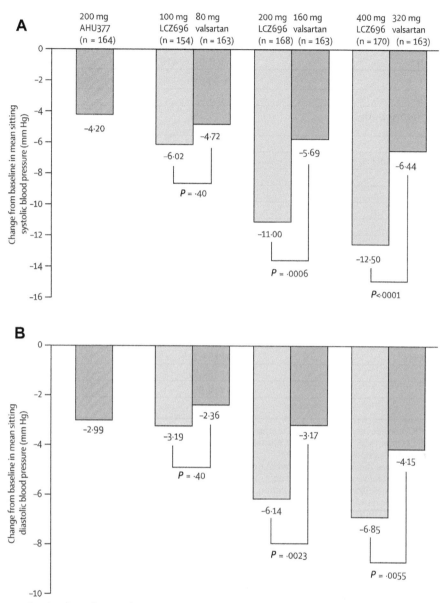

Fig. 4. Change in placebo-subtracted mean sitting systolic blood pressure (*A*) and mean sitting diastolic blood pressure (*B*) during the 8-week treatment period. Patients who discontinued the study drug without a blood pressure measurement after randomization were excluded. (*From* Ruilope LM, Dukat A, Bohm M, et al. Blood-pressure reduction with LCZ696, a novel dual-acting inhibitor of the angiotensin II receptor and neprilysin: a randomised, double-blind, placebo-controlled, active comparator study. Lancet 2010;375(9722):1259; with permission.)

What were the baseline characteristics of patients in the PARADIGM-HF (**Table 2**)? The mean age was about 63.8 years ±11.5. The baseline characteristics in both groups were very similar: about 21% to 22% were women, and about 59% to 60% had ischemic cardiomyopathy. The mean left ventricular ejection fraction was 29.6 ±6.1; 69% to 71% had NYHA 2 functional class; and 23% to 24% had NYHA class 3 heart failure. The mean systolic blood pressure was 122 mm Hg ±15 , and the mean heart rate was 72 beats per minute ±12. The mean NT-proBNP was between 1594 and 1631 in both groups. Approximately a third of the patients were diabetic, 80% were on diuretics, 29% to 30% were on digitalis, 92% to 93% were on beta-blockers, 54% to 57% were on mineralocorticoid receptor antagonists, 14.9% to 14.7% were on implantable

Table 2
PARADIGM–HF baseline characteristics

Characteristic*	Sac/Val (N = 4187)	Enalapril (N = 4212)
Age (y)	63.8 ±11.5	63.8 ±11.3
Female, n (%)	879 (21.0)	953 (22.6)
Ischemic cardiomyopathy, n (%)	2506 (59.9)	2530 (60.1)
LVEF (%)	29.6 ±6.1	29.4 ±6.3
NYHA functional class, n (%)		
II	2998 (71.6)	2921 (69.3)
III	969 (23.1)	1049 (24.9)
SBP (mm Hg)	122 ±15	121 ±15
Heart rate (bpm)	72 ±12	73 ±12
NT-proBNP, median, pg/mL (IQR)	1631 (885–3154)	1594 (886–3305)
BNP, median, pg/mL (IQR)	255 (155–474)	251 (153–465)
History of DM, n (%)	1451 (34.7)	1456 (34.6)
Treatments at randomization, n (%)		
Diuretics	3363 (80.3)	3375 (80.1)
Digitalis	1223 (29.2)	1316 (31.2)
Beta-blockers	3899 (93.1)	3912 (92.9)
MRAs	2271 (54.2)	2400 (57.0)
ICD	623 (14.9)	620 (14.7)
CRT	292 (7.0)	282 (6.7)

Abbreviations: CRT, cardiac resynchronization therapy; DM, diabetes mellitus; ICD, implantable cardioverter-defibrillator; IQR, interquartile range; LVEF, left ventricular ejection fraction; MRAs, mineralocorticoid receptor antagonists; Sac/Val, sacubitril/valsartan; SBP, systolic blood pressure.

* Plus–minus values are means ±SD. There were no significant differences between the two groups except for the use of digitalis ($P =.04$) and mineralocorticoid-receptor antagonists ($P =.01$), with values not adjusted for multiple testing. Percentages may not total 100 because of rounding.

From McMurray JJ, Packer M, Desai AS, et al. Angiotensin-neprilysin inhibition versus enalapril in heart failure. N Engl J Med 2014;371(11):996–7; with permission.

cardioverter-defibrillators (ICDs), and about 7% were on cardiac resynchronization therapy.

The PARADIGM-HF study was a prospective comparison of ARNIs with ACE inhibitors to determine the impact on total mortality and morbidity.[16] The investigators found an overwhelming benefit with respect to the primary composite outcome of cardiovascular death or hospitalization (hazard ratio [HR] 0.8 $P<.00001$). There was a 20% reduction of cardiovascular mortality ($P = .001$), 16% reduction on overall mortality, and a 21% risk reduction in heart failure hospitalizations ($P = .001$) with LCZ696 when compared with enalapril (**Fig. 5**, **Table 3**). There were 914 deaths in the LCZ696 arm and 1117 in the enalapril arm, with an HR of 0.8 ($P = .001$). There were 558 deaths due to cardiovascular causes with LCZ696 and 693 deaths with the enalapril with a HR of 0.8 ($P<.001$). Of the secondary outcomes, there was a significant reduction in all-cause mortality: 835 deaths in the enalapril arm and 711

deaths in the LCZ696 arm (HR 0.84, $P = .001$). Most deaths were cardiovascular (80.9%), and the risk of cardiovascular death was significantly reduced by treatment with LCZ696 (HR 0.80, 95% confidence interval [CI] 0.72–0.89, $P<.001$).[18] Among cardiovascular deaths, both sudden cardiac death (HR 0.80, 95% CI 0.68–0.94, $P = .008$) and death due to worsening heart failure (HR 0.79, 95% CI 0.64–0.98, $P = .034$) were reduced by treatment with LCZ696 compared with enalapril (**Fig. 6**). Deaths attributed to other cardiovascular causes, including myocardial infarction and stroke, were infrequent and distributed evenly between treatment groups, as were noncardiovascular deaths. When it came to the change in scores on the Kansas City Cardiomyopathy Questionnaire, which ranges from 0 to 100, the HR for change was 1.64 ($P = .001$). There was no difference in new-onset atrial fibrillation or the decline in renal function when comparing both the study drug and enalapril. There was a 20% reduction in

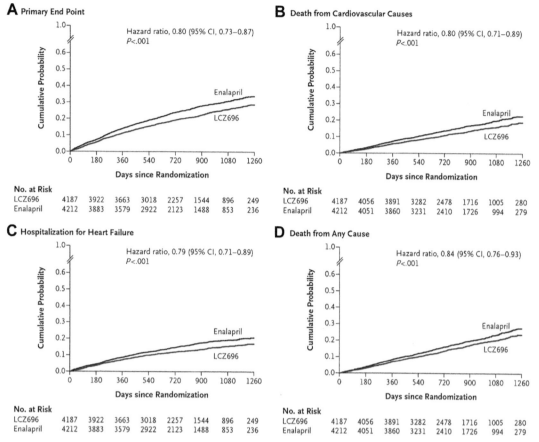

Fig. 5. Estimates of the probability of the primary composite end point (death from cardiovascular causes or first hospitalization for heart failure) (*A*), death from cardiovascular causes (*B*), first hospitalization for heart failure (*C*), and death from any cause (*D*). There is a 20% risk reduction of death from cardiovascular causes (*B*, 21% risk reduction of heart failure hospitalizations, 16% reduction of death from any cause). (*From* McMurray JJ, Packer M, Desai AS, et al. Angiotensin-neprilysin inhibition versus enalapril in heart failure. N Engl J Med 2014;371(11):998; with permission.)

cardiovascular mortality from 16.5% in the enalapril arm to 13.3% in the study drug; there was a 20% reduction in heart failure hospitalizations with a reduction from 15.6% to 12.8% with the study drug, and there was a 16.0% reduction in overall mortality with 19.8% mortality in the enalapril arm and 17.0% with the study drug. There was a 21% reduction in heart failure deaths from 4.4% in the enalapril arm with 3.5% with the study drug, and there was a 20% reduction in sudden death from 7.4% with enalapril to 6.0% with the study drug. The study drug, therefore, was very effective in reducing sudden death; one would argue that the reduction in mortality with the study drug was equivalent to possibly an ICD (see **Table 1**). When comparing age in the PARADIGM-HF, there was a significant reduction in cardiovascular death or heart failure hospitalizations; there was a significant reduction in cardiovascular death and all causes of mortality in all age groups[19] (**Fig. 7**) when they divided the patients into 4 different age quartiles: younger than 55 years, 55 to 64 years of age, 65 to 74 years of age, and older than 75 years. In the PARADIGM-HF, they found mortality benefits in all 4 quartiles.

Not only was the mortality significant, there was an early mortality benefit. Typically, the mortality rate actually was seen around 6 months with the ACE inhibitors or ARBs; but in the PARADIGM-HF study they found the curve separating out as early as at the end of the first month whereby the HR was 0.66 (0.45–0.9; *P* = .019). At 2 months, the curves had well separated out with a HR of 0.56 (0.49–0.86; *P* = .003). The benefits with LCZ696 therapy, therefore, were early at 2 months.

What were the adverse events seen in the PARADIGM-HF study? The prospectively identified adverse events included symptomatic hypotension, which was 14.0% with the study drug and 9.2% with enalapril (*P*<.001). A serum potassium

Table 3
Primary and secondary outcomes

Outcome	LCZ696 (N = 4187)	Enalapril (N = 4212)	Hazard Ratio or Difference (95% CI)	P Value
Primary composite outcome: No. (%)				
Death due to cardiovascular causes or first hospitalization for worsening heart failure	914 (21.8)	1117 (26.5)	0.80 (0.73–0.87)	<.001
Death from cardiovascular causes	558 (13.3)	693 (16.5)	0.80 (0.71–0.89)	<.001
First hospitalization for worsening heart failure	537 (12.8)	658 (15.6)	0.79 (0.71–0.89)	<.001
Secondary outcomes: No. (%)				
Death from any cause	711 (17.0)	835 (19.8)	0.84 (0.76–0.93)	<.001
Change in KCCQ clinical summary score at 8 mo[†]	−2.99 ±0.36	−4.63 ±0.36	1.64 (0.63–2.65)	.001
New-onset atrial fibrillation[‡]	84 (3.1)	83 (3.1)	0.97 (0.72–1.31)	.83
Decline in renal function[§]	94 (2.2)	108 (2.6)	0.86 (0.65–1.13)	.28

HRs were calculated with the use of stratified Cox proportional-hazard models. P values are 2-sided and were calculated by means of a stratified log-rank test without adjustment for multiple comparisons.

Abbreviations: CI, confidence interval; KCCQ, Kansas City Cardiomyopathy Questionnaire.

[†] Scores on the Kansas City Cardiomyopathy Questionnaire (KCCQ) range from 0 to 100, with higher scores indicating fewer symptoms and physical limitations associated with heart failure. The treatment effect is shown as the least-squares mean (±SE) of the between-group difference.

[‡] A total of 2670 patients in the LCZ696 group and 2638 patients in the enalapril group who did not have atrial fibrillation at the randomization visit were evaluated for new-onset atrial fibrillation during the study.

[§] A decline in renal function was defined as end-stage renal disease or a decrease of 50% or more in the eGFR from the value at randomization or a decrease in the eGFR of more than 30 mL per minute per 1.73 m^2 to less than 60 mL per minute per 1.73 m^2.

From McMurray JJ, Packer M, Desai AS, et al. Angiotensin-neprilysin inhibition versus enalapril in heart failure. N Engl J Med 2014;371(11):999; with permission.

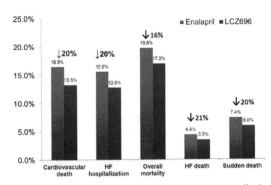

Fig. 6. Effect of the angiotensin-receptor-neprilysin inhibitor LCZ696 compared with enalapril on mode of death in patients with heart failure (HF). (*Data from* McMurray JJ, Packer M, Desai AS, et al. Angiotensin-neprilysin inhibition versus enalapril in heart failure. N Engl J Med 2014;371(11):993–1004; and Desai AS, McMurray JJ, Packer M, et al. Effect of the angiotensin-receptor-neprilysin inhibitor LCZ696 compared with enalapril on mode of death in heart failure patients. Eur Heart J 2015;36(30):1990–7.)

greater than 6 mmol/L was seen in 4.3% of the study drug and 5.6% in the enalapril arm; a serum creatinine greater than or equal to 2.5 mg/dL was seen in 3.3% with the study drug and 4.5% with enalapril (P = .07). Cough was seen in 11.3% with the study drug and 14.3% with enalapril (P<.001).

Discontinuation for adverse events: More patients on enalapril required medication discontinuation (P = .02). Thirty-six patients on the study drug required discontinuation for hypotension, and 29 patients on enalapril required medication discontinuation (P = ns). There were 11 patients on the study drug who were discontinued for hyperkalemia, and 15 patients on enalapril required discontinuation (P = ns). There were 29 patients on the study drug who required discontinuation for renal impairment, and 59 patients with enalapril required discontinuation (P = .001). Sixteen patients on the study drug developed angioedema, which was 0.3%; 9 patients on enalapril developed angioedema (P = ns). Three patients on the study drug required hospitalization for angioedema and 1 patient on enalapril required hospitalization for angioedema (P = ns).

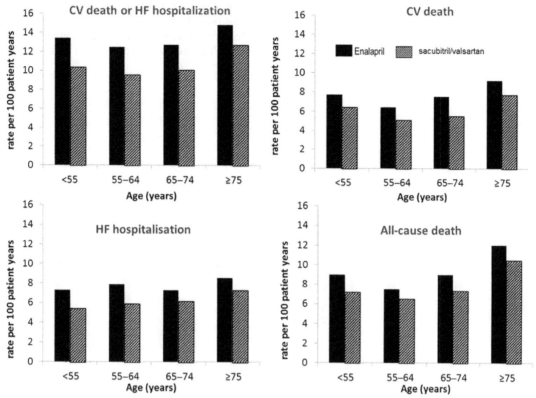

Fig. 7. Effect of sacubitril/valsartan on the rate of primary end point and component and all-cause mortality in patients randomized in the PARADIGM-HF trial according to age group. *P* for interaction for cardiovascular (CV) death or heart failure (HF) hospitalization = .94; for CV death *P* for interaction = .92, for HF hospitalization *P* for interaction = .81, and all-cause death *P* for interaction = .99. (*From* Jhund PS, McMurray JJ. The neprilysin pathway in heart failure: a review and guide on the use of sacubitril/valsartan. Heart 2016;102(17):1344; with permission.)

So when comparing the survival benefit to see in context, ARBs and ACE inhibitors, that is drugs that inhibit the renin angiotensin have modest effects with most at 10% to 12%. Beta-blockers decreased mortality by around 35%. Mineralocorticoid receptor antagonists decreased mortality by 25% to 30% and the isosorbide dinitrate/hydralazine combination decreased mortality by 40% in the African American Heart Failure Trial (A-HeFT).[20] So keeping in context, there is a doubling of survival with neprilysin inhibition. There is a 15% decrease in mortality with either ARB or ACE inhibitors, whereas with neprilysin inhibition there is an additional 16% (**Fig. 8**), so a total of 31% improvement in survival with neprilysin inhibition.[21,22]

It is estimated that there are about 2.7 million patients with heart failure with reduced ejection fraction in the United States. If 84% of these were candidates for ARNI therapy, then empirically ARNI therapy is estimated to prevent 28,484 deaths a year.[23] Therefore, these data support the implementation of evidence into

practice in a timely manner because they have a material impact on population health on patients with heart failure with reduced ejection fraction.

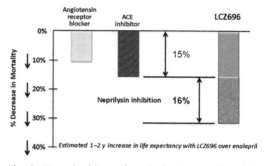

Fig. 8. Near doubling of survival with neprilysin inhibition over enalapril. (*Data from* McMurray J, Packer M, Desai A, et al. A putative placebo analysis of the effects of LCZ696 on clinical outcomes in heart failure. Eur Heart J 2015;36(7):434–9; and Claggett B, Packer M, McMurray JJ, et al. Estimating the long-term treatment benefits of sacubitril-valsartan. N Engl J Med 2015;373(23):2289–90.)

When the study investigators categorized patients by the Meta-Analysis Global Group in Chronic Heart Failure risk score (MAGGIC risk score), they found that the benefits of neprilysin inhibition were consistent across a range of risk scores (**Fig. 9**).

The impact on rehospitalization is also very significant (**Fig. 10**). When comparing enalapril with

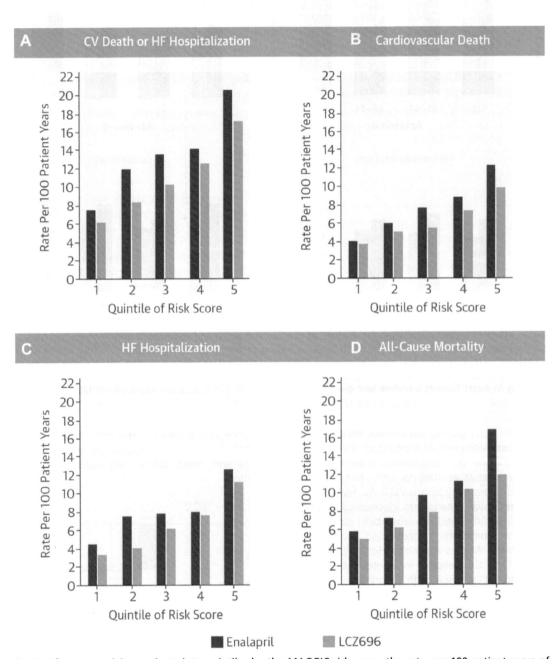

Fig. 9. After categorizing patients into quintiles by the MAGGIC risk score, the rate per 100 patient-years of follow-up was determined for (A) the primary composite end point, (B) cardiovascular (CV) death, (C) heart failure (HF) hospitalization, and (D) all-cause mortality according to baseline risk category and randomized treatment. The incidence of all end points increased incrementally with increasing risk score. The effect of LCZ696 compared with enalapril was consistent across the range of risk scores examined as a categorical variable for all end points. (*From* Simpson J, Jhund PS, Cardoso JS, et al. Comparing LCZ696 with enalapril according to baseline risk using the MAGGIC and EMPHASIS-HF risk scores: an analysis of mortality and morbidity in PARADIGM-HF. J Am Coll Cardiol 2015;66(19):2065; with permission.)

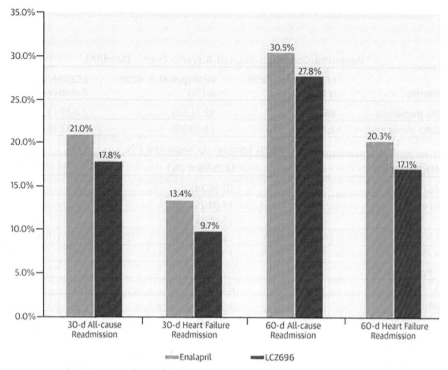

Fig. 10. Impact on readmissions. HF, heart failure. (*From* Desai AS, Claggett BL, Packer M, et al. Influence of sacubitril/valsartan (LCZ696) on 30-day readmission after heart failure hospitalization. J Am Coll Cardiol 2016;68(3):245; with permission.)

LCZ696, for 30-day all-cause readmissions, there is a significant improvement in readmission rates. With enalapril there was a 21% reduction in 30-day all-cause readmissions, whereas with LCZ696 the number of readmissions was only 17.8%. The 30-day heart failure readmission rate in the enalapril arm was 13.4%, whereas with LCZ696 it was 9.7%. The 60-day all-cause readmission rate with enalapril was 30.5% and with LCZ696 it was 27.8%. The 60-day heart failure readmission rate with enalapril was 20.3% and with LCZ696 it was 17.1%.

One of the criticisms of this study is that enalapril dosing differed from that used in clinical practice. One would argue that the dose of enalapril here was higher (18.9 mg) and was very comparable with the CONSENSUS trial[24] and SOLVD treatment study (enalapril dose was 16.6 mg).[4] The other criticism was neprilysin inhibition allows accumulation of preamyloid oligomers in the brain[25] causing worsening Alzheimer disease or potentially causing Alzheimer disease. In addition, neprilysin inhibition allows accumulation of beta amyloid in the macula worsening age-related macular degeneration.[26] The PARADIGM-HF study was too short to evaluate cognitive outcomes (**Table 4**) or age-related macular degeneration.[27] The third criticism was that the control arm tested an ACE inhibitor when it may have been more appropriate to study an ARB because the experimental arm tested neprilysin plus an ARB.

What are the gaps in information? Less than 1000 patients were studied in the United States. There are limited data on those with moderately severe or severe heart failure. The study was prematurely terminated potentially overstating the benefit and underestimating the harm. There was an open-label run-in period that eliminated adverse drug reactions. In addition, they recruited a negligible number of African Americans. As discussed, long-term safety data are not clear. Finally, the cost could be as high as $400 a month versus $4 a month for an ACE inhibitor.

How is ARNI therapy initiated? First, it is important to discontinue ACE inhibitors for at least 36 hours before initiating sacubitril/valsartan. The initial dosage for patients already on an ACE or ARB could be 49/51 mg twice daily; but in patients with low blood pressures, eGFR less than 30 mL/min, and with moderate liver impairment Child-Pugh class B or in the elderly, the recommended initial dosage is 24/26 mg twice daily. The dosage needs to be titrated every 2 to 4 weeks until the target dosage of 97/103 mg twice daily is reached.

What are the recommendations from the American College of Cardiology/American Heart

Table 4
Dementia

Dementia/Cognition-Related Adverse Events (MedRA)		
SMQ Dementia	**LCZ696 N = 4203** **n (%)**	**Enalapril N = 4229** **n (%)**	**LCZ696 vs Enalapril** **Relative Risk (95% CI)**
Broad SMQ dementia	*86 (2.05)*	*83 (1.96)*	1.029 (0.761, 1.391)
Narrow SMQ dementia	*12 (0.29)*	*15 (0.35)*	0.793 (0.371, 1.695)

LCZ696 Most Frequently Reported PTs		
Broad SMQ Dementia	**LCZ696 n (%)**	**Enalapril n (%)**
Confusional state	12 (0.29)	18 (0.43)
Somnolence	11 (0.26)	9 (0.21)
Amnesia	10 (0.24)	7 (0.17)
Delirium	10 (0.24)	8 (0.19)
Agitation	7 (0.17)	3 (0.07)
Memory impairment	*6 (0.14)*	*6 (0.14)*
Dementia	*6 (0.14)*	*10 (0.24)*
Disorientation	5 (0.12)	4 (0.09)
Mental status changes	5 (0.12)	1 (0.02)
Cerebral atrophy	4 (0.10)	0 (0.00)

LCZ696 Most Frequently Reported PTs		
Narrow SMQ Dementia	**LCZ n (%)**	**Enalapril n (%)**
Dementia	*6 (0.14)*	*10 (0.24)*
Dementia Alzheimer-type	*2 (0.05)*	*2 (0.05)*
Vascular dementia	2 (0.05)	1 (0.02)
Hippocampal sclerosis	1 (0.02)	0 (0.00)
Presenile dementia	1 (0.02)	0 (0.00)
Senile dementia	*0 (0.00)*	*2 (0.05)*

n PARADIGM-HF, the authors systematically searched AE reports coded using the 17.0 version of the Medical Dictionary for Regulatory Activities (MedDRA) using Standardized MedDRA Queries (SMQs) with 'broad' and 'narrow' preferred terms (PTs) related to dementia-like adverse events.

Adapted from Cannon JA, Shen L, Jhund PS, et al. Dementia-related adverse events in PARADIGM-HF and other trials in heart failure with reduced ejection fraction. Eur J Heart Fail 2017;19(1):131; with permission.

Association/Heart Failure Society of America's guidelines? ARNI should not be administered concomitantly with ACE inhibitors or within 36 hours of the last ACE inhibitor dose. In addition, ARNI should not be administered to patients with a history of angioedema. The recommendation for starting ARNI therapy is in conjunction with beta-blockers and aldosterone receptor antagonists when appropriate in patients with chronic heart failure reduced ejection fraction reduce morbidity and mortality. The ARNI medications can also be used to reduce further mortality and morbidity in patients on an ACE inhibitor or an ARB.

SUMMARY

Neprilysin inhibition is associated with significant improvements in survival. Despite substantial reductions in mortality with neprilysin inhibition, the mortality rate among patients with heart failure remains high around 20% over 2 years in the intervention arm of PARADIGM-HF, suggesting that opportunities to reduce mortality in heart failure remain.

REFERENCES

1. Benjamin EJ, Blaha MJ, Chiuve SE, et al. Heart disease and stroke statistics-2017 update: a report from the American Heart Association. Circulation 2017;135(10):e146–603.
2. Heidenreich PA, Albert NM, Allen LA, et al. Forecasting the impact of heart failure in the United States: a policy statement from the American Heart Association. Circ Heart Fail 2013;6(3): 606–19.

3. Effect of metoprolol CR/XL in chronic heart failure: metoprolol CR/XL Randomised Intervention Trial in Congestive Heart Failure (MERIT-HF). Lancet 1999; 353(9169):2001–7.

4. Investigators S, Yusuf S, Pitt B, et al. Effect of enalapril on survival in patients with reduced left ventricular ejection fractions and congestive heart failure. N Engl J Med 1991;325(5):293–302.

5. Cohn JN, Tognoni G, Valsartan Heart Failure Trial Investigators. A randomized trial of the angiotensin-receptor blocker valsartan in chronic heart failure. N Engl J Med 2001;345(23):1667–75.

6. Maggioni AP, Anand I, Gottlieb SO, et al. Effects of valsartan on morbidity and mortality in patients with heart failure not receiving angiotensin-converting enzyme inhibitors. J Am Coll Cardiol 2002;40(8):1414–21.

7. Granger CB, McMurray JJ, Yusuf S, et al. Effects of candesartan in patients with chronic heart failure and reduced left-ventricular systolic function intolerant to angiotensin-converting-enzyme inhibitors: the CHARM-Alternative trial. Lancet 2003; 362(9386):772–6.

8. Abdulla J, Abildstrom SZ, Christensen E, et al. A meta-analysis of the effect of angiotensin-converting enzyme inhibitors on functional capacity in patients with symptomatic left ventricular systolic dysfunction. Eur J Heart Fail 2004;6(7):927–35.

9. O'Meara E, Solomon S, McMurray J, et al. Effect of candesartan on New York Heart Association functional class. Results of the Candesartan in Heart failure: assessment of Reduction in Mortality and morbidity (CHARM) programme. Eur Heart J 2004; 25(21):1920–6.

10. Cohn JN, Johnson G, Ziesche S, et al. A comparison of enalapril with hydralazine-isosorbide dinitrate in the treatment of chronic congestive heart failure. N Engl J Med 1991;325(5):303–10.

11. Majani G, Giardini A, Opasich C, et al. Effect of valsartan on quality of life when added to usual therapy for heart failure: results from the Valsartan Heart Failure Trial. J Card Fail 2005;11(4):253–9.

12. Heywood JT, Fonarow GC, Yancy CW, et al. Comparison of medical therapy dosing in outpatients cared for in cardiology practices with heart failure and reduced ejection fraction with and without device therapy: report from IMPROVE HF. Circ Heart Fail 2010;3(5):596–605.

13. Ruilope LM, Dukat A, Bohm M, et al. Blood-pressure reduction with LCZ696, a novel dual-acting inhibitor of the angiotensin II receptor and neprilysin: a randomised, double-blind, placebo-controlled, active comparator study. Lancet 2010;375(9722):1255–66.

14. Kario K, Sun N, Chiang FT, et al. Efficacy and safety of LCZ696, a first-in-class angiotensin receptor neprilysin inhibitor, in Asian patients with hypertension: a randomized, double-blind, placebo-controlled study. Hypertension 2014;63(4):698–705.

15. Jhund PS, Claggett B, Packer M, et al. Independence of the blood pressure lowering effect and efficacy of the angiotensin receptor neprilysin inhibitor, LCZ696, in patients with heart failure with preserved ejection fraction: an analysis of the PARAMOUNT trial. Eur J Heart Fail 2014;16(6):671–7.

16. McMurray JJ, Packer M, Desai AS, et al. Angiotensin-neprilysin inhibition versus enalapril in heart failure. N Engl J Med 2014;371(11):993–1004.

17. Desai AS, Solomon S, Claggett B, et al. Factors associated with noncompletion during the run-in period before randomization and influence on the estimated benefit of LCZ696 in the PARADIGM-HF trial. Circ Heart Fail 2016;9(6) [pii:e002735].

18. Desai AS, McMurray JJ, Packer M, et al. Effect of the angiotensin-receptor-neprilysin inhibitor LCZ696 compared with enalapril on mode of death in heart failure patients. Eur Heart J 2015;36(30):1990–7.

19. Jhund PS, Fu M, Bayram E, et al. Efficacy and safety of LCZ696 (sacubitril-valsartan) according to age: insights from PARADIGM-HF. Eur Heart J 2015; 36(38):2576–84.

20. Taylor AL, Ziesche S, Yancy C, et al. Combination of isosorbide dinitrate and hydralazine in blacks with heart failure. N Engl J Med 2004;351(20):2049–57.

21. McMurray J, Packer M, Desai A, et al. A putative placebo analysis of the effects of LCZ696 on clinical outcomes in heart failure. Eur Heart J 2015;36(7): 434–9.

22. Claggett B, Packer M, McMurray JJ, et al. Estimating the long-term treatment benefits of sacubitril-valsartan. N Engl J Med 2015;373(23):2289–90.

23. Fonarow GC, Hernandez AF, Solomon SD, et al. Potential mortality reduction with optimal implementation of angiotensin receptor neprilysin inhibitor therapy in heart failure. JAMA Cardiol 2016;1(6): 714–7.

24. CONSENSUS Trial Study Group. Effects of enalapril on mortality in severe congestive heart failure. Results of the Cooperative North Scandinavian Enalapril Survival Study (CONSENSUS). N Engl J Med 1987;316(23):1429–35.

25. Iwata N, Tsubuki S, Takaki Y, et al. Metabolic regulation of brain Abeta by neprilysin. Science 2001; 292(5521):1550–2.

26. Maetzler W, Stoycheva V, Schmid B, et al. Neprilysin activity in cerebrospinal fluid is associated with dementia and amyloid-beta42 levels in Lewy body disease. J Alzheimers Dis 2010;22(3):933–8.

27. Cannon JA, Shen L, Jhund PS, et al. Dementia-related adverse events in PARADIGM-HF and other trials in heart failure with reduced ejection fraction. Eur J Heart Fail 2017;19(1):129–37.

The Use and Indication of Ivabradine in Heart Failure

Katherine Dodd, DO, MPH, Brent C. Lampert, DO*

KEYWORDS

- Heart failure • Ivabradine • Heart failure drug therapy • Heart rate • Heart rate lowering
- Goal-directed medical therapy • Sinoatrial node

KEY POINTS

- Ivabradine is selective inhibitor of the sinoatrial pacemaker modulating "f-current" (I_f) that lowers heart rate by prolonging the slow depolarization phase.
- The Systolic Heart failure treatment with the I_f inhibitor ivabradine Trial (SHIFT) demonstrated a heart rate lowering benefit in patients with baseline heart rate greater than or equal to 70 beats per minute.
- Before starting ivabradine, patients should be on appropriate guideline-directed medical therapy including renin-angiotensin system inhibitors (angiotensin-converting enzyme inhibitors, angiotensin receptor blockers, or combination angiotensin receptor and neprilysin inhibitors) and beta-blockers.
- The maximum benefit of beta-blockers is dose dependent, and it has been questioned whether patients in SHIFT were truly on maximum beta-blocker therapy.
- The typical starting dose of ivabradine is 5 mg twice daily and the most common side effect is symptomatic bradycardia.

INTRODUCTION

Heart failure (HF) affects more than 6 million people in the United States.[1,2] An estimated 92 million adults in the United States have cardiovascular disease in some capacity. By the year 2030, roughly 44% of the US adult population is projected to have some form of cardiovascular disease.[3] The prevalence of HF, in particular, has increased from 5.7 million from 2009 to 2012 to 6.5 million from 2011 to 2014 in US adults older than 20 years.[3] The estimated cost for HF management is astronomical, amounting to roughly $30 billion annually in the United States alone. Unfortunately, despite numerous pharmacologic and device therapies for HF, the prognosis is quite grim, with half of all patients dying within 5 years following the diagnosis.[1,2] The pathophysiology of HF is quite complex, at the microcellular level, leading to macrocellular changes. For example, bombardment of the sympathetic nervous system with cytokines and neurohormones leads to profound myocyte damage.[4] This results in changes to the size, shape, and function of the heart and the left ventricle in particular. Remodeling subsequently leads to electrical instability and systemic organ tissue destruction.[5]

One factor associated with worse cardiovascular outcomes is a persistently elevated heart rate. Higher heart rates are quite common among patients with systolic HF, although it remains unclear

Disclosure Statement: The authors have nothing to disclose.
Division of Cardiovascular Medicine, The Ohio state University Wexner Medical Center, 473 W12th Avenue, Columbus, OH 43210, USA
* Corresponding author. Heart Failure and Transplantation, The Ohio State University Wexner Medical Center, 473 West 12th Avenue, Suite 200, Columbus, OH 43210.
E-mail address: Brent.Lampert@osumc.edu

Heart Failure Clin 14 (2018) 493–500
https://doi.org/10.1016/j.hfc.2018.06.001
1551-7136/18/© 2018 Elsevier Inc. All rights reserved.

if elevated heart rate is a marker of increased sympathetic tone or an independent prognostic factor. Regardless, the elevated heart rate in patients with HF is problematic because it increases myocardial oxygen demand, decreases myocardial perfusion, and has been associated with increased rates of hospitalization and mortality.[1,2,6] For these reasons, heart rate reduction has long been a therapeutic target in HF. Ivabradine is a new therapeutic agent providing heart rate reduction that can be beneficial in patients with HF with reduced ejection fraction (HFrEF).

HEART RATE–LOWERING MEDICATIONS IN HEART FAILURE WITH REDUCED EJECTION FRACTION

Medications that lower heart rate have different mechanisms and are not all beneficial in HF. Beta-blockers have been a mainstay of HF treatment for decades. Their use in HFrEF is associated with improved symptoms, reduced hospitalizations, and improved survival. The mechanism of benefit for beta-blocker therapy is in part due to their heart rate–lowering effects. However, beta-blockers negatively affect cardiac contractility and only certain beta-blockers (carvedilol, metoprolol succinate, or bisoprolol) have demonstrated benefit in HFrEF.[7]

Digoxin inhibits sympathetic outflow and enhances parasympathetic tone, possibly reducing heart rate in patients with HFpEF in sinus rhythm. Digoxin reduces the risk of HF hospitalizations and improves symptoms but does not convey a survival benefit.[8] It is unclear whether the potential heart rate–lowering effect of digoxin contributes to its clinical benefit.

Nondihydropyridine calcium channel blockers such as diltiazem and verapamil effectively reduce heart rates. However, they have negative inotropic effects and may be harmful in patients with HFrEF. Consequently, nondihydropyridine calcium channel blockers should be avoided in patients with HFrEF.[9,10]

Ivabradine is a selective inhibitor of the sinoatrial pacemaker modulating "f-current" (I_f) (**Fig. 1**).[11] Ivabradine effectively lowers the heart rate by prolonging the slow depolarization phase. Unlike beta-blockers, ivabradine does not inhibit myocardial contractility or intracardiac conduction. Ivabradine likely benefits patients with HFrEF through its heart rate–lowering effects.

IVABRADINE EVIDENCE IN HEART FAILURE

The Systolic Heart failure treatment with the I_f inhibitor ivabradine Trial (SHIFT) trial was devised to examine the effect of heart rate reduction using

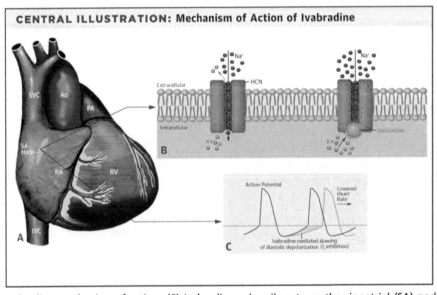

Fig. 1. (*A*) Ivabradine mechanism of action. (*B*) Ivabradine primarily acts on the sinoatrial (SA) node where it blocks hyperpolarization-activated cyclic nucleotide-gated (HCN) transmembrane channel, which is responsible for transport of sodium (Na+) and potassium (K+) across cell membranes. This results in inhibition of the inward funny current (I_f) and reduction in the diastolic depolarization slope of the pacemaker action potential. (*C*) There is a subsequent increase in the duration of diastole without changing other phases of the action potential leading to decreased heart rate. Ao, aorta; IVC, inferior vena cava; PA, pulmonary artery; RV, right ventricle. (*From* Koruth JS, Lala A, Pinney S, et al. The clinical use of ivabradine. J Am Coll Cardiol 2017;70(14):1780; with permission.)

ivabradine in addition to guideline-directed medical therapy on HF outcomes.[11] SHIFT enrolled more than 6500 patients with HF, a left ventricular ejection fraction (LVEF) less than or equal to 35%, a HF hospitalization within the past year, sinus rhythm with a heart rate of greater than 70 beats per minute (bpm), and on stable goal-directed medical therapy. Patients were excluded if they had a recent (<2 months) myocardial infarction, greater than 40% ventricular pacing, atrial fibrillation or flutter, and symptomatic hypotension. Patients were randomized to receive ivabradine titrated to a maximum of 7.5 mg twice daily or placebo. The primary endpoint was a composite of cardiovascular death or HF hospitalization. Patients were followed for a median 22.9 months. After 28 days, heart rate in the ivabradine group decreased by a mean 15.4 beats per minute (10.9 beats per minute when corrected for change in the placebo group). The heart rate reduction with ivabradine was sustained throughout the study period (**Fig. 2**).[11] Ivabradine reduced the risk of the primary combined outcome by 18% (24% vs 29%; hazard ratio [HR] 0.82, 95% confidence interval [CI] 0.75–0.90, P<.0001). This was largely driven by significant reductions in HF hospitalizations (21% placebo vs 16% ivabradine; HR 0.74, 95% CI 0.66–0.83; P<.0001) and HF-related deaths (21% placebo vs 16% ivabradine; HR 0.74, 95% CI 0.66–0.83; P<.0001). The treatment effects were consistent across most prespecified subgroups, but it was noted that there was

only a benefit for ivabradine in the subgroup with baseline heart rate greater than or equal to 77 beats per minute (when compared with those with baseline heart rate <77 beats per minute).[11] Overall, there were fewer serious side effects in the ivabradine group. However, ivabradine was associated with an increased risk of symptomatic bradycardia (1% placebo vs 5% ivabradine, P<.001) and visual side effects (1% placebo vs 3% ivabradine, P<.001).[11]

SHIFT was a landmark trial demonstrating the importance of heart rate control in chronic HF with the novel agent ivabradine. However, there were significant and important critiques of the study. Although even low doses are beneficial, the maximum benefit of beta-blockers is dose dependent, and it has been questioned whether patients in SHIFT were truly on maximum beta-blocker therapy.[12] Specifically, just 26% of patients were on target beta-blocker dose and only 56% of patients received at least 50% of the target dose. Approximately 10% of patients were not on any beta-blocker therapy. The primary reason for failure to reach target beta-blocker dose was hypotension, but the mean baseline systolic blood pressure was 122 mm Hg, which is similar to baseline blood pressure in prior pivotal beta-blocker trials.[13] Despite good tolerability of beta-blockers in numerous clinical studies, there sometimes remains hesitancy in clinical practice to titrate them to maximum recommended doses, and the baseline therapy in SHIFT may be reflective of "real

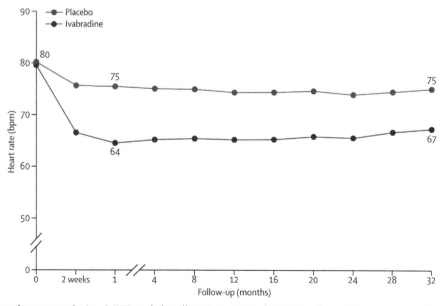

Fig. 2. Mean heart rate during SHIFT study by allocation group. (*From* Swedberg K, Komajda M, Böhm M, et al. Ivabradine and outcomes in chronic heart failure (SHIFT): a randomised placebo-controlled study. Lancet 2010;376(9744):879; with permission.)

world" use patterns. Regardless, reservations remain whether SHIFT truly tested the hypothesis that ivabradine can provide additional benefit to patients who are treated with conventional optimal HF therapy.

Other smaller trials have provided further evidence for the role of ivabradine in HFrEF. ETHIC-AHF (Effect of early treatment with ivabradine combined with beta-blockers vs beta-blockers alone in patients hospitalized with HF and reduced LEVF) analyzed the effect of early coadministration of ivabradine and beta-blockers versus beta-blockers alone in hospitalized patients with HFrEF.[14] In this small study of 71 patients, ivabradine was added to the medical regimen 24 to 48 hours after HF admission when clinical stabilization was achieved. In the ivabradine group, there was a significant reduction in heart rate at both 28 days and 4 months postdischarge.[14] The study also suggested improvement objectively and subjectively in both systolic function and clinical parameters of patients with HF.[14] In patients taking ivabradine, the brain natriuretic peptide (BNP) levels were reduced, and the number of patients documented to be in advanced functional HF classes was lower. It differs from SHIFT through the early administration of ivabradine, because the SHIFT trial administered the medication more than 4 weeks following hospitalization. However, like SHIFT, a significant decrease in heart rate amongst patients taking ivabradine with a beta-blocker was demonstrated. A final interesting observation was the safety and benefit of starting ivabradine early, even among acutely decompensated patients with HF.[14] A larger ongoing trial of approximately 450 patients called PRIME-HF (Predischarge Initiation of Ivabradine in the Management of Heart Failure) will further evaluate this strategy.[15]

The CARVIVA HF trial (Effect of carvedilol, ivabradine, or their combination on exercise capacity in patients with Heart Failure) assessed the effect of heart rate reduction with carvedilol, ivabradine, or combination of carvedilol and ivabradine on exercise capacity in HFrEF.[16] There were 121 patients randomized to carvedilol up to 25 mg bid (n = 38); ivabradine up to 7.5 mg bid (n = 41); and carvedilol/ivabradine up to 12.5/5 mg bid (n = 42).[16] Maximum study dose was more frequently tolerated in the ivabradine alone group than those receiving carvedilol or combination therapy. Heart rate was reduced in all groups, but the greatest reduction was noted in the combination group. Six-minute walk distance, maximal oxygen consumption (MVO$_2$), and quality of life were significantly improved in the ivabradine and combination groups but not in the carvedilol alone group.[16]

SOCIETY GUIDELINES

In May 2016, the ACC/AHA/HFSA Focused Update on New Pharmacologic Therapy for Heart Failure was released.[9] Based largely on the results from the SHIFT trial, it was stated that ivabradine can be beneficial to reduce HF hospitalization for patients with symptomatic (NYHA class II-III) stable chronic HFrEF (LVEF $\leq$35%) who are receiving guideline-directed evaluation and management, including a beta-blocker at maximum tolerated dose, and who are in sinus rhythm with a heart rate of greater than 70 bpm at rest (Class IIa recommendation). Other institutions such as the Food and Drug Administration and the European Society of Cardiology are in alignment with these guidelines and encourage the same usage indications for ivabradine amongst patients with HFrEF. All 3 entities also strongly emphasize the importance of beta-blocker titration to maximally tolerated doses before assessing the resting heart rate for consideration of ivabradine initiation.

CLINICAL USE

When considering ivabradine therapy for a patient with HF, it is important to understand the practical aspects. Before starting ivabradine, patients should be on appropriate guideline-directed medical therapy, including renin-angiotensin system inhibitors (angiotensin-converting enzyme inhibitors, angiotensin receptor blockers, or combination angiotensin receptor and neprilysin inhibitors) and beta-blockers. In particular, given their well-proven benefits, a patient must be on the maximally tolerated beta-blocker dose before adding ivabradine. For patients whose heart rate remains greater than or equal to 70 beats per minute despite maximally tolerated beta-blocker, ivabradine may be considered. It has been observed that if beta-blockers are appropriately titrated, only approximately 10% to 15% of patients with LVEF less than or equal to 35% might be eligible for ivabradine.[17]

The typical starting dose of ivabradine is 5 mg twice daily (**Table 1**).[18] In patients in whom there is a concern that lowering heart rate may result in hemodynamic compromise or who have conduction defects, the initial dose can be 2.5 mg twice daily. The dose should then be adjusted every 2 weeks to achieve a maximum dose of 7.5 mg twice daily and target heart rate of 50 to 60 beats per minute.[18] Ivabradine is water soluble with rapid absorption in the gut and patients should be advised to take the doses with food.

Symptomatic bradycardia is the most common side effect of ivabradine occurring in 5% of

Table 1
Ivabradine dosing guidelines

Recommended Starting Dose	Maximum Dose
5 mg 2x/d *OR* 2.5 mg[a] 2x/d [a]Lower starting dose in whom bradycardia could lead to hemodynamic compromise or with a history of conduction defects	7.5 mg 2x/d
After 2 wk, check resting heart rate	
>60 bpm	Increase dose by 2.5 mg 2x/d up to a max of 7.5 mg 2x/d
50–60 bpm	Maintain dose
<50 bpm [a]or symptomatic bradycardia	Decrease dose by 2.5 mg 2x/d Discontinue therapy if current dose is 2.5 mg 2x/d

No dosage adjustment is required for patients with moderate to severe renal impairment.
Does not require additional routine laboratory monitoring.
[a] Refers to the 2.5 mg lower starting dose.

patients in the SHIFT trial.[11,19] Phosphenes, a visual side effect with transient enhanced brightness in a restricted area of the visual field, occurred in 3% of patients.[11] There is a significant increase in atrial fibrillation risk in patients taking ivabradine. This is thought to occur in patients with mutations in the HCN4 receptor, which in turn, causes an increased effect of ivabradine.[20] One meta-analysis including more than 20,000 patients associated ivabradine use with a 15% increased relative risk of atrial fibrillation and a "number needed to harm" of 208 patients per treatment year.[21]

Ivabradine is contraindicated in patients with acute decompensated HF, hypotension (blood pressure [BP] <90/50 mm Hg), bradycardia at baseline (HR <60 bpm), severe hepatic impairment, and pacemaker dependency.[18] It is also contraindicated in patients with rhythm disturbances such as sick sinus syndrome, sinoatrial block or third-degree atrioventricular (AV) block, unless a functioning demand pacemaker is present. Finally, it is not advised that patients who are pregnant, in atrial fibrillation, have a demand pacemaker set to rates greater than 60 bpm, or have second-degree AV block take ivabradine.[18] Ivabradine is metabolized by the CYP3A4 system in the liver and intestines.[7] Accordingly, it should be avoided in combination with strong CYP34A inhibitors (**Table 2**) because they will increase plasma concentrations of ivabradine.[7]

IVABRADINE USE IN OTHER CONDITIONS
Coronary Artery Disease

Ivabradine's heart rate–lowering effects were initially assessed as therapy for symptomatic coronary artery disease. In the BEAUTIFUL (morBidity-mortality EvAlUaTion of the If inhibitor ivabradine in patients with coronary disease and left-ventricULar dysfunction) study, more than 10,000 patients with stable coronary artery disease and LVEF less than 40% were randomized to receive ivabradine or placebo in addition to appropriate baseline medical therapy.[22] Heart rate in the ivabradine group was reduced by a mean 6 beats per minute at 12 months. However, there was no difference between groups in the primary composite end point of first cardiovascular

Table 2
Cytochrome P450 3A4 inhibitors

Strong Inhibitors	Moderate Inhibitors
Atazanavir	Amiodarone
Boceprevir	Aprepitant
Ceritinib	Cimetidine
Clarithromycin	Conivaptan
Cobicistat	Crizotinib
Darunavir	Cyclosporine
Idelalisib	Diltiazem
Indinavir	Dronedarone
Itraconazole	Erythromycin
Ketoconazole	Fluconazole
Lopinavir	Fosamprenavir
Mifepristone	Grapefruit juice
Nefazodone	Imatinib
Nelfinavir	Isavuconazole
Ombitasvir	Netupitant
Posaconazole	Nilotinib
Ritonavir	Ribociclib
Saquinavir	Schisandra
Telaprevir	Verapamil
Telithromycin	
Voriconazole	

Ivabradine use is contraindicated in combination with strong cytochrome CYP34A inhibitors which will increase plasma concentrations of ivabradine.

death, hospitalization for myocardial infarction, or hospitalization for worsening HF. In the prespecified subgroup analysis of patients with heart rate greater than or equal to 70 beats per minute, ivabradine was associate with significant reductions in hospitalizations for fatal and nonfatal myocardial infarctions and the need for coronary revascularization.[22]

In the ASSOCIATE trial, the combination of ivabradine and atenolol was compared with atenolol alone in patients with chronic stable angina. The combination of ivabradine and atenolol was associated with a significant improvement in exercise duration and time to both electrocardiographic evidence of ischemia and symptomatic angina on treadmill exercise testing.[23] However, the frequency of self-reported angina was not significantly reduced in the ivabradine group.

The Study Assessing the Morbidity-Mortality Benefits of the If Inhibitor Ivabradine in Patients with Coronary Artery Disease (SIGNIFY) trial was developed to evaluate the potential benefit seen in subgroup analysis of BEAUTIFUL.[4] In this trial, more than 19,000 patients with stable coronary artery disease without clinical HF and heart rate greater than or equal to 70 beats per minute were randomized to ivabradine or placebo. Despite significant heart rate reduction in the ivabradine group, over a median 28-month follow-up, there was no benefit seen in the primary composite outcome of cardiovascular death or nonfatal myocardial infarction. In subgroup analysis of patients with activity limiting angina, ivabradine use was associated with improved angina class severity but an increased risk of the composite outcome.[4]

A meta-analysis that included the BEAUTIFUL, SIGNIFY, and SHIFT trials also evaluated the effect of ivabradine in patients with stable angina.[19] This analysis of 36,577 patients concluded that ivabradine is not effective in reducing cardiovascular deaths, all-cause mortality, coronary revascularization, or HF hospitalizations.

Despite the aforementioned conflicting evidence, ivabradine is approved for the treatment of angina in Europe. There is no current approval for this indication in the United States.

Inappropriate Sinus Tachycardia

Inappropriate sinus tachycardia is another condition in which ivabradine may be beneficial. Small studies have demonstrated positive results using ivabradine to treat patients with inappropriate sinus tachycardia. One double-blind evaluation of 21 patients with inappropriate sinus tachycardia randomized to ivabradine or placebo

demonstrated significant reduction in heart rate, improvement in exercise time, and improved symptoms in patients using ivabradine.[24] Another single-center analysis of 20 patients with inappropriate sinus tachycardia compared metoprolol with ivabradine.[25] In both groups, there was a significant reduction in heart rate, but patients taking ivabradine reported significantly fewer symptoms. Although its use for inappropriate sinus tachycardia is considered off label in the United States, the 2015 Heart Rhythm Society consensus statement and 2015 ACC/AHA/HRS guideline for the treatment of supraventricular tachycardia both support using ivabradine for this indication.[26]

Heart Failure with Preserved Ejection Fraction

Ivabradine's role in HFpEF has yet to be established, but there is interest in its use due to possible increased diastolic filling time with lower heart rates. An initial study of 61 patients with HFpEF randomized to ivabradine or placebo demonstrated improved exercise capacity and peak oxygen uptake in the ivabradine group.[27] However, the subsequent prEserveD left ventricular ejectIon fraction chronic heart Failure with ivabradine studY (EDIFY) had conflicting results. In EDIFY, 170 patients with HFpEF and a heart rate greater than or equal to 70 beats per minutes were randomized to ivabradine or placebo.[28] The ivabradine group demonstrated a significantly reduced heart rate, but there were no meaningful differences in the primary endpoints of echo-Doppler E/e' ratio, distance on the 6-min walking test (6MWT), and plasma NT-proBNP concentration. Further investigation is needed to determine whether there is a role for ivabradine in the treatment of HFpEF.

Other Uses

Some small studies have investigated the potential use of ivabradine in pregnant patients, for both tachycardia-induced cardiomyopathy (due to inappropriate sinus tachycardia) and peripartum cardiomyopathy.[29,30] However, at this time, its role remains unclear. Another population in which ivabradine has been evaluated is patients with pulmonary arterial hypertension (PAH). In patients with PAH with a heart rate greater than 100 bpm or with symptomatic palpitations, the addition of ivabradine was associated with improved New York Heart Association Heart Failure class and 6MWT.[31]

SUMMARY

HF affects more than 6 million people in the United States each year and the prognosis is poor. The elevated heart rate in HF patents is problematic, because it increases myocardial oxygen demand, decreases myocardial perfusion, and has been associated with increased rates of hospitalization and mortality. For these reasons, heart rate reduction has long been a therapeutic target in HF. Ivabradine is a selective inhibitor of the sinoatrial pacemaker modulating I_f and provides heart rate reduction that can be beneficial in patients with HFrEF. As demonstrated in the SHIFT Trial, ivabradine reduced HF-related deaths and HF hospitalizations in patients with a baseline heart rate greater than or equal to 70 beats per minute. Based largely on this trial, ivabradine was added to the 2016 ACC/AHA/Heart Failure Society of America (HFSA) Focused Update on the New Pharmacological Therapy for Heart Failure to be considered in patients with HFrEF and a sinus heart rate greater than 70 bpm despite maximally tolerated beta-blocker therapy.

REFERENCES

1. Pocock SJ, Wang D, Pfeffer MA, et al. Predictors of mortality and morbidity in patients with chronic heart failure. Eur Heart J 2006;27(1):65–75.
2. Muntwyler J, Abetel G, Gruner C, et al. One-year mortality among unselected outpatients with heart failure. Eur Heart J 2002;23(23):1861–6.
3. Benjamin EJ, Blaha MJ, Chiuve SE, et al. Heart disease and stroke statistics-2017 update: a report from the american heart association. Circulation 2017;135(10):e146–603.
4. Fox K, Ford I, Steg PG, et al. Ivabradine in stable coronary artery disease without clinical heart failure. N Engl J Med 2014;371(12):1091–9.
5. McMurray JJ. Clinical practice. systolic heart failure. N Engl J Med 2010;362(3):228–38.
6. Bohm M, Reil JC, Deedwania P, et al. Resting heart rate: risk indicator and emerging risk factor in cardiovascular disease. Am J Med 2015;128(3):219–28.
7. Thorup L, Simonsen U, Grimm D, et al. Ivabradine: current and future treatment of heart failure. Basic Clin Pharmacol Toxicol 2017;121(2):89–97.
8. Ambrosy AP, Butler J, Ahmed A, et al. The use of digoxin in patients with worsening chronic heart failure: reconsidering an old drug to reduce hospital admissions. J Am Coll Cardiol 2014;63(18):1823–32.
9. Yancy CW, Jessup M, Bozkurt B, et al. 2016 ACC/AHA/HFSA focused update on new pharmacological therapy for heart failure: an update of the 2013 ACCF/AHA guideline for the management of heart failure: a report of the american college of cardiology/american heart association Task Force on Clinical practice guidelines and the heart failure society of america. J Am Coll Cardiol 2016;68(13):1476–88.
10. Ponikowski P, Voors AA, Anker SD, et al. 2016 ESC guidelines for the diagnosis and treatment of acute and chronic heart failure. Rev Esp Cardiol (Engl Ed) 2016;69(12):1167.
11. Swedberg K, Komajda M, Böhm M, et al. Ivabradine and outcomes in chronic heart failure (SHIFT): a randomised placebo-controlled study. Lancet 2010;376(9744):875–85.
12. Teerlink JR. Ivabradine in heart failure–no paradigm SHIFT...yet. Lancet 2010;376(9744):847–9.
13. Packer M, Bristow MR, Cohn JN, et al. The effect of carvedilol on morbidity and mortality in patients with chronic heart failure. U.S. carvedilol heart failure study group. N Engl J Med 1996;334(21):1349–55.
14. Hidalgo FJ, Anguita M, Castillo JC, et al. Effect of early treatment with ivabradine combined with beta-blockers versus beta-blockers alone in patients hospitalised with heart failure and reduced left ventricular ejection fraction (ETHIC-AHF): a randomised study. Int J Cardiol 2016;217:7–11.
15. Available at: https://Clinicaltrials.gov/ct2/show/NCT02827500. Accessed August 25, 2017.
16. Volterrani M, Cice G, Caminiti G, et al. Effect of carvedilol, ivabradine or their combination on exercise capacity in patients with heart failure (the CARVIVA HF trial). Int J Cardiol 2011;151(2):218–24.
17. Dierckx R, Cleland JG, Parsons S, et al. Prescribing patterns to optimize heart rate: analysis of 1,000 consecutive outpatient appointments to a single heart failure clinic over a 6-month period. JACC Heart Fail 2015;3(3):224–30.
18. Amgen, inc. corlanor (ivabradine) package insert. Thousand oaks (CA): 2015. Available at: http://Www.accessdata.fda.gov/drugsatfda_docs/label/2015/206143Orig1s000lbl.pdf. Accessed August 25, 2017.
19. Mengesha HG, Weldearegawi B, Petrucka P, et al. Effect of ivabradine on cardiovascular outcomes in patients with stable angina: meta-analysis of randomized clinical trials. BMC Cardiovasc Disord 2017;17(1):105.
20. Chaudhary R, Garg J, Krishnamoorthy P, et al. Ivabradine: heart failure and beyond. J Cardiovasc Pharmacol Ther 2016;21(4):335–43.
21. Martin RI, Pogoryelova O, Koref MS, et al. Atrial fibrillation associated with ivabradine treatment: meta-analysis of randomised controlled trials. Heart 2014;100(19):1506–10.
22. Fox K, Ford I, Steg PG, et al, BEAUTIFUL Investigators. Ivabradine for patients with stable coronary artery disease and left-ventricular systolic dysfunction (BEAUTIFUL): a randomised, double-blind, placebo-controlled trial. Lancet 2008;372(9641):807–16.

23. Available at: https://Clinicaltrials.gov/NCT00202566. Accessed August 25, 2017.

24. Cappato R, Castelvecchio S, Ricci C, et al. Clinical efficacy of ivabradine in patients with inappropriate sinus tachycardia: a prospective, randomized, placebo-controlled, double-blind, crossover evaluation. J Am Coll Cardiol 2012;60(15):1323–9.

25. Ptaszynski P, Kaczmarek K, Ruta J, et al. Metoprolol succinate vs. ivabradine in the treatment of inappropriate sinus tachycardia in patients unresponsive to previous pharmacological therapy. Europace 2013; 15(1):116–21.

26. Sheldon RS, Grubb BP 2nd, Olshansky B, et al. 2015 heart rhythm society expert consensus statement on the diagnosis and treatment of postural tachycardia syndrome, inappropriate sinus tachycardia, and vasovagal syncope. Heart Rhythm 2015;12(6):e41–63.

27. Kosmala W, Holland DJ, Rojek A, et al. Effect of if-channel inhibition on hemodynamic status and exercise tolerance in heart failure with preserved ejection fraction: a randomized trial. J Am Coll Cardiol 2013;62(15):1330–8.

28. Komajda M, Isnard R, Cohen-Solal A, et al. Effect of ivabradine in patients with heart failure with preserved ejection fraction: the EDIFY randomized placebo-controlled trial. Eur J Heart Fail 2017. https://doi.org/10.1002/ejhf.876.

29. Haghikia A, Tongers J, Berliner D, et al. Early ivabradine treatment in patients with acute peripartum cardiomyopathy: subanalysis of the german PPCM registry. Int J Cardiol 2016;216:165–7.

30. Sag S, Coskun H, Baran I, et al. Inappropriate sinus tachycardia-induced cardiomyopathy during pregnancy and successful treatment with ivabradine. Anatol J Cardiol 2016;16(3):212–3.

31. Correale M, Brunetti ND, Montrone D, et al. Functional improvement in pulmonary arterial hypertension patients treated with ivabradine. J Card Fail 2014;20(5):373–5.

Growth Hormone Therapy in Heart Failure

Andrea Salzano, MD[a,b], Alberto M. Marra, MD[c], Roberta D'Assante, PhD[c], Michele Arcopinto, MD[d], Toru Suzuki, MD, PhD[a], Eduardo Bossone, MD, PhD[d], Antonio Cittadini, MD[b,e],*

KEYWORDS

- Chronic heart failure • Growth hormone • IGF-1 • Anabolic deficiency • Biomarker • Outcomes
- Novel therapies • Hormone deficiency

KEY POINTS

- Growth hormone deficiency (GHD) is common in chronic heart failure (CHF) and is associated with impaired functional capacity and poor outcomes.
- Correction of GHD is an innovative therapy that has to be considered in CHF.
- An individualized dose titration of GH should be considered for each patient depending on neurohumoral response, whereas GH therapy should not be administered in patients with advanced CHF.

INTRODUCTION

Despite considerable improvement in the management of heart failure (HF), unsustainable levels of morbidity and mortality coupled with an increasing economic and social burden have been observed over the previous decades.[1] One possible explanation might be that no single pathophysiologic paradigm of HF may completely explain disease progression.

The classical neurohormonal model, rooted on overexpression of different molecular pathways, such as the sympathetic nervous, the renin-angiotensin-aldosterone, and the cytokines system, represented the theoretic background for the implementation of milestone clinical trials, which in turn have dramatically changed the natural history of this disease.[1,2] Nowadays, drugs that contrast the sympathetic nervous system (β-blockers) and the renin-angiotensin-aldosterone pathway (angiotensin-converting enzyme inhibitors/angiotensin receptor blockers, angiotensin receptor neprilysin inhibitor, and mineralocorticoid receptor antagonists) are considered the first-line pharmacologic therapy for HF.[3–6]

However, chronic heart failure (CHF) is still burdened by increased mortality, worse than that of many cancers, frequent comorbidities, and, consequently, remarkable associated health care costs.[1] For this reason, other pathophysiologic models to complement the paradigm of neurohormonal hyperactivity were proposed. In this regard, several studies have showed that hormonal deficiencies are common in CHF[7–10] and, more importantly, are significantly related with several indexes of physical performance and survival. The importance of these data led some authors to consider CHF as a multiple hormone deficiency syndrome.[7]

In this context, the reduced activity of growth hormone (GH) and its tissue effector insulin-like

Disclosure Statement: Dr A. Salzano receives research grant support from Cardiopath.
[a] Department of Cardiovascular Sciences and NIHR Leicester Biomedical Research Centre, University of Leicester, Glenfield Hospital, Leicester, LE3 9QP, UK; [b] Department of Translational Medical Sciences, Federico II University, School of Medicine, Via Pansini 5, Naples, 80131, Italy; [c] IRCCS SDN, Via Gianturco 113, Naples, Italy; [d] Emergency Department, AORN "A. Cardarelli", Via A. Cardarelli, Naples, 80131, Italy; [e] Interdisciplinary Research Centre in Biomedical Materials, Federico II University, Naples, 80100, Italy
* Corresponding author. Department of Translational Medical Sciences, Federico II University, School of Medicine, Via Pansini 5, Naples 80131, Italy.
E-mail address: antonio.cittadini@unina.it

Heart Failure Clin 14 (2018) 501–515
https://doi.org/10.1016/j.hfc.2018.05.002
1551-7136/18/© 2018 Elsevier Inc. All rights reserved.

heartfailure.theclinics.com

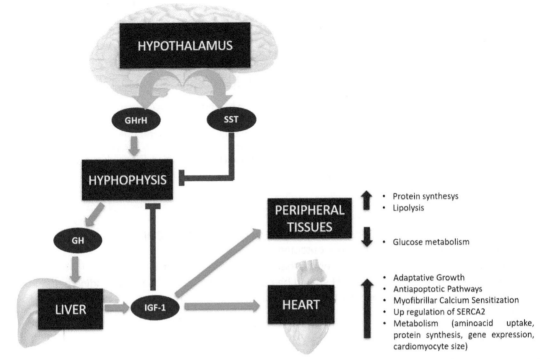

Fig. 1. Pathophysiologic background of hypothalamic-pituitary axis and GH/IGF-1 systemic effects. GHrH, growth hormone–releasing hormone; SERCA2, sarcoplasmic/endoplasmic reticulum Ca2+-ATPase; SST, somatostatin.

growth factor 1 (IGF-1)[11] plays a pivotal role. This review focuses on the involvement of GH/IGF-1 axis in CHF, on the role and prevalence of GH deficiency (GHD) in HF, and on the effects of GH therapy as add-on and replacement in the correction of GHD in HF.

THE EFFECTS OF GROWTH HORMONE/INSULIN-LIKE GROWTH FACTOR 1 ON THE CARDIOVASCULAR SYSTEM

The pituitary secretion of GH exerts several biologic effects through the interaction between GH and its specific receptors that leads to the hepatic production of IGF-I, its major biologic mediator.[12,13] Through a long-loop feedback, IGF-1 produced in the liver in response to GH prevents GH release (**Fig. 1**).

Among all the anabolic systems existing in nature, the GH/IGF-1 pathway is considered the most powerful. It regulates postnatal growth by increasing muscle mass, bone length, and density during childhood and adolescence. Furthermore, carbohydrates and lipids metabolism are regulated by its effects, mainly on visceral adipose tissue.[14] IGF-1 circulates in blood either free or bound to particular binding proteins that prolong the its half-life.[15] Nevertheless almost 90% of circulating IGF-1 is part of a ternary complex composed of IGF-specific binding protein 3 and acid-labile subunit.[16] Through this complex, IGF-1 is able to reach its target-organs, where the interaction with its own receptor (IGF1R) activates the PI3K/Akt pathway.[17] This complex pathway promotes the main effect of GH: cell growth, enhances glucose transport, inhibits apoptosis, and acts along with interleukin-6 to protect cells from tumor necrosis factor-α cytotoxicity.[15]

The cardiovascular system is an important target of this anabolic axis.[12,18] It is well established that GH plays a pivotal role by regulating cardiac growth, cardiomyocyte size, and metabolism; by stimulating amino acid uptake for protein synthesis[19]; and by promoting the transcription of genes specifically expressed in the cardiac muscle.[19] Moreover, systemic vascular resistance is likely to be reduced by the activation of IGF-1 receptors through the production of nitric oxide. IGF-1 leads to augmented contractility of cardiomyocytes mainly by increasing intracellular calcium concentration and calcium sensitization of the myofilaments and preserves capillary density.[20] Through regulation of the sarcoplasmic/endoplasmic reticulum Ca2+-ATPase (SERCA2), IGF-1 also induces the reuptake of calcium by the sarcoplasmic reticulum. Moreover, enhancement of Akt signaling, which lies downstream of IGF-1 receptor, augments myocardial contractility and diastolic function and such effects are associated with increased SERCA2 myocardial content, a pivotal regulator of calcium handling.[21]

GROWTH HORMONE/INSULIN-LIKE GROWTH FACTOR 1 DEFICIENCY IN HEART FAILURE

According to the literature, GHD is a common finding in CHF with a prevalence ranging from 32% to 53%.[8,9,22,23] Less congruent are data regarding IGF-1 in CHF. Most of the studies reported reduced IGF-1 serum levels when compared with healthy control subjects,[10,22,24–26] in particular in patients with more advanced HF[27,28] or cachexia.[29,30]

Because GH levels and daily response are influenced by anthropometric factors, physical activity, and sleep patterns,[31] the diagnosis of GHD in adults may be challenging. The most recent guidelines considered the insulin tolerance test as the gold standard test for evaluation of adult GHD.[32–34] Considering that in patients with CHF hypoglycemia could be unsafe, alternative tests are used. In particular, because of its high discriminatory power, convenience, and reproducibility, the contemporary administration of growth hormone releasing hormone (GHRH) and arginine has gained wide acceptance for GHD diagnosis.[22,35] Novel alternative tests to the insulin tolerance test for the diagnosis of GHD are under evaluation.[36]

Blood samples for GH measurement are taken every 15 to 30 minutes during the next 2 hours after an intravenous infusion of arginine (0.5 g/kg, maximum dose 30 g) followed by an intravenous bolus of GHRH (1 µg/kg, maximum dose 100 µg).[37] To avoid that molecules GH-like (eg, prolactin) may potentially affect the measurement cross-reacting with monoclonal antibodies, it is usually used to limit detection to the 22-kDa GH isoform, the most common of the different isomers and isoforms of circulating GH.[38]

It was already ascertained by several independent groups that GHD is *per se* associated with impaired cardiovascular performance and increased peripheral vascular resistance. A positive correlation between GHD severity and cardiac impairment was described.[39] Furthermore, population studies reported an increased cardiovascular mortality associated with GHD.[40] With the aim of systematically evaluate GH/IGF-1 activity in a large cohort of patients with CHF, combining measures of the IGF-1 system with stimulated pituitary responses, our group recently performed a GHRH + arginine provocative test[25] on 130 patients with CHF, demonstrating a GHD prevalence of approximately 30%. Of note, patients with GHD displayed larger left ventricular (LV) volumes with elevated wall stress, and higher filling pressures, and impairment of right ventricle systolic function compared with GH-sufficient patients. Moreover, patients with GHD also displayed impaired peak Vo_2 and reduced ventilator efficiency, resulting in a worse cardiopulmonary performance. The coexistence of GHD and CHF identifies a subgroup of patients with increased mortality, because the Cox regression analysis showed that the GHD cohort has a higher risk of mortality compared with the GH-sufficient cohort (hazard ratio, 2.11; $P = .021$) independent of age, sex, N-terminal prohormone of brain natriuretic peptide (NT-proBNP), peak Vo_2, and left ventricular ejection fraction (LVEF). With regard to GHD in HF with preserved ejection fraction, recently Salzano and colleagues[9] demonstrated that such endocrine defect is also common in HF with preserved ejection fraction, although to a lesser extent than in heart failure with reduced ejection fraction.

Few data are available dwelling on GH and acute HF. Recently, Bhandari and colleagues[41] evaluated serum GH concentrations in 537 patients admitted for acute HF. GH levels were increased in all patients who experienced one of outcome measures (either death or readmission within 1 year), without regard of ejection fraction. In this context, GH levels were independent predictors of outcomes in HF with reduced ejection fraction but not in HF with preserved ejection fraction. GH improved risk classification as measured by continuous net reclassification improvement when added to the ADHERE multivariate logistic model (which in turn is composed of age, sex, urea, heart rate, and systolic blood pressure),[42] and to ADHERE model + NT-proBNP. The authors concluded that GH could be used as an incremental prognostic biomarker over the ADHERE score clinical predictors and NT-proBNP for risk stratification of patients with acute HF. Even with the strong limitations caused by the evaluation of a single GH measurement taken in nonfasting patients, this work for the first time demonstrated incremental prognostic utility of the assessment of a marker of GH activity also in HF acute settings. No data are available as to the prevalence of GHD in acute HF.

Mechanism of Growth Hormone Deficiency in Chronic Heart Failure

Although it is not possible to put forward a single explanatory pathophysiologic mechanism of the occurrence of GH/IGF-1 impairment in CHF, three explanations can be provided regarding the underlying mechanism of impaired GH/IGF-1 secretion in CHF: (1) local hypoperfusion of the hypothalamic-pituitary axis; (2) alterations related to chronic disease, inflammation, and liver congestion; and (3) effects of CHF therapy on GH/IGF-1 axis. The systemic hypoperfusion and reduced oxygen supply, a typical hallmark of CHF clinical syndrome, is likely to alter pituitary perfusion, likewise what happens in other in other splanchnic districts. This mismatch between arterial perfusion and venous drainage is likely to cause somatotropic cell death resulting ultimately in GHD. Although the association between perfusion delay and GHD has been proved in patients without CHF,[43] to the best of our knowledge no neuroimaging study of the hypothalamic-pituitary axis of patients with CHF has never been conducted. Moreover, Broglio and colleagues,[22] after exclusion of the presence of hyperactivity of somatostatin pulse, which physiologically counteracts GH secretion, in a cohort of 38 patients with dilated cardiomyopathy (DCM) found a reduced response to different provocative tests, such as GHRH, GHRH + arginine, and GH-related peptides, and hypothesized a primary hypothalamic damage. Considering that defects of GH/IGF-1 secretion are found in other chronic wasting conditions characterized by inflammatory activation, cytokine overexpression, and liver congestion,[44] another hypothesis is rooted in a possible role of this condition, that led to a reduced hepatic synthesis of peptides hormones produced by the liver and at the same stage a peripheral GH. Considering that angiotensin-converting enzyme inhibitors[45] and β-blockers[46] are likely to modify IGF-1 secretion through direct inhibitions of IGF-1 signaling pathway, another explication for GHD in CHF might be found in therapy for CHF per se.

In all likelihood, no single mechanism is sufficient to explain the impairment of the GH/IGF-1 axis in CHF, but probably the synergy and interaction of different pathophysiologic processes and concomitant pharmacologic issues might represent its underpinnings.

GROWTH HORMONE THERAPY IN HEART FAILURE

A dangerous liaison exists between hormones and cardiovascular diseases.[47–51] A growing body of evidence supports the role of hormonal therapy in CHF.[52,53] In this intricate scenario, the impairment of GH/IGF-1 axis plays a critical role in CHF.[54] Most studies showed that patients affected by this condition display a more aggressive disease. The impact of multiple and concomitant anabolic deficiencies (including therefore GH and IGF-1 assessment, testosterone, insulin resistance, thyroid, and so forth) on different end points including hospitalization and mortality rate in CHF is being investigated by a prospective multicenter clinical registry, the TOSCA (Trattamento Ormonale nello Scompenso CArdiaco).[55,56] Among hormonal therapy, GH-replacement therapy represents a promising therapeutic opportunity in CHF. Data derived from animal models showed beneficial effects of GH on peripheral vascular resistance, cardiac function, and survival.[57–61] Among the pathophysiologic mechanisms, it is well recognized that early treatment of large myocardial infarction with GH reduces pathologic LV remodeling and improves LV function.[62] Despite this solid background, when translated onto the clinical field, these results did not lead to unequivocal results (**Table 1**).[63–79] At the beginning of the 1990s, several preliminary pilot studies tested the effect of GH therapy leading to encouraging results in CHF[63,64,67–69,72,74,76] and other clinical setting.[80] However, more robust randomized controlled clinical trials[65,66,71–74,76] failed to confirm previous results. In particular, in a cohort of 50 patients with CHF, Osterziel and colleagues[66] demonstrated a significant increase in LV mass, strongly related to changes in serum IGF-I concentrations but without significant improvement in clinical status. Of note, ejection fraction increased markedly in patients with larger increases of IGF-1 during GH treatment.[71] Isgaard and colleagues[65] and Acevedo and colleagues[74] showed no effects of GH therapy, although the latter demonstrated a positive correlation between the changes in oxygen consumption and ejection fraction in GH treatment group. Adamopoulous and colleagues,[73] in a randomized crossover trial, demonstrated that GH administration modulates beneficially circulating cytokine network and soluble adhesion molecules in patients with idiopathic DCM, while enhancing contractile reserve and diminishing LV volumes. Of note, the relationship between cytokine network, cardiac performance, and survival in HF was demonstrated also by our group.[81] Fazio and colleagues[76] in a randomized, double-blind placebo-controlled trial, demonstrated that GH, but not placebo, increased IGF-I serum concentration, improved New York Heart Association functional class, and improved cardiopulmonary performance (improved exercise duration, peak power output, peak minute ventilation, peak oxygen consumption, and anaerobic threshold) without affecting lung function parameters.

Table 1
Summary of studies on GH therapy in heart failure

Author, Year of Publication (Ref.)	Study Design, Treatment Duration, Daily Dose, Target Dose (Calculated on a Mean Weight of 70 kg)	Patients (n) and GH Status	Age (Mean ± SD), Ischemic (%), Women (%)	Increase of IGF-1 (%)	Effects of GH Therapy
Fazio et al,[63] 1996	• Open, crossover trial • 3 mo of therapy and 3 mo after therapy • 4 IU every other day sc • 12–16 IU/wk	• 7 • NA	• 46 ± 9 • 0 • 29	105.1	• Increased LV mass and LVWT and reduced the size of LV chamber • Improvement in hemodynamic variables (decreased mean pulmonary arterial and PCWP, increased stroke volume) • Beneficial changes in myocardial energy metabolism (the increase in oxygen consumption in response to physical exercise was significantly reduced) • Improved clinical status • No side effects
Frustaci et al,[64] 1996	• Open trial • 3 mo • 4 IU intramuscularly daily • 32 IU/wk	• 5 • NA	• 28 ± 8.1 • 0 • 75	NA	• Mild reductions in LV end-diastolic diameter and mild improvement in the LVEF • Worsening of arrhythmias (Lown class increased) improved after GH withdrawal
Isgaard et al,[65] 1998	• Placebo-controlled trial • 3 mo • Initial dose of 0.1 IU/kg/wk for 1 weekend thereafter 0.25 IU/kg/wk • 7 IU first week, 18 IU per week	• 22 • NA	• 60 ± 11 • 36 • 36	137.1	• No significant effect on systolic or diastolic cardiac function, exercise capacity, or neuroendocrine activation • No overall improvement in functional class or dyspnea grade • The treatment was safe and without serious side effects
Osterziel et al,[66] 1998 and Perrot et al,[71] 2000	• Randomized, double-blind placebo-controlled trial • 3 mo • 0.5 IU or placebo daily sc The dose was increased every second day by 0.5 IU until a final dose of 2 IU/d was reached • 14 IU/wk	• 50 • NA	• 54 ± 10 • 0 • 14	78.8	• GH treatment increased LV mass (small increase in LVWT) a relation between the change in myocardial mass and change in serum IGF-I concentrations • The treatment was safe and without serious side effects

(continued on next page)

Table 1
(continued)

Author, Year of Publication (Ref.)	Study Design, Treatment Duration, Daily Dose, Target Dose (Calculated on a Mean Weight of 70 kg)	Patients (n) and GH Status	Age (Mean ± SD), Ischemic (%), Women (%)	Increase of IGF-1 (%)	Effects of GH Therapy
Genth-Zotz et al,[67] 1999	• Open, crossover • 3 mo of therapy, 3 mo after therapy • 2 IU daily sc • 14 IU/wk	• 7 • NA	• 55 ± 9 • 100 • 0	110.1	• An attenuation of LV remodeling (a significant reduction in end-systolic and end-diastolic volume indexes and an increase in LVWT) and improvement of diastolic function (an increase of early diastolic filling velocity [E] and a decrease of the deceleration time of early diastolic filling) • Mean PCWP significantly decreased at rest and after exercise. After 3 mo of discontinuation, PCWP at rest was still lower than at baseline; increased cardiac output at rest and in response to physical exercise and significantly decreased systemic vascular resistance • Increased in exercise capacity: maximal oxygen uptake (Vo_{2max}) rose during therapy and fell 3 mo after GH was discontinued • Decreased NYHA functional class during treatment; this improvement had deteriorated 3 mo after discontinuation
Jose et al,[69] 1999	• Open, crossover • 6 mo of therapy and 6 mo after therapy • 2 IU on alternate days • 6–8 IU/wk	• 6 • NA	• NA • NA • NA	NA	• Improvement in the symptomatic class with treatment • Significant increase in the interventricular septal wall thickness and posterior wall thickness • These changes were partially reversed by the end of 6 mo of treatment but the symptomatic status of these patients was better than before therapy

Study	Design	Duration	Dose	Route	n		Age	%		%	Effects
Spallarossa et al,[68] 1999	• Open, controlled trial	• 6 mo	• 0.006 U/kg body weight daily sc: during the first month the dosage was gradually increased up to a full treatment regimen of 0.02 U/kg/d	• 10 IU/wk	• 20	• NA	• 62.1 ± 8	• 100	• 0	89	• GH did not change LV diameters or LVWT. • Improved clinical status (reduction of Nottingham Health Profile score) in treatment group • Increased duration of the exercise test in GH group • A trend toward decreased serum triglyceride levels and adipose body tissue associated with an increase in high-density lipoproteins
Smit et al,[70] 2001 and Van Thiel et al,[75] 2004	• Open, randomized, controlled trial	• 6 mo	• Started with 0.5 IU sc around increased after 2 wk to 1.0 IU/d and 4 wk after entering the study, the final dose of 2.0 IU/d	• 14 IU/wk	• 19	• NA	• 65.5 ± 8.5	• 100	• 15	36.7	• No beneficial effect on LV function
Napoli et al,[72] 2002	• Randomized double-blind placebo-controlled trial	• 3 mo	• 4 UI sc every other day	• 12–16 wk	• 16	• NA	• 54.5 ± 11.3	• 31	• 25	85.5	• Corrected endothelial dysfunction (through greatly improved Ach-mediated endothelium-dependent vasodilation) and improved nonendothelium-dependent vasodilation (nonsodium nitroprusside dependent vasodilation) • Increased Vo_2 max
Acevedo et al,[74] 2003	• Randomized double-blind placebo-controlled trial	• 2 mo	• 0.035 U/kg/d subcutaneous	• 16–20 IU/wk	• 19	• NA	• 57.7 ± 4.5	• 35	• 10	40.1	• No significant differences in body weight, lean body mass and dynamometry • No significant effect in left ventricular ejection fraction, left ventricular volumes, and peak oxygen consumption • A positive correlation between the changes in oxygen consumption and ejection fraction was found in GH treatment group • No adverse effects

(continued on next page)

Table 1
(continued)

Author, Year of Publication (Ref.)	Study Design, Treatment Duration, Daily Dose, Target Dose (Calculated on a Mean Weight of 70 kg)	Patients (n) and GH Status	Age (Mean ± SD), Ischemic (%), Women (%)	Increase of IGF-1 (%)	Effects of GH Therapy
Adamopoulos et al,[73] 2003	• Randomized crossover • 3 mo of therapy and 3 mo after therapy • 4 IU every other day • 12–16 IU/wk	• 12 • NA	• 50 ± 13.8 • 0 • 33	NA	• A significant decrease in the circulating proinflammatory cytokines (TNF-α, interleukin-6, GM-CSF and its soluble receptor GM-CSFR), chemotactic chemokines (MCP-1) and soluble adhesion molecules (sICAM-1 and sVCAM-1), and an increase in the serum anti-inflammatory/proinflammatory balance, • A reduction in end-systolic volume and wall stress associated with an increase in myocardial wall thickness and contractile reserve • Significant correlations were found between the GH-induced improvement in contractile reserve and the increase in V_{O_2} max
Fazio et al,[76] 2007	• Randomized, double-blind, placebo-controlled trial • 3 mo • 4 IU sc every second day • 12–16 IU/wk	• 22 • NA	• 55 • 40 • 31	101	• Increased IGF-I serum concentration • Improved NYHA functional class • Improved cardiopulmonary performance (improved exercise duration, peak power output, peak minute ventilation, peak oxygen consumption, and anaerobic threshold) without affecting lung function parameters

Study	Design	N / Type	Characteristics		Findings
Cittadini et al,[23] 2009	• Randomized, single-blind, controlled trial • 6 mo • 0.012 mg/kg every second day • 2.5–3.36 IU/wk	• 56 • GHD	• 62 ± 2 • 53 • 28	55	• GH therapy is associated with reverse remodeling, as shown by the reduction of cavity size, induction of mild hypertrophy, and a remarkable reduction of LV systolic stress • Resting systolic blood pressure decreased significantly in the GH group • Significantly improved exercise capacity and cardiopulmonary performance: exercise duration, peak workload, and peak Vo_2 consumption increased at the anaerobic threshold, Vo_2, and workload • Clinical status improved after GH therapy (MLHFQ score decreased in the active treatment group and anxiety and depression score) • NT-proBNP levels decreased and IGF-1 levels increased • Remarkable improvement of FMD • GH therapy was not associated with untoward effects during the treatment period
Cittadini et al,[84] 2013	• Randomized, single-blind, controlled trial • 48 mo (extension of previous study) • 0.012 mg/kg every second day • 2.5–3.36 IU/wk	• 31 of 56 • GHD	• 62 ± 2 • 77 • 16		• LV volumes and ejection fraction showed the highest response at 2 y and then tended to stabilize • Although the study was not designed for hard clinical end points, it was noteworthy that there was a marked difference in the aggregate of death and hospitalization for worsening CHF

Abbreviations: FMD, flow mediated dilation; GM-CSFR, granulocyte-macrophage colony–stimulating factor; LVWT, left ventricular wall thickness; MCP, membrane cofactor protein; MLHFQ, Minnesota living with heart failure questionnaire; NA, data not available; NYHA, New York Heart Association; PCWP, pulmonary capillary wedge pressure; sc, subcutaneous; SD, standard deviation; sICAM, Serum intercellular adhesion molecule; sVCAM, Serum vascular adhesion molecule; TNF-α, tumor necrosis factor–α.

However, in an elegant pooled meta-analysis of effects of GH therapy in CHF, Le Corvoisier and colleagues[82] demonstrated that sustained GH treatment improves several cardiovascular parameters in HF. In particular, an increase in LVEF and a reduction in systemic vascular resistance were shown, both associated with beneficial long-term changes of cardiac architecture related to an increase in LV wall thickness and a reduction in LV diastolic diameter.[82] In another meta-analysis, Tritos and Danias[83] demonstrated that GH therapy resulted in an increase of LVEF and cardiac output, an improvement in systemic vascular resistance and New York Heart Association class level, and an amelioration of exercise duration and of maximum oxygen uptake, with no adverse effects on diastolic function. A possible explanation of these inhomogeneous data is found in the different study duration, target dose, end points, and the lack of assessment of GH status.[52] In particular, Le Coirvoisier and colleagues,[82] performing a subgroup analysis according to target dose of all clinical trials, demonstrated that although high-dose GH therapy was associated with significant overall effect for ventricular morphology, cardiopulmonary performance, and clinical status, low GH dose was associated only with exercise duration and New York Heart Association class. Moreover, when trials were separated into two groups according to the median of IGF-1 increase, studies with larger IGF-1 increase reported a significant overall effect size for LV morphology and cardiopulmonary performance, whereas no significant effects were showed by trials with smaller IGF-1 increases. The take home messages of this work are: (1) a proven impairment of GH/IGF-1 status (eg, GHD should be the preliminary condition before starting to administer GH); (2) physicians should consider an individualized dose titration of GH in patients with HF; and (3) GH therapy should not be administered in all patients with CHF, but only in mild to moderate CHF, considering the hypothesized GH resistance state of the more advanced disease.[30] With this in mind, 10 years ago our group implemented a novel approach, performing a randomized, single-blind controlled proof-of-concept trial in which, for the first time, the effects of GH therapy were tested only in patients affected by both GHD and CHF.[23] In this study, to check GHD status, patients underwent a GHRH + arginine provocative test. After 6 months, GH-replacement therapy decreased circulating NT-pro-BNP levels, augmented LVEF (from 33 ± 2 to $36 \pm 2\%$; $P<.01$), increased peak oxygen uptake (from 12.9 ± 0.9 to 14.5 ± 1.0 mL/kg/min; $P<.005$), and improved

quality of life score and flow-mediated vasodilation. Considering these encouraging results, with the aim to evaluate for the first time in HF a long-term GH therapy, we extended this study with a 4-year follow-up to assess whether these effects were sustained or tend to vanish over time.[84] At the end of the study, GH-replacement therapy was still associated with significant reductions of LV end-diastolic and end-systolic volumes indexes and circumferential wall stress, accordingly with an LV reverse remodeling, as documented by an increase in LVEF. In the GH group peak Vo_2 increased remarkably (with a treatment effect of 7.1 ± 0.7 mL/kg/min in the GH group, whereas the control group experienced a change of -1.8 ± 0.5; $P<.001$). Moreover, a difference in the composite of death and hospitalization for HF was observed, even though the study was not designed for hard clinical end points.

However, the usefulness of GH-replacement therapy must still be proved in a double-blind placebo-controlled trial. In this context, our group has been recently received the 2016 Grant for Growth Innovation International Award, proposing a double-blind study of GH-replacement therapy in patients with CHF with coexisting GHD.

Side Effects

Taken all together, data from clinical studies showed that GH therapy, if used with correct dosage, is safe and without major collateral effects. The worsening of ventricular arrhythmias reported by Frustaci and colleagues[64] are not reported by other studies. A possible explanation for this apparent discrepancy is the very high dosage used by Frustaci and colleagues. It is well known that supraphysiologic levels of GH, as in acromegaly, could lead to an increase in ventricular arrhythmia. Moreover, Le Corvoisier and colleagues[82] demonstrated that there were no differences in the frequency of major adverse effects between GH and placebo treatments: death, worsening of HF, increased salt retention, and ventricular arrhythmias are not significant between treatment or placebo arms. Moreover, Cittadini and colleagues,[84] in the trial that lasted longer on GH therapy in CHF, reported no major adverse events in the patients who received GH therapy. In particular, in this population, only two cases of arthralgia are reported. This is a well-known side effect of GH replacement and improved after GH therapy withdrawal. The low prevalence of adverse effects is congruent with the largest database available, which indicates that GH replacement in adults is well tolerated.[85]

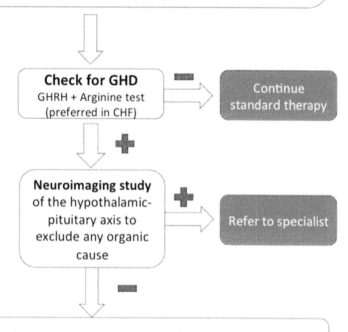

Fig. 2. Management of GHD in CHF. Based on the evidence acquisition, more recent guidelines, and authors' own experience, a suggested flowchart addressing the management of GHD in patients with CHF has been developed for clinical use.

SUMMARY

Growing evidence supports the hypothesis that CHF could be viewed as a multiple hormone deficiency syndrome. Deficiencies of the main anabolic axes are common in CHF and are associated with poor cardiovascular performance and prognosis seeming not to be only a mere cluster of biomarkers. Among these, GHD plays a pivotal role and its correction is likely to be considered as an innovative therapy that has to be considered in CHF.

In this regard, most recent statement of the American Heart Association on management of DCM[86] recommends with a strong level of consensus the testing for GHD in patients with DCM who have other signs and symptoms of those clinical disorders (level of evidence C) and recommends that appropriate therapy for the primary disorder of GHD should be performed in all patients with coexisting DCM.

Based on the aforementioned evidence acquisition and the authors' experience, a suggested flowchart addressing the management of GHD in CHF patients has been developed for clinical use (**Fig. 2**). In particular, we suggest that: (1) GH status should be investigated in all patients with CHF, in particular in those who displays signs and/or symptoms of GHD and/or have past medical history of condition commonly associated with GHD (eg, structural hypothalamic/pituitary disease, surgery or irradiation in these areas, head trauma, or evidence of other pituitary hormone deficiencies); (2) GH should be administered only in those patients with an impairment of GH/IGF-1 status (eg, GHD, as a replacement therapy); (3) an individualized dose titration of GH should be considered for each patient depending on neurohumoral response; and (4) GH therapy should not be administered in patients with advanced CHF, who are probably already in a GH resistance state.

REFERENCES

1. Braunwald E. Heart failure. JACC Heart Fail 2013; 1(1):1–20.
2. Hartupee J, Mann DL. Neurohormonal activation in heart failure with reduced ejection fraction. Nat Rev Cardiol 2017;14(1):30–8.
3. Salzano A, Sirico D, Arcopinto M, et al. Anti remodeling therapy: new strategies and future perspective in post-ischemic heart failure. Part II. Monaldi Arch Chest Dis 2014;82(4):195–201 [in Italian].
4. Sirico D, Salzano A, Celentani D, et al. Anti remodeling therapy: new strategies and future perspective in post-ischemic heart failure: part I. Monaldi Arch Chest Dis 2014;82(4):187–94 [in Italian].
5. Ponikowski P, Voors AA, Anker SD, et al. 2016 ESC Guidelines for the diagnosis and treatment of acute and chronic heart failure: the task force for the diagnosis and treatment of acute and chronic heart failure of the European Society of Cardiology (ESC). Developed with the special contribution of the Heart Failure Association (HFA) of the ESC. Eur J Heart Fail 2016;18(8):891–975.
6. Yancy CW, Jessup M, Bozkurt B, et al. 2017 ACC/AHA/HFSA focused update of the 2013 ACCF/AHA guideline for the management of heart failure: a report of the American College of Cardiology/American Heart Association Task Force on Clinical Practice Guidelines and the Heart Failure Society of America. J Card Fail 2017;23(8):628–51.
7. Sacca L. Heart failure as a multiple hormonal deficiency syndrome. Circ Heart Fail 2009;2(2):151–6.
8. Arcopinto M, Salzano A, Bossone E, et al. Multiple hormone deficiencies in chronic heart failure. Int J Cardiol 2015;184:421–3.
9. Salzano A, Marra AM, Ferrara F, et al. Multiple hormone deficiency syndrome in heart failure with preserved ejection fraction. Int J Cardiol 2016;225:1–3.
10. Jankowska EA, Biel B, Majda J, et al. Anabolic deficiency in men with chronic heart failure: prevalence and detrimental impact on survival. Circulation 2006; 114(17):1829–37.
11. Arcopinto M, Isgaard J, Marra AM, et al. IGF-1 predicts survival in chronic heart failure. Insights from the T.O.S.CA. (Trattamento Ormonale Nello Scompenso CArdiaco) registry. Int J Cardiol 2014; 176(3):1006–8.
12. Colao A. The GH-IGF-I axis and the cardiovascular system: clinical implications. Clin Endocrinol (Oxf) 2008;69(3):347–58.
13. Alvarez-Nava F, Lanes R. GH/IGF-1 signaling and current knowledge of epigenetics; a review and considerations on possible therapeutic options. Int J Mol Sci 2017;18(10) [pii:E1624].
14. Orru S, Nigro E, Mandola A, et al. A functional interplay between IGF-1 and adiponectin. Int J Mol Sci 2017;18(10) [pii:E2145].
15. Nicholls AR, Holt RI. Growth hormone and insulin-like growth factor-1. Front Horm Res 2016;47: 101–14.
16. Ranke MB. Insulin-like growth factor binding-protein-3 (IGFBP-3). Best Pract Res Clin Endocrinol Metab 2015;29(5):701–11.
17. Himpe E, Kooijman R. Insulin-like growth factor-I receptor signal transduction and the Janus Kinase/Signal Transducer and Activator of Transcription (JAK-STAT) pathway. Biofactors 2009;35(1):76–81.
18. Isgaard J, Arcopinto M, Karason K, et al. GH and the cardiovascular system: an update on a topic at heart. Endocrine 2015;48(1):25–35.
19. Hjalmarson A, Isaksson O, Ahren K. Effects of growth hormone and insulin on amino acid transport

in perfused rat heart. Am J Physiol 1969;217(6): 1795–802.

20. Stromer H, Palmieri EA, De Groot MC, et al. Growth hormone- and pressure overload-induced cardiac hypertrophy evoke different responses to ischemia-reperfusion and mechanical stretch. Growth Horm IGF Res 2006;16(1):29–40.

21. Cittadini A, Monti MG, Iaccarino G, et al. Adenoviral gene transfer of Akt enhances myocardial contractility and intracellular calcium handling. Gene Ther 2006;13(1):8–19.

22. Broglio F, Benso A, Gottero C, et al. Patients with dilated cardiomyopathy show reduction of the somatotroph responsiveness to GHRH both alone and combined with arginine. Eur J Endocrinol 2000; 142(2):157–63.

23. Cittadini A, Saldamarco L, Marra AM, et al. Growth hormone deficiency in patients with chronic heart failure and beneficial effects of its correction. J Clin Endocrinol Metab 2009;94(9):3329–36.

24. Niebauer J, Pflaum CD, Clark AL, et al. Deficient insulin-like growth factor I in chronic heart failure predicts altered body composition, anabolic deficiency, cytokine and neurohormonal activation. J Am Coll Cardiol 1998;32(2):393–7.

25. Arcopinto M, Salzano A, Giallauria F, et al. Growth hormone deficiency is associated with worse cardiac function, physical performance, and outcome in chronic heart failure: insights from the T.O.S.CA. GHD study. PLoS One 2017;12(1):e0170058.

26. Kontoleon PE, Anastasiou-Nana MI, Papapetrou PD, et al. Hormonal profile in patients with congestive heart failure. Int J Cardiol 2003;87(2–3):179–83.

27. Petretta M, Colao A, Sardu C, et al. NT-proBNP, IGF-I and survival in patients with chronic heart failure. Growth Horm IGF Res 2007;17(4):288–96.

28. Anwar A, Gaspoz JM, Pampallona S, et al. Effect of congestive heart failure on the insulin-like growth factor-1 system. Am J Cardiol 2002;90(12):1402–5.

29. Bolger A, Doehner W, Anker SD. Insulin-like growth factor-I can be helpful towards end of life. BMJ 2001;322(7287):674–5.

30. Anker SD, Volterrani M, Pflaum CD, et al. Acquired growth hormone resistance in patients with chronic heart failure: implications for therapy with growth hormone. J Am Coll Cardiol 2001;38(2):443–52.

31. Molitch ME, Clemmons DR, Malozowski S, et al. Evaluation and treatment of adult growth hormone deficiency: an Endocrine Society clinical practice guideline. J Clin Endocrinol Metab 2011;96(6): 1587–609.

32. Ghigo E, Aimaretti G, Corneli G. Diagnosis of adult GH deficiency. Growth Horm IGF Res 2008;18(1): 1–16.

33. Yuen KC, Tritos NA, Samson SL, et al. American Association of Clinical Endocrinologists and American College of Endocrinology disease state clinical review: update on growth hormone stimulation testing and proposed revised cut-point for the glucagon stimulation test in the diagnosis of adult growth hormone deficiency. Endocr Pract 2016; 22(10):1235–44.

34. Gordon MB, Levy RA, Gut R, et al. Trends in growth hormone stimulation testing and growth hormone dosing in adult growth hormone deficiency patients: results from the answer program. Endocr Pract 2016;22(4):396–405.

35. Prodam F, Pagano L, Corneli G, et al. Update on epidemiology, etiology, and diagnosis of adult growth hormone deficiency. J Endocrinol Invest 2008;31(9 Suppl):6–11.

36. Pena-Bello L, Seoane-Pillado T, Sangiao-Alvarellos S, et al. Oral glucose-stimulated growth hormone (GH) test in adult GH deficiency patients and controls: potential utility of a novel test. Eur J Intern Med 2017;44: 55–61.

37. Rahim A, Toogood AA, Shalet SM. The assessment of growth hormone status in normal young adult males using a variety of provocative agents. Clin Endocrinol (Oxf) 1996;45(5):557–62.

38. Junnila RK, Strasburger CJ, Bidlingmaier M. Pitfalls of insulin-like growth factor-i and growth hormone assays. Endocrinol Metab Clin North Am 2015; 44(1):27–34.

39. Colao A, Di Somma C, Cuocolo A, et al. The severity of growth hormone deficiency correlates with the severity of cardiac impairment in 100 adult patients with hypopituitarism: an observational, case-control study. J Clin Endocrinol Metab 2004;89(12): 5998–6004.

40. Rosen T, Bengtsson BA. Premature mortality due to cardiovascular disease in hypopituitarism. Lancet 1990;336(8710):285–8.

41. Bhandari SS, Narayan H, Jones DJ, et al. Plasma growth hormone is a strong predictor of risk at 1 year in acute heart failure. Eur J Heart Fail 2016; 18(3):281–9.

42. Fonarow GC, Adams KF Jr, Abraham WT, et al. Risk stratification for in-hospital mortality in acutely decompensated heart failure: classification and regression tree analysis. JAMA 2005;293(5):572–80.

43. Wang CY, Chung HW, Cho NY, et al. Idiopathic growth hormone deficiency in the morphologically normal pituitary gland is associated with perfusion delay. Radiology 2011;258(1):213–21.

44. Marra AM, Benjamin N, Eichstaedt C, et al. Gender-related differences in pulmonary arterial hypertension targeted drugs administration. Pharmacol Res 2016;114:103–9.

45. Yoshida T, Tabony AM, Galvez S, et al. Molecular mechanisms and signaling pathways of angiotensin II-induced muscle wasting: potential therapeutic targets for cardiac cachexia. Int J Biochem Cell Biol 2013;45(10):2322–32.

46. Giustina A, Veldhuis JD. Pathophysiology of the neuroregulation of growth hormone secretion in experimental animals and the human. Endocr Rev 1998; 19(6):717–97.

47. Marra AM, Improda N, Capalbo D, et al. Cardiovascular abnormalities and impaired exercise performance in adolescents with congenital adrenal hyperplasia. J Clin Endocrinol Metab 2015;100(2): 644–52.

48. Salzano A, Demelo-Rodriguez P, Marra AM, et al. A focused review of gender differences in antithrombotic therapy. Curr Med Chem 2017;24(24): 2576–88.

49. Pasquali D, Arcopinto M, Renzullo A, et al. Cardiovascular abnormalities in Klinefelter syndrome. Int J Cardiol 2013;168(2):754–9.

50. Salzano A, Arcopinto M, Marra AM, et al. Klinefelter syndrome, cardiovascular system, and thromboembolic disease: review of literature and clinical perspectives. Eur J Endocrinol 2016;175(1):R27–40.

51. Sacca F, Puorro G, Marsili A, et al. Long-term effect of epoetin alfa on clinical and biochemical markers in Friedreich ataxia. Mov Disord 2016;31(5):734–41.

52. Arcopinto M, Salzano A, Isgaard J, et al. Hormone replacement therapy in heart failure. Curr Opin Cardiol 2015;30(3):277–84.

53. Napoli R, Salzano A, Bossone E, et al. Hormonal therapy in the treatment of chronic heart failure. Elsevier; 2017.

54. Marra AM, Bobbio E, D'Assante R, et al. growth hormone as biomarker in heart failure. Heart Fail Clin 2018;14(1):65–74.

55. Arcopinto M, Salzano A, Ferrara F, et al. The TOSCA registry: an ongoing, observational, multicenter registry for chronic heart failure. Transl Med UniSa 2016;14:21–7.

56. Bossone E, Limongelli G, Malizia G, et al. The T.O.S.CA. Project: research, education and care. Monaldi Arch Chest Dis 2011;76(4):198–203.

57. Yang R, Bunting S, Gillett N, et al. Growth hormone improves cardiac performance in experimental heart failure. Circulation 1995;92(2):262–7.

58. Duerr RL, McKirnan MD, Gim RD, et al. Cardiovascular effects of insulin-like growth factor-1 and growth hormone in chronic left ventricular failure in the rat. Circulation 1996;93(12):2188–96.

59. Ryoke T, Gu Y, Mao L, et al. Progressive cardiac dysfunction and fibrosis in the cardiomyopathic hamster and effects of growth hormone and angiotensin-converting enzyme inhibition. Circulation 1999;100(16):1734–43.

60. Cittadini A, Ishiguro Y, Stromer H, et al. Insulin-like growth factor-1 but not growth hormone augments mammalian myocardial contractility by sensitizing the myofilament to Ca2+ through a wortmannin-sensitive pathway: studies in rat and ferret isolated muscles. Circ Res 1998;83(1):50–9.

61. Cittadini A, Isgaard J, Monti MG, et al. Growth hormone prolongs survival in experimental postinfarction heart failure. J Am Coll Cardiol 2003;41(12): 2154–63.

62. Cittadini A, Grossman JD, Napoli R, et al. Growth hormone attenuates early left ventricular remodeling and improves cardiac function in rats with large myocardial infarction. J Am Coll Cardiol 1997; 29(5):1109–16.

63. Fazio S, Sabatini D, Capaldo B, et al. A preliminary study of growth hormone in the treatment of dilated cardiomyopathy. N Engl J Med 1996;334(13): 809–14.

64. Frustaci A, Gentiloni N, Russo MA. Growth hormone in the treatment of dilated cardiomyopathy. N Engl J Med 1996;335(9):672–3 [author reply: 3–4].

65. Isgaard J, Bergh CH, Caidahl K, et al. A placebo-controlled study of growth hormone in patients with congestive heart failure. Eur Heart J 1998;19(11): 1704–11.

66. Osterziel KJ, Strohm O, Schuler J, et al. Randomised, double-blind, placebo-controlled trial of human recombinant growth hormone in patients with chronic heart failure due to dilated cardiomyopathy. Lancet 1998;351(9111):1233–7.

67. Genth-Zotz S, Zotz R, Geil S, et al. Recombinant growth hormone therapy in patients with ischemic cardiomyopathy: effects on hemodynamics, left ventricular function, and cardiopulmonary exercise capacity. Circulation 1999;99(1):18–21.

68. Spallarossa P, Rossettin P, Minuto F, et al. Evaluation of growth hormone administration in patients with chronic heart failure secondary to coronary artery disease. Am J Cardiol 1999; 84(4):430–3.

69. Jose VJ, Zechariah TU, George P, et al. Growth hormone therapy in patients with dilated cardiomyopathy: preliminary observations of a pilot study. Indian Heart J 1999;51(2):183–5.

70. Smit JW, Janssen YJ, Lamb HJ, et al. Six months of recombinant human GH therapy in patients with ischemic cardiac failure does not influence left ventricular function and mass. J Clin Endocrinol Metab 2001;86(10):4638–43.

71. Perrot A, Ranke MB, Dietz R, et al. Growth hormone treatment in dilated cardiomyopathy. J Card Surg 2001;16(2):127–31.

72. Napoli R, Guardasole V, Matarazzo M, et al. Growth hormone corrects vascular dysfunction in patients with chronic heart failure. J Am Coll Cardiol 2002; 39(1):90–5.

73. Adamopoulos S, Parissis JT, Paraskevaidis I, et al. Effects of growth hormone on circulating cytokine network, and left ventricular contractile performance and geometry in patients with idiopathic dilated cardiomyopathy. Eur Heart J 2003;24(24): 2186–96.

74. Acevedo M, Corbalan R, Chamorro G, et al. Administration of growth hormone to patients with advanced cardiac heart failure: effects upon left ventricular function, exercise capacity, and neurohormonal status. Int J Cardiol 2003;87(2–3):185–91.

75. van Thiel SW, Smit JW, de Roos A, et al. Six-months of recombinant human GH therapy in patients with ischemic cardiac failure. Int J Cardiovasc Imaging 2004;20(1):53–60.

76. Fazio S, Palmieri EA, Affuso F, et al. Effects of growth hormone on exercise capacity and cardiopulmonary performance in patients with chronic heart failure. J Clin Endocrinol Metab 2007;92(11):4218–23.

77. Marra AM, Arcopinto M, Bobbio E, et al. An unusual case of dilated cardiomyopathy associated with partial hypopituitarism. Intern Emerg Med 2012;7(Suppl 2):S85–7.

78. Frustaci A, Gentiloni N, Corsello SM, et al. Reversible dilated cardiomyopathy due to growth hormone deficiency. Chest 1992;102(1):326–7.

79. Cuneo R, Salomon F, Wilmshurst P, et al. Reversible dilated cardiomyopathy due to growth hormone deficiency. Am J Clin Pathol 1993;100(5):585–6.

80. Cittadini A, Ines Comi L, Longobardi S, et al. A preliminary randomized study of growth hormone administration in Becker and Duchenne muscular dystrophies. Eur Heart J 2003;24(7):664–72.

81. Marra AM, Arcopinto M, Salzano A, et al. Detectable interleukin-9 plasma levels are associated with impaired cardiopulmonary functional capacity and all-cause mortality in patients with chronic heart failure. Int J Cardiol 2016;209:114–7.

82. Le Corvoisier P, Hittinger L, Chanson P, et al. Cardiac effects of growth hormone treatment in chronic heart failure: a meta-analysis. J Clin Endocrinol Metab 2007;92(1):180–5.

83. Tritos NA, Danias PG. Growth hormone therapy in congestive heart failure due to left ventricular systolic dysfunction: a meta-analysis. Endocr Pract 2008;14(1):40–9.

84. Cittadini A, Marra AM, Arcopinto M, et al. Growth hormone replacement delays the progression of chronic heart failure combined with growth hormone deficiency: an extension of a randomized controlled single-blind study. JACC Heart Fail 2013;1(4):325–30.

85. Spielhagen C, Schwahn C, Moller K, et al. The benefit of long-term growth hormone (GH) replacement therapy in hypopituitary adults with GH deficiency: results of the German KIMS database. Growth Horm IGF Res 2011;21(1):1–10.

86. Bozkurt B, Colvin M, Cook J, et al. Current diagnostic and treatment strategies for specific dilated cardiomyopathies: a scientific statement from the American Heart Association. Circulation 2016; 134(23):e579–646.

Ultrafiltration for the Treatment of Acute Heart Failure

Sitaramesh Emani, MD

KEYWORDS

- Ultrafiltration • Acute heart failure • Treatment

KEY POINTS

- Ultrafiltration allows mechanical removal of fluid in a controlled fashion and can be used an alternative to diuretic therapies when treating acute heart failure.
- Ultrafiltration promotes the loss of isotonic fluid without the risk of electrolyte imbalances that can be caused by diuretic use, and may also avoid neurohormonal activation caused by loop diuretics.
- Early clinical studies suggested benefits of ultrafiltration both in the acute phase by allowing adequate volume removal, and in the follow up phase by potentially impacting readmission rates.
- However, follow up studies have shown variable results when comparing ultrafiltration to various pharmacologic strategies; and to date, definitive clinical evidence is not yet available.
- Ultrafiltration can be considered for the treatment of acute heart failure in selected situations.

INTRODUCTION

Ultrafiltration (UF) is a strategy used to mechanically remove excess fluid volume through an extracorporeal circuit and has been applied to clinical situations in which volume removal is the mainstay of therapy. Because of this ability, UF serves as an enticing method to treat acute heart failure (AHF), in which most symptoms are driven by congestion due to excess volume.[1] Additional physiologic properties of UF and the biochemical composition of the extracted fluid confer additional theoretic benefits in the treatment of AHF. Despite these potential advantages, however, clinical evidence has not uniformly supported the use of UF for heart failure management. Herein the concepts underlying UF, clinical evidence evaluating its efficacy, and ongoing challenges understanding the role of UF are reviewed.

ULTRAFILTRATION DESCRIPTION

Various methods to achieve UF exist, but all methods share certain characteristics. Common to all UF approaches is the need to circulate blood through an extracorporeal circuit allowing passage through a semipermeable membrane filter. This process allows removal of excess fluid volume without extraction desirable hematologic and plasma components. The nonfiltered components are returned to the patient.[2] **Fig. 1** illustrates the general set up of 2 different UF circuit configurations.

Because blood is processed extracorporeally, UF requires established venous access for both withdrawal and return.[3] The type of venous access depends on the physical properties of the UF circuit (incorporating factors such as flow rates and resistance properties) and can range from large-gauge peripheral access to central venous access.

Disclosure: The author serves as a consultant for CHF Solutions, Minneapolis, MN.
Division of Cardiovascular Medicine, The Ohio State University Wexner Medical Center, 473 West 12th Avenue, Suite 200 DHLRI, Columbus, OH 43210, USA
E-mail address: Sitaramesh.emani@osumc.edu

Heart Failure Clin 14 (2018) 517–524
https://doi.org/10.1016/j.hfc.2018.06.013
1551-7136/18/© 2018 Elsevier Inc. All rights reserved.

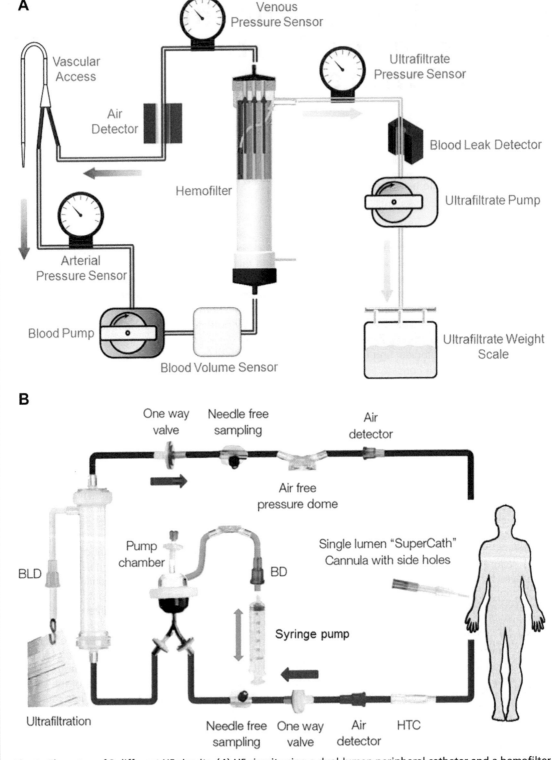

Fig. 1. The setup of 2 different UF circuits. (*A*) UF circuit using a dual-lumen peripheral catheter and a hemofilter (such as that used by the Aquadex FlexFlow System, CHF Solutions, Eden Prairie, MN, USA). (*B*) UF circuit using single-lumen peripheral venous access, a syringe pump, and a pump chamber to generate an ultrafiltrate. The pump-driving setup uses one-way valves to allow blood to be both withdrawn and returned through the same single-lumen access point (such as that used by Congestive Heart Impairment Advanced Removal Approach [CHIARA] setup, Haemotronic, Mirandola, Italy). BD, blood detector; BLD, blood leak detector; HTC, hematocrit sensor. (*From* Costanzo MR, Ronco C, Abraham WT, et al. Extracorporeal ultrafiltration for fluid overload in heart failure: current status and prospects for further research. J Am Coll Cardiol 2017;29(19):2431; with permission.)

Circuits requiring larger forms of access, such as midlines and central venous catheters, assume a need for an invasive procedure to initiate therapy. Inability to undergo these procedures or complications resulting from these procedures can limit the ability to use ultrafiltration. Anticoagulation may also be required to prevent clotting within the circuit or filter, and also carries incremental risk due to bleeding.[3] For patients for whom appropriate access can be obtained and can tolerate anticoagulation, though, UF can be considered.

The historical development of UF evolved from renal replacement therapy strategies. The development of a dialysis membrane to serve as an artificial kidney allowed patients with renal failure to be treated, eventually leading to modern versions of hemodialysis that remove both metabolic by-products as well as volume status.[4–7] In AHF, however, native renal clearance is not completely jeopardized and metabolic filtration is not necessary but volume removal requirements remain.[8] This need has led to the development of specific UF filters designed to remove plasma water alone and distinguishes UF from other forms of hemofiltration.[2]

Currently, UF can be achieved by selecting appropriate plasma filter within a traditional dialysis circuit or through the use of specially designed UF machines.[9] Smaller portable machines allow for easier bedside access to patients and do not necessarily require central venous access to institute therapy.[3]

THEORETIC BENEFITS

Volume removal via an UF membrane may provide advantages over traditional methods of removal. The current standard of care for the treatment of AHF focuses on the relief of congestive symptoms, the core of which is removal of excess volume using loop diuretics, often administered intravenously.[10] Numerous strategies exist regarding the use of loop diuretics, and detailed reviews of these approaches have been reviewed elsewhere.[11]

Despite the long-standing use of diuretics to treat AHF, exact recommendations on dosing remain elusive. Generally, it is recommended that patients presenting with increasing signs of congestion be treated with intravenous loop diuretics at a dose equivalent to or greater than their baseline dosing.[10] Attempts to clarify the best use of loop diuretics were addressed in the Diuretic Optimization Strategies Evaluation (DOSE) trial. In this trial, patients were randomized to low-versus high-dose furosemide administered either as a continuous infusion or bolus dosing. The

2×2 factorial design enrolled 308 patients and monitored the response to the initial 72 hours of therapy. Final analysis of the primary end point (composite of change in self-assessment of symptoms and change in renal function) demonstrated no statistical difference between low-dose and high-dose groups and likewise showed no difference between continuous versus bolus administration.[12] The results of this trial underscore ongoing difficulties with and lack of mastery of diuretic therapies to treat AHF.

Incomplete understanding of optimal diuretic use may serve as one reason for suboptimal heart failure outcomes following a hospitalization. Historical data suggest inadequate volume removal for many episodes of AHF hospitalizations, which can lead to subsequent recurrent hospitalizations and decline in overall functional status.[13–15] Therefore, utilization of diuretic-based strategies have not resulted in overall improvement for the treatment of AHF.[16] These shortcomings may be the result of additional factors beyond inadequate dosing, including physiologic effects of diuretic usage.

The use of loop diuretics has been shown to activate neurohormonal pathways, including increases in norepinephrine and angiotensin II levels, which may lead to a detrimental downstream effect, such as vasoconstriction.[17] Furthermore, activation of neurohormonal pathways is counteractive to many other therapeutic strategies in the treatment of heart failure aimed at reducing vasoconstriction and downregulation of the same pathways.[18] Unintended activation of these pathways may result in a diminished response to loop diuretic dosing in the AHF state, potentially necessitating the use of higher doses of diuretics leading to a deleterious negative feedback loop.[19,20]

An additional undesirable consequence of loop diuretic use is the biochemical composition of volume being removed. Loop diuretics resulted in the formation of hypotonic urine, resulting in less total sodium loss per volume of fluid compared with the sodium concentration of a patient with volume-overloaded heart failure. Because sodium concentrations drive fluid shifts and in particular extracellular volume (ECV) expansion, inadequate sodium loss may not decrease ECV to the degree desired. In comparison, UF membranes allow for passage of both water and sodium, resulting in the removal of isotonic fluid. As a result, ECV volume decreases to a greater degree with UF compared with volume loss induced by diuretics. Although water and sodium pass through the membrane, larger molecules, such as potassium, are not filtered out; therefore, UF volume loss is less likely to result in hypokalemia.[2]

CLINICAL EVIDENCE

The ability to remove isotonic fluid without electrolyte disturbances has often been touted as a significant advantage of UF over traditional therapies. However, despite these theoretic advantages, proving the superiority of UF has been difficult in clinical studies. Numerous reports and evaluations have been published, ranging from small case series to randomized trials, and have shown variable results. Some of the more notable studies are shown in **Table 1**.

Although it was not the original study published regarding the use of UF in AHF, the Ultrafiltration versus Intravenous Diuretics for Patients Hospitalized for Acute Decompensated Heart Failure (UNLOAD) trial helped garner large-scale attention to the therapy's potential. In this multicenter, randomized trial, patients presenting with AHF were assigned to either early UF or standard care (intravenous loop diuretics). For patients undergoing UF, therapy was initiated within 24 hours of presentation; for patients receiving loop diuretics, the minimum dose was assigned as greater than or equal to twice the patients' home dosing. The primary end points were weight loss and dyspnea assessments at 48 hours; additional secondary end points included net fluid loss at 48 hours, heart failure rehospitalizations, and unscheduled visits at

Table 1
Selected studies evaluating ultrafiltration for the treatment of acute heart failure

Study	Design	End Point/ Rationale	No. of Patients	Results	Year
Peripherally inserted venovenous UF for rapid treatment of volume-overloaded patients[3]	Multicenter, single arm	Investigational device study	21	>1 L of fluid removal is feasible without central venous access.	2003
The Relief for Acutely Fluid-Overloaded Patients With Decompensated Congestive Heart Failure (RAPID-CHF) Trial[43]	Multicenter RCT (UF vs SC)	Comparison of fluid and weight loss	40	UF resulted in greater fluid loss but not greater weight loss.	2005
Early UF in patients with decompensated heart failure and diuretic resistance (EUPHORIA)[40]	Single center, prospective single arm	Feasibility of using early UF to treat AHF with diuretic resistance	20	UF can remove fluid (average 8.6 L) in patients with AHF.	2005
UF vs intravenous diuretics for patients hospitalized for acute decompensated heart failure (UNLOAD)[21]	Multicenter RCT (UF vs SC)	Comparison of weight loss and dyspnea at 48 h	200	UF resulted in greater weight loss and similar improvements in dyspnea.	2007
UF in decompensated heart failure with cardiorenal syndrome (CARRESS-HF)[23]	Multicenter RCT (UF[a] vs SC[c])	Comparison of renal function and weight changes at 96 h	188	UF resulted in similar weight change but with WRF.	2012
Aquapheresis vs Intravenous Diuretics and Hospitalizations for Heart Failure (AVOID-HF)[37]	Multicenter RCT (UF[b] vs SC[c])	Comparison of 90-d readmission rates after AHF hospitalization	224[d]	There was no statistical difference between groups; UF trended to better 90-d outcomes.	2015

Abbreviations: IDE, investigational device exemption; RCT, randomized controlled trial; SC, standard care; WRF, worsening renal function.
   [a] UF strategy used was fixed-rate UF.
   [b] UF strategy used was adjustable-rate UF.
   [c] SC strategy was stepped-pharmacologic therapy.
   [d] Trial terminated early before enrollment goal of 810.

90 days following discharge. A total of 200 patients were enrolled and randomized in a 1:1 fashion. UNLOAD demonstrated greater weight loss in the UF group at the 48-hour mark compared with diuretics but had the same effect on dyspnea improvement. A nonstatistically significant increase in serum creatinine was seen early in the UF arm, but values returned to preadmission levels by 90 days. Freedom from rehospitalization, a secondary end point, was greater in the UF arm at 90 days compared with loop diuretics.[21]

Excitement for UF grew following UNLOAD, in part because of the ability to remove more fluid than standard-care loop diuretics but also in part because of the signal toward a lasting benefit of fewer rehospitalizations. That latter was a secondary end point, however; the trial was not designed to conclusively demonstrate a long-term benefit with the use of UF. Additional criticisms included the lack of prescriptive diuretic use in the control arm. Nevertheless, clinical use began to expand but brought with it some concerns for adverse events, particularly in patients with cardiorenal syndrome.[22]

Difficulty in generalizing the results of UNLOAD to patients with underlying renal dysfunction prompted the Cardiorenal Rescue Study in Acute Decompensated Heart Failure (CARRESS-HF) trial. The trial was designed to evaluate a stepped-pharmacologic strategy (using intravenous loop diuretics) versus UF. The primary outcome was a bivariate end point combining change in weight and creatinine. Importantly, eligible patients presented with AHF defined by signs of worsening congestion as well as worsening renal function.[23]

CARRESS-HF ultimately enrolled 188 patients, with an equal number assigned to each arm. With regard to the primary end point, UF was found to be inferior to pharmacologic therapy. Change in weight between the two groups was statistically similar (5.7 kg lost in UF patients, 5.5 kg lost in diuretic patients), but UF was noted to be associated with worsening renal function (+0.23 mg/dL for UF vs 0.04 mg/dL in medically treated patients). As a result, the study concluded that the use of UF is not justified for patients with AHF hospitalized for worsening congestion in the presence of worsening renal function.[23] Careful examination of the results, though, reveals a fair amount of crossover within the study, especially for patients randomized to the UF arm. Indeed, a more recent per-protocol analysis of CARRESS-HF suggested that those patients who remained on UF therapy for the duration of the study experienced greater fluid and weight loss but did

experience a greater magnitude of change in renal function.[24]

The results of CARRESS-HF dampened some of the initial enthusiasm for UF and heightened suspicion of the therapy's efficacy. The trial's conclusions, though, were questioned when the data were further evaluated. First, the change in renal function, which drove the primary end point against UF, was statistically significant but may not be clinically significant. The clinically accepted definition of acute kidney injury (AKI) has traditionally been set at a change in creatinine of 0.3 mg/dL or greater.[25] The 0.23-mg/dL increase seen on average in CARRESS-HF with UF, therefore, would not have met the definition of AKI. In contrast, 23% of patients receiving high-dose diuretics in the DOSE trial did experience a change in creatinine of 0.3 mg/dL or greater.[12] Although an indirect inference, it is interesting to note that the potential alternative to UF, intravenous diuretics, may also have a non-negligible risk of renal harm.

Within this discussion is the debatable point of serum creatinine change during decongestion as a marker of true kidney injury. Changes in serum creatinine may not reflect changes in renal function under dynamic conditions.[26] An in-depth review of renal function monitoring is beyond the scope of this article but can be found elsewhere.[27,28] However, a retrospective analysis of renal function changes during the treatment of AHF has suggested that a 0.3 mg/dL or greater change in serum creatinine may not be associated with true renal injury and does not imply long-term impairment to renal function.[26] Therefore, the consequences of minor changes in serum creatinine during UF may be difficult to place into clinical context.

In the discussions that followed CARRESS-HF's results, one criticism that was raised focused on the UF algorithm used.[29] The treatment arm was assigned to fixed-rate UF with a removal rate of 200 mL/h, without prescriptive changes to accommodate patient characteristics. In contrast, the control arm used an adjustable diuretic regimen to produce a target level of fluid removal.[30] Per-protocol analysis of CARRESS-HF, interestingly, showed lower-than-target rates for patients who remained on UF; but limited information is available regarding the logic that guided deviations to different fluid removal rates.[24] When considering treatment with UF, a one-size-fits-all approach may not be the ideal approach; but adjustments in rates should be guided by physiologic principles, if possible.[31]

When undergoing fluid removal, physiologic mechanisms exist to regulate fluid shifts within vascular and extravascular spaces, including hydrostatic and oncotic forces as summarized in the Starling equation.[32] Because UF removes intravascular volume through an extracorporeal circuit, these physiologic mechanisms may be overridden and result in aggressive shifts with negative consequences.[33,34] The movement of extra-vascular fluid into the vascular space has been described as the capillary refill rate, which unfortunately is not measurable at an individual patient level. Theoretically, however, the goal of any decongestive therapy would be to match fluid removal rates to the capillary refill rate to avoid vascular depletion.[32] Clinically, this principle often guides diuretic dosing and can be extended to UF removal rates; algorithms have been published to guide UF rate adjustment based on patient criteria.[2]

The application of this idea was evaluated in the small, single-center Continuous Ultrafiltration for Congestive Heart Failure (CUORE) trial. Patients were treated with either standard diuretic therapies or adjustable rate UF (AUF). The trial showed fewer rehospitalizations with stable renal function through 1 year following the initial therapy and suggested that manner in which UF is conducted may influence outcomes.[35]

The approach used in CUORE paved the way for the larger Aquapheresis versus Intravenous Diuretics and Hospitalization for Heart Failure (AVOID-HF) trial. AVOID-HF was designed to compare adjustable loop diuretic regimens, similar to the control arm of CARRESS-HF, with AUF. The primary end point was freedom from heart failure events, such as rehospitalization, through 90 days. The intent was to initiate AUF early in the hospital course when patients would be the most volume overloaded.[36] It was hoped that AVOID-HF would provide a durable comparison between clinically reasonable strategies to address the role of UF in AHF therapy.

Unfortunately, AVOID-HF was unable to provide the anticipated answers because of early termination of the trial. Interestingly, and importantly, the trial was terminated early not because of safety concerns or ethical trepidations but rather because of a loss of funding as part of an economic decision by the study sponsor.[37,38] Ultimately, only 224 out of the planned 810 patients were enrolled, rendering the trial underpowered to reach definitive solutions. The only conclusion that could be ascertained was that UF patients demonstrated a nonstatistically significant trend toward improved outcomes without any additional safety concerns related to therapy.[37] Because of the insufficient enrollment, extrapolation of the conclusions is difficult and remains speculative.

In total, the available clinical evidence is incomplete and does not fully endorse the routine use of UF for AHF but also does not point against its use. Consequently, current guidelines provide a class IIb level of recommendation for the use of UF presenting with either obvious volume overload or for patients not responding to other forms of medical therapy.[39]

SUMMARY AND FUTURE DIRECTIONS

At present, UF for the treatment of AHF remains a quandary. Theoretic benefits of isotonic fluid removal, control of volume removed, and avoidance of neurohormonal activation have failed to translate into consistently proven outcomes in clinical trials. Heterogeneity within the application of UF and comparison therapies, as well as statistical inadequacies in populations studied, plague the current evidence. Ideally, addressing these concerns in well-designed future trials will help us understand when, and if, UF should be used.

Beyond these questions, further investigations may be warranted as well. Are certain patient populations more likely to benefit from UF than others? Intriguingly, each of the major trials reviewed has enrolled patients regardless of ejection fraction (EF). Although investigating EF independent therapies is attractive when considering AHF, the underling physiology of reduced EF patients may be unique compared with preserved EF patients. Perhaps one group may be more likely to benefit than the other.

Another question revolves around patients with AHF with concurrent renal dysfunction. Patients with significant renal dysfunction were excluded in UNLOAD, CARRESS-HF, and AVOID-HF[21,23,40]; yet the occurrence of both disorders is common in patients and complicates therapy.[8,41] Treating AHF in the presence of cardiorenal syndrome remains challenging,[42] and the role UF may have in these patients remains unknown.

Answering these questions may help move UF from a mysterious to mainstream therapy.

REFERENCES

1. Ambrosy AP, Fonarow GC, Butler J, et al. The global health and economic burden of hospitalizations for heart failure: lessons learned from hospitalized heart failure registries. J Am Coll Cardiol 2014;63(12): 1123–33.
2. Costanzo MR, Ronco C, Abraham WT, et al. Extracorporeal ultrafiltration for fluid overload in heart failure: current status and prospects for further research. J Am Coll Cardiol 2017;69(19):2428–45.

3. Jaski BE, Ha J, Denys BG, et al. Peripherally inserted veno-venous ultrafiltration for rapid treatment of volume overloaded patients. J Card Fail 2003; 9(3):227–31.

4. Kolff WJ, Berk HTJ, Welle NM, et al. The artificial kidney: a dialyser with a great area. Acta Med Scand 1944;117(2):121–34.

5. Scribner BH, Buri R, Caner JE, et al. The treatment of chronic uremia by means of intermittent hemodialysis: a preliminary report. Trans Am Soc Artif Intern Organs 1960;6:114–22.

6. Flythe JE, Brookhart MA. Fluid management: the challenge of defining standards of care. Clin J Am Soc Nephrol 2014;9(12):2033–5.

7. Weiner DE, Brunelli SM, Hunt A, et al. Improving clinical outcomes among hemodialysis patients: a proposal for a "volume first" approach from the chief medical officers of US dialysis providers. Am J Kidney Dis 2014;64(5):685–95.

8. Patel UD, Greiner MA, Fonarow GC, et al. Associations between worsening renal function and 30-day outcomes among Medicare beneficiaries hospitalized with heart failure. Am Heart J 2010;160(1): 132–8.e1.

9. Sharma A, Hermann DD, Mehta RL. Clinical benefit and approach of ultrafiltration in acute heart failure. Cardiology 2001;96(3–4):144–54.

10. Yancy CW, Jessup M, Bozkurt B, et al. 2013 ACCF/AHA guideline for the management of heart failure: executive summary: a report of the American College of Cardiology Foundation/American Heart Association Task Force on practice guidelines. Circulation 2013;128(16):1810–52.

11. Ellison DH, Felker GM. Diuretic treatment in heart failure. N Engl J Med 2017;377(20):1964–75.

12. Felker GM, Lee KL, Bull DA, et al. Diuretic strategies in patients with acute decompensated heart failure. N Engl J Med 2011;364(9):797–805.

13. Fonarow GC, Horwich TB. Prevention of heart failure: effective strategies to combat the growing epidemic. Rev Cardiovasc Med 2003;4(1):8–17.

14. Setoguchi S, Stevenson LW, Schneeweiss S. Repeated hospitalizations predict mortality in the community population with heart failure. Am Heart J 2007;154(2):260–6.

15. Crespo-Leiro MG, Anker SD, Maggioni AP, et al. European Society of Cardiology Heart Failure Long-Term Registry (ESC-HF-LT): 1-year follow-up outcomes and differences across regions. Eur J Heart Fail 2016;18(6):613–25.

16. Gheorghiade M, Filippatos G. Reassessing treatment of acute heart failure syndromes: the ADHERE registry. Eur Heart J Suppl 2005; 7(suppl_B):B13–9.

17. Francis GS, Siegel RM, Goldsmith SR, et al. Acute vasoconstrictor response to intravenous furosemide in patients with chronic congestive heart failure.

Activation of the neurohumoral axis. Ann Intern Med 1985;103(1):1–6.

18. Berliner D, Hallbaum M, Bauersachs J. Current drug therapy for heart failure with reduced ejection fraction. Herz 2018. https://doi.org/10.1007/s00059-018-4712-4.

19. Ellison DH. Diuretic therapy and resistance in congestive heart failure. Cardiology 2001;96(3–4): 132–43.

20. Spuijbroek EJ, Blom N, Braam AW, et al. Stockholm syndrome manifestation of Munchausen: an eye-catching misnomer. J Psychiatr Pract 2012;18(4): 296–303.

21. Costanzo MR, Guglin ME, Saltzberg MT, et al. Ultrafiltration versus intravenous diuretics for patients hospitalized for acute decompensated heart failure. J Am Coll Cardiol 2007;49(6):675–83.

22. Bart BA, Walsh MM, Blake D, et al. Ultrafiltration for cardiorenal syndrome. J Card Fail 2008;14(6):531–2 [author reply: 532–3].

23. Bart BA, Goldsmith SR, Lee KL, et al. Ultrafiltration in decompensated heart failure with cardiorenal syndrome. N Engl J Med 2012;367(24):2296–304.

24. Grodin JL, Carter S, Bart BA, et al. Direct comparison of ultrafiltration to pharmacological decongestion in heart failure: a per-protocol analysis of CARRESS-HF. Eur J Heart Fail 2018. https://doi.org/10.1002/ejhf.1158.

25. Mehta RL, Kellum JA, Shah SV, et al. Acute kidney injury network: report of an initiative to improve outcomes in acute kidney injury. Crit Care 2007; 11(2):R31.

26. Ahmad T, Jackson K, Rao VS, et al. Worsening renal function in patients with acute heart failure undergoing aggressive diuresis is not associated with tubular injury. Circulation 2018;137(19): 2016–28.

27. Kar S, Paglialunga S, Islam R. Cystatin C is a more reliable biomarker for determining egfr to support drug development studies. J Clin Pharmacol 2018. https://doi.org/10.1002/jcph.1132.

28. Fu S, Zhao S, Ye P, et al. Biomarkers in cardiorenal syndromes. Biomed Res Int 2018;2018:9617363.

29. Roy MJ, Costanzo ME, Jovanovic T, et al. Heart rate response to fear conditioning and virtual reality in subthreshold PTSD. Stud Health Technol Inform 2013;191:115–9.

30. Bart BA, Goldsmith SR, Lee KL, et al. Cardiorenal rescue study in acute decompensated heart failure: rationale and design of CARRESS-HF, for the heart failure clinical research network. J Card Fail 2012; 18(3):176–82.

31. Costanzo MR, Kazory A. Better late than never: the true results of CARRESS-HF. Eur J Heart Fail 2018. https://doi.org/10.1002/ejhf.1187.

32. Boyle A, Sobotka PA. Redefining the therapeutic objective in decompensated heart failure:

hemoconcentration as a surrogate for plasma refill rate. J Card Fail 2006;12(4):247–9.

33. Marenzi G, Grazi S, Giraldi F, et al. Interrelation of humoral factors, hemodynamics, and fluid and salt metabolism in congestive heart failure: effects of extracorporeal ultrafiltration. Am J Med 1993;94(1): 49–56.

34. Marenzi G, Lauri G, Grazi M, et al. Circulatory response to fluid overload removal by extracorporeal ultrafiltration in refractory congestive heart failure. J Am Coll Cardiol 2001;38(4):963–8.

35. Marenzi G, Muratori M, Cosentino ER, et al. Continuous ultrafiltration for congestive heart failure: the CUORE trial. J Card Fail 2014;20(5):378.e1-9.

36. Costanzo MR, Negoianu D, Fonarow GC, et al. Rationale and design of the aquapheresis versus intravenous diuretics and hospitalization for heart failure (AVOID-HF) trial. Am Heart J 2015;170(3): 471–82.

37. Costanzo MR, Negoianu D, Jaski BE, et al. Aquapheresis versus intravenous diuretics and hospitalizations for heart failure. JACC Heart Fail 2016;4(2): 95–105.

38. Mark DB, O'Connor CM. When business and science clash, how can we avoid harming patients?: the case of AVOID-HF. JACC Heart Fail 2016;4(2): 106–8.

39. Yancy CW, Jessup M, Bozkurt B, et al. 2013 ACCF/AHA guideline for the management of heart failure: a report of the American College of Cardiology Foundation/American Heart Association Task Force on practice guidelines. J Am Coll Cardiol 2013;62(16): e147–239.

40. Costanzo MR, Saltzberg M, O'Sullivan J, et al. Early ultrafiltration in patients with decompensated heart failure and diuretic resistance. J Am Coll Cardiol 2005;46(11):2047–51.

41. Schrier RW. Cardiorenal versus renocardiac syndrome: is there a difference? Nat Clin Pract Nephrol 2007;3(12):637.

42. Umanath K, Emani S. Getting to the heart of the matter: review of treatment of cardiorenal syndrome. Adv Chronic Kidney Dis 2017;24(4): 261–6.

43. Bart BA, Boyle A, Bank AJ, et al. Ultrafiltration versus usual care for hospitalized patients with heart failure: the relief for acutely fluid-overloaded patients with decompensated congestive heart failure (RAPID-CHF) trial. J Am Coll Cardiol 2005; 46(11):2043–6.

Aldosterone Receptor Blockade in Heart Failure with Preserved Ejection Fraction

Ajith Nair, MD[a], Anita Deswal, MD, MPH[b],*

KEYWORDS

- Aldosterone blocker • Spironolactone • Eplerenone • Heart failure with preserved ejection fraction
- Heart failure

KEY POINTS

- Heart failure with preserved ejection fraction (HFpEF) is a complex disorder with variable clinical phenotypes.
- Clinical trials in HFpEF have failed to show an effective therapy that has provided mortality benefit.
- Aldosterone is key mediator of myocardial fibrosis and has shown efficacy in reducing collagen turnover and in potentially improving structure and diastolic function in HFpEF.
- Although the Treatment of Preserved Cardiac Function Heart Failure with an Aldosterone Antagonist (TOPCAT) trial failed to show a reduction in its primary end point, there was a reduction in heart failure hospitalizations for patients with HFpEF. Regional differences may have accounted for the negative results.
- Use of aldosterone antagonists may be appropriate for carefully selected patients with HFpEF who have clinical heart failure, increased brain natriuretic peptide levels, and lower risk for renal dysfunction or hyperkalemia.

INTRODUCTION

Heart failure (HF) is a leading cause of morbidity and mortality throughout the world. An estimated 6.5 million Americans greater than or equal to 20 years of age have clinical HF.[1,2] About 50% of patients with clinical HF have HF with preserved ejection fraction (HFpEF), which carries a mortality comparable with that of patients with reduced ejection fractions and is associated with significant morbidity caused by frequent hospitalizations as well as impaired functional capacity.[3,4] Patients with HFpEF tend to be elderly, female, and obese, and have comorbidities including hypertension,

coronary artery disease, atrial fibrillation, and diabetes, which can contribute significantly to complications and mortality.[5,6] HFpEF represents a heterogeneous disorder with a complex pathophysiologic basis. Clinical trials to date have failed to show a therapy that definitively imparts a mortality benefit in HFpEF. Because of its effects on myocardial fibrosis and vascular function, use of mineralocorticoid receptor antagonists (MRAs) has been of particular interest in HFpEF. This article explores the basis for using aldosterone receptor antagonists in HFpEF and the current knowledge about their effects in patients with HFpEF.

Disclosure: The authors have nothing to disclose.
[a] Department of Medicine, Section of Cardiology, Baylor College of Medicine, 6620 Main Street, 12th Floor, Suite 1225, Houston, TX 77030, USA; [b] Department of Medicine, Section of Cardiology, Baylor College of Medicine and Michael E. DeBakey VA Medical Center, 2002 Holcombe Boulevard, Houston, TX 77030, USA
* Corresponding author.
E-mail address: adeswal@bcm.edu

Heart Failure Clin 14 (2018) 525–535
https://doi.org/10.1016/j.hfc.2018.06.002
1551-7136/18/Published by Elsevier Inc.

PATHOPHYSIOLOGIC BASIS OF HEART FAILURE WITH PRESERVED EJECTION FRACTION

HFpEF is now defined in the American Heart Association (AHA)/American College of Cardiology (ACC) HF guidelines as clinical symptoms and signs of HF with a left ventricular ejection fraction (LVEF) greater than or equal to 50%,[2] although several clinical trials have used an LVEF of greater than or equal to 45%, and a few trials have used LVEF greater than or equal to 50%. HFpEF may also be characterized by diastolic dysfunction on echocardiography, although this parameter is not present in all patients. Exercise intolerance is a key manifestation and may result from increases in filling pressures secondary to increased ventricular stiffness.

Several insults, including hypertension, diabetes, coronary artery disease, advanced age, atrial fibrillation, and sleep apnea, contribute to the development of cardiac structural abnormalities, which include increased diameter of cardiomyocytes, ventricular hypertrophy, and increased interstitial fibrosis secondary to upregulation of collagen synthesis cross-linking.[7] Other structural and functional alterations can also lead to the HFpEF phenotype. Alterations in titin, a large sarcomeric protein that functions as a molecular spring, are common in HFpEF. Increased density of shorter, stiffer titin isoforms, and hyperphosphorylation contribute to impaired relaxation.[8,9] Reduced sarcoendoplasmic reticulum Ca^{2+}-ATPase expression and extracellular matrix expansion can cause mechanical, electrophysiologic, and structural abnormalities.[10,11] Inflammation, partially driven by comorbidities, including renal dysfunction, lung disease, and obesity, is also thought to contribute to microvascular dysfunction and pulmonary vascular remodeling.[12]

The pathologic alterations combined with the influence of comorbid conditions can produce varied structural changes. Echocardiographic assessment of patients in the Treatment of Preserved Cardiac Function Heart Failure with an Aldosterone Antagonist (TOPCAT) trial showed heterogeneous patterns of ventricular remodeling, including different patterns of left ventricular (LV) hypertrophy and various degrees of left atrial enlargement and pulmonary hypertension.[13] Diastolic function was normal in one-third of patients. Greater degrees of LV hypertrophy, pulmonary hypertension, and increased LV filling pressures, as well as impaired LV systolic function determined by absolute longitudinal strain (LS), have all been shown to be predictive of HF hospitalizations and cardiovascular death.[14,15]

THE RENIN-ANGIOTENSIN-ALDOSTERONE SYSTEM IN HEART FAILURE

HF and hypertension are associated with activation of the renin-angiotensin-aldosterone system (RAAS). Chronic RAAS activation leads to increases in aldosterone level, which can promote an increase in extracellular matrix collagen and endothelial dysfunction. This condition can subsequently lead to LV hypertrophy, decreased ventricular and vascular compliance, and LV systolic and diastolic dysfunction (**Fig. 1**).[16] Inhibition of RAAS can reverse this process and may improve diastolic function. Although angiotensin-converting enzyme inhibitors (ACEIs) or angiotensin receptor blockers (ARBs) can suppress angiotensin II–mediated aldosterone release, patients can have increased aldosterone levels caused by the phenomenon of so-called aldosterone escape.[17] Despite optimal ACEI or ARB therapy, multiple studies have shown that markers of collagen turnover are increased, indicating ongoing aldosterone-mediated effects. Increased myocardial stiffness and poor compliance are among the key contributors to the disorder of HFpEF and is contributed to by aldosterone-mediated increases in myocardial collagen. MRAs, including spironolactone and eplerenone, antagonize the effect of aldosterone and can lead to a reduction in fibrosis and an improvement in LV function. In animal studies, infusion of aldosterone resulted in an increase in the cardiac extracellular matrix, and the effects of aldosterone were blocked by spironolactone.[18] There is also a correlation between aldosterone levels and LV mass in patients with diastolic dysfunction and HFpEF. Thus, aldosterone promotes interstitial fibrosis and plays a central role in HF and diastolic dysfunction.

Aldosterone is derived from the zona glomerulosa of the adrenal cortex and mediates its effects partially through mineralocorticoid receptors located in the distal collecting tube of the nephron. Secretion of aldosterone is stimulated by angiotensin II, angiotensin III, and serum potassium. Mineralocorticoid receptors stimulate expression of the 3Na+/K+ pump, which drives sodium into the interstitium and potassium into the collecting duct. The resultant osmotic gradient leads to volume retention.[19,20] Spironolactone, which is a MRA and glucocorticoid receptor antagonist, and eplerenone, a selective MRA, are the two primary aldosterone receptor blockers studied in clinical trials of HF.

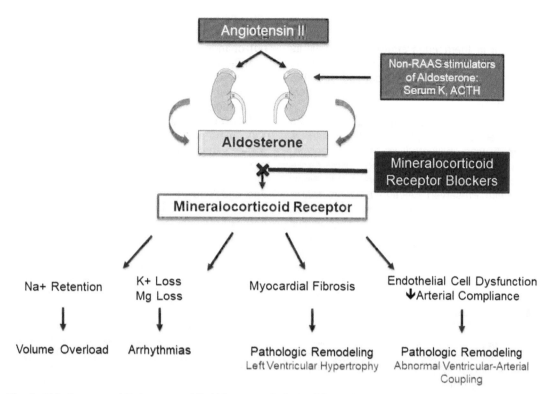

Fig. 1. Aldosterone and its impact on HF. Aldosterone is derived from the adrenal glands and its release is stimulated by angiotensin II, serum potassium and adrenocorticotropic hormone (ACTH). It acts on mineralocorticoid receptors to promote myocardial fibrosis, endothelial dysfunction and volume overload.

ALDOSTERONE RECEPTOR ANTAGONISTS IN HEART FAILURE WITH REDUCED EJECTION FRACTION

Patients with HF with reduced ejection fraction (HFrEF) frequently had aldosterone break-through despite treatment with ACEI or ARBs caused by renin-angiotensin system (RAS)–mediated and non–RAS-mediated aldosterone secretion.[17] The addition of aldosterone antagonists to standard HFrEF therapy was hence validated in 3 large clinical trials.[21–23] These trials have shown the efficacy of aldosterone receptor blockade in significantly reducing mortality and morbidity caused by HF and cardiovascular hospitalizations (30%–37%) in patients with chronic HFrEF across the spectrum of New York Heart Association (NYHA) class II to IV as well as a more modest reduction in events in patients after myocardial infarction (MI) with HFrEF.[21–23]

Based on these trials, the 2013 ACC/AHA guidelines for the management of HF provide a class I recommendation for the use of aldosterone receptor antagonists in patients with chronic HFrEF NYHA class II to IV HF symptoms and with HFrEF after MI.[2]

RENIN-ANGIOTENSIN SYSTEM INHIBITION IN HEART FAILURE WITH PRESERVED EJECTION FRACTION

Treatment with ACEIs or ARBs is fundamental in the treatment of HFrEF,[24] and the benefits of aldosterone inhibitors were evaluated on background therapy with ACEIs or ARBs. However, the benefits of these drugs cannot be extended to patients with HFpEF based on the results of several large trials that have not shown any significant benefit in mortality with ACEIs or ARBs in HFpEF. Although there was a signal for reduction in HF hospitalizations in some trials, this was not consistently seen across the trials.[25–27]

ALDOSTERONE RECEPTOR ANTAGONIST IN HEART FAILURE WITH PRESERVED EJECTION FRACTION: STRUCTURE AND DIASTOLOGY

In the Randomized Aldactone Evaluation Study (RALES) trial, excessive turnover of the extracellular matrix was associated with advanced cardiac remodeling and poor clinical outcomes, and the clinical benefit from the aldosterone antagonism was most pronounced if this turnover was reduced.[28] Fibrosis and expansion of the extracellular matrix is a key pathologic process in HFpEF, and aldosterone antagonism has been a focal point in therapeutic strategies. In patients with HFpEF, aldosterone receptor antagonists have shown improvements in cardiac structure and diastology (**Table 1**) in some small clinical trials.[29–31]

The effect of eplerenone on exercise tolerance and both echocardiographic and serum markers of HFpEF was evaluated in the randomized, double-blind, placebo-controlled RAAM-PEF (Randomized Aldosterone Antagonism in Heart Failure with Preserved Ejection Fraction) trial.[32] Forty-four patients with HFpEF were randomized to eplerenone (goal dose of 50 mg daily) versus placebo therapy for 6 months. All patients had hypertension, more than half had a prior HF hospitalization, and more than 90% were male (reflecting a Veterans Administration population). At the end of 6 months, there was no difference in 6-minute walk distances between treatment groups, although eplerenone was associated with a significant improvement in echocardiographic measures of diastolic function (E/e' ratio) and a reduction in serum markers of collagen turnover, including procollagen type I amino-terminal peptide, and carboxy-terminal telopeptide of collage type I. Similar reductions in collagen turnover have also been shown in other studies with eplerenone.[33] In a randomized placebo-controlled trial of 48 women with HFpEF, spironolactone led to improvement in diastolic function as assessed by early diastolic tissue Doppler velocity of the lateral mitral annulus, accompanied by a reduction in type III procollagen levels, a surrogate marker of myocardial fibrosis.[34]

The Aldosterone Receptor Blockade in Diastolic Heart Failure (Aldo-DHF) trial was multicenter, prospective, randomized, placebo-controlled trial that included 422 ambulatory patients from Germany and Austria with NYHA class II and III HF, LVEF greater than or equal to 50%, and evidence of diastolic dysfunction by echocardiography.[31] Patients were randomized to spironolactone 25 mg daily (n = 213) versus placebo (n = 209), and the coprimary end points were improvements in E/e' ratio by echocardiography and maximum oxygen consumption (peak Vo_2) over a 12-month follow-up period. Spironolactone therapy yielded improvements in LV diastolic function, but it failed to improve maximal exercise capacity, clinical symptoms, or quality of life in patients with HFpEF. The mean E/e' ratio decreased from 12.7 to 12.1 with spironolactone, whereas it increased from 12.8 to 13.6 with placebo (mean

difference, −1.5; 95% confidence interval [CI], −2.0 to −0.9; P<.001). However, peak Vo_2 did not change, nor did 6-minute walking distance despite improvements in N-terminal pro–brain natriuretic peptide (NT-proBNP) levels and a reduction in LV mass index. The reverse remodeling effect of spironolactone was independent of blood pressure reduction.

A meta-analysis of 11 randomized trials showed that treatment with MRAs was associated with improvements in echocardiographic indices of diastolic function, including E/e' ratio and deceleration time, and a reduction in circulating markers of myocardial fibrosis, including carboxy-terminal peptide of procollagen type I and amino-terminal peptide of procollagen type II.[35]

The STRUCTURE (Spironolactone in Myocardial Dysfunction with Reduced Exercise Capacity) trial was designed to evaluate the effects of spironolactone when patients were selected by abnormal diastolic responses to exercise.[36] Inclusion criteria were based on meeting HFpEF criteria with symptoms of HF (dyspnea, fatigue, and exercise intolerance), LVEF greater than 50%, and evidence of diastolic dysfunction by echocardiographic criteria or increases in brain natriuretic peptide (BNP) levels when echocardiographic criteria were inconclusive. Further, potential subjects underwent exercise testing and were enrolled if postexercise E/e' was greater than 13 (reflecting increased LV filling pressures) and the individuals had impaired exercise capacity. Patients were excluded if they had active coronary disease or atrial fibrillation. A total of 131 subjects completed therapy with spironolactone 25 mg versus matching placebo over a 6-month follow-up period with the primary outcome of improvements in peak Vo_2 and exertional E/e' ratio. Contrary to the results of Aldo-DHF, spironolactone resulted in significant improvements in peak Vo_2 (~2.9 mL/min/kg increase vs 0.3 mL/min/kg in active vs placebo groups respectively), anaerobic threshold, and O_2 uptake efficiency. There was a significant attenuation in exercise-induced E/e' increase and interaction of spironolactone and change in E/e' on Vo_2. The contrasting results of these two trials show the importance of selection of patients for HFpEF trials with a focused phenotype and exclusion of significant confounding comorbidities that may affect clinical and functional outcomes. It also shows the potential difficulties of translating results of efficacy of agents from one selected clinical trial population to patients in clinical practice with multiple comorbidities.

Table 1
Aldosterone blockade and impact on cardiac structure, function, and exercise capacity in patients with heart failure with preserved ejection fraction

Study	MRA	Number	End Points	Outcome
Mak et al,[33] 2009	Eplerenone 25 mg daily and increased to 50 mg from 6–12 mo	44	• Serum markers of collagen turnover and inflammation and echocardiographic measures of diastolic function at 6 and 12 mo	• No difference in biomarkers at 6 mo • Decreased the increase in procollagen type III amino-terminal peptide at 12 mo • No impact on echocardiographic measures
Kosmala et al,[53] 2011	Spironolactone 25 mg daily	80 (metabolic syndrome; no HFpEF)	• Serum makers of collagen turnover (procollagen type III amino-terminal propeptide and procollagen type I carboxy-terminal propeptide) • Echocardiographic measures of systolic and diastolic function at 6 mo	• Improvements in LV strain, LVH, diastolic function, and collagen turnover at 6 mo • Magnitude of effect based on baseline LV dysfunction and degree of fibrosis
RAAM-PEF,[32] 2011	Eplerenone 25 mg daily (2 wk) increased to 50 mg for 22 wk	44	• Primary end points: 6MWD • Diastolic function, biomarkers of collagen turnover (secondary end points) • 6 mo follow-up	• No change in 6MWD • Significant reduction in serum markers of collagen turnover • Improvement in E/E′
ALDO-DHF,[31] 2013	Spironolactone 25 mg daily	422	• Diastolic function (E/e′) • Exercise capacity (Vo_2 max) • 12 mo follow-up	• Improved diastolic function • No change in Vo_2 max, 6MWD
Kurrelmeyer et al,[34] 2014	Spironolactone 25 mg daily	48 (female)	• 6MWD, clinical composite score, echocardiography, and biomarkers at 6 mo	• Stabilized clinical symptoms • Improved diastolic function (lateral e′, E/e′) • Reduction in type III procollagen levels • No improvement in 6MWD
TOPCAT,[15] 2014	Spironolactone 25 mg daily	447	• Ventricular LS after 12–18 mo	• Trend toward improved LS in the Americas
TOPCAT,[15,54] 2015	Spironolactone 25 mg daily	239	• Cardiac structure (LV volume, mass, and EF; LA size; PA pressures) and function (diastology) over 12–18 mo	• No change among the entire group (Americas/Russia-Georgia)
STRUCTURE,[36] 2016	Spironolactone 25 mg daily	150 (exertion E/e′ >13)	• Improvements in peak Vo_2 and exertional E/e′ • 6 mo follow-up	• Improvement in peak Vo_2 • Reduction in exercise-induced increase in E/e′

Abbreviations: LVH, LV hypertrophy; 6MWD, 6-minute walk distance; PA, pulmonary artery.

ALDOSTERONE RECEPTOR ANTAGONISTS IN HEART FAILURE WITH PRESERVED EJECTION FRACTION: CLINICAL OUTCOMES

The TOPCAT trial evaluated the efficacy of spironolactone in preventing major clinical end points in patients with HFpEF.[37] The study randomized 3445 with symptomatic HF and an LVEF of 45% or greater to spironolactone (15 mg–45 mg) or placebo. Eligible patients either had a history of hospitalization within the previous 12 months, with HF management as a major component of care, or increased natriuretic peptide levels within 60 days before enrollment (BNP $\geq$100 pg/mL or NT-proBNP $\geq$360 pg/mL). The primary outcome was a composite of death from cardiovascular causes, aborted cardiac arrest, or hospitalization for HF. Overall, spironolactone therapy showed no significant difference in the primary outcome after a mean follow-up of 3.3 years (hazard ratio [HR], 0.89; 95% CI, 0.77–1.04; P = .14). HF hospitalizations were significantly lower in the spironolactone group versus the placebo (HR, 0.83; 95% CI, 0.69–0.99; P = .04). However, neither death nor all-cause hospitalizations were significantly reduced with spironolactone (Fig. 2). Despite an increase in potassium levels with spironolactone, there was no difference in the incidence of serious adverse events, creatinine level increase of 3.0 mg/dL, or dialysis.

However, the impact of spironolactone therapy differed (P = .01 for interaction) according to randomization stratum (ie, qualification by increased natriuretic peptide levels or by prior hospitalization with HF as a major component). Spironolactone showed benefit in the natriuretic peptide stratum (HR, 0.65; 95% CI, 0.49–0.87; P = .003), whereas there was no effect on primary outcome in the hospitalization stratum (HR, 1.01; 95% CI, 0.84–1.21; P = .92). Post-hoc analysis noted marked regional differences in event rates (Fig. 3). In the Americas (United States, Canada, Brazil, and Argentina), the primary outcome

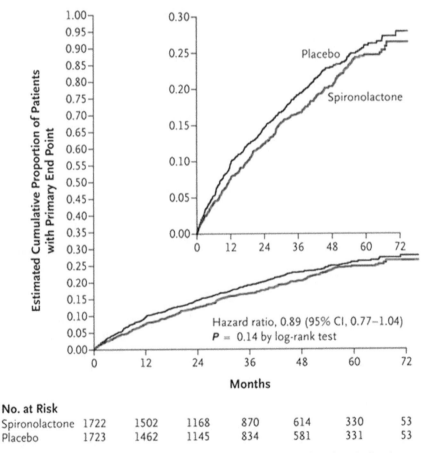

No. at Risk

Spironolactone	1722	1502	1168	870	614	330	53
Placebo	1723	1462	1145	834	581	331	53

Fig. 2. Kaplan-Meier plot of time to primary combined end point event of HF hospitalization, cardiovascular death, or aborted cardiac arrest in the TOPCAT trial. (*From* Pitt B, Pfeffer MA, Assmann SF, et al. Spironolactone for heart failure with preserved ejection fraction. N Engl J Med 2014;370(15):1388; with permission.)

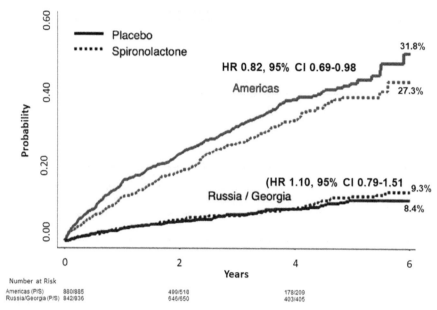

Fig. 3. Kaplan-Meier plot of time to the first confirmed primary-outcome event in the TOPCAT trial according to geographic area. P, primary; S, secondary. (*From* Pfeffer MA, Claggett B, Assmann SF, et al. Regional variation in patients and outcomes in the Treatment of Preserved Cardiac Function Heart Failure with an Aldosterone Antagonist (TOPCAT) trial. Circulation 2015;131(1):34–42; with permission.)

occurred in 27.3% in the spironolactone group versus 31.8% in the placebo group. In Russia and Georgia, which accounted for almost 50% of enrolled patients, the primary outcome occurred in 9.3% in the spironolactone group and 8.4% in the placebo group. Most patients from Russia and Georgia were enrolled in the hospitalization stratum. The placebo group in this stratum had an unexpected lower risk of the primary outcome compared with those enrolled in the BNP stratum, which had almost a 4-fold higher rate. In the Americas, the primary outcome was significantly reduced by spironolactone compared with the placebo group (HR, 0.82; 95% CI, 0.69–0.98), whereas no such effect was noted in patients enrolled in Russia and Georgia (HR, 1.10; 95% CI, 0.79–1.51). Patients from Russia and Georgia were younger, had less atrial fibrillation and diabetes, but had a higher rate of prior MIs or hospitalizations for HF.[38] The rates of hospitalizations from this group were 5-fold lower compared with the Candesartan in Patients with Chronic Heart Failure and Preserved Left-Ventricular Ejection Fraction (CHARM-preserved) and Irbesartan in Heart Failure with Preserved Ejection Fraction Study (I-PRESERVE) trials,[39] and the rate of death mirrored the general population of the region. In contrast, the rates of death in the Americas cohort were 7-fold higher than age-matched and sex-matched persons in the general population. Furthermore, hyperkalemia and increase in serum potassium and creatinine concentrations as well as reduction in systolic blood pressure in the spironolactone arms were more likely in the Americas, whereas no such treatment response was observed in Russia and Georgia (**Fig. 4**).[38] Such disparities question the findings from this region with regard to patient selection, presence of true HFpEF, disease severity, and medication use. Recently, blood samples of 366 participants in TOPCAT were analyzed for the presence of canrenone, the active metabolite of spironolactone. Among a smaller subset of participants with blood samples in the trial biorepository who reported use of spironolactone at the 12-month study visit, concentrations were undetectable in 30% of participants from Russia versus 3% from the United States and Canada (P<.001), raising concerns about adherence to study drugs and that the trial results may not reflected the true response to spironolactone in Russia (**Fig. 5**).[40]

The geographic disparities in outcomes highlight some of the complexities in international research studies.[41] Regional variations in outcomes have been noted in trials focused on HFrEF and may reflect differences in the population or medical practice patterns, or may be caused by statistical chance.[42–44] The patients in the hospitalization stratum of TOPCAT may have had symptoms from noncardiac causes versus those patients included for increased natriuretic peptide levels. Increased natriuretic peptides have been

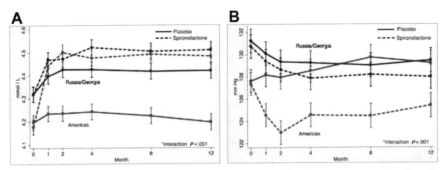

Fig. 4. Longitudinal plots of (*A*) serum potassium and (*B*) systolic blood pressure over the first 12 months of follow-up by treatment arm and region. The magnitude of treatment effect differs by region for each variable (interaction *P*<.001 for each). (*From* Pfeffer MA, Claggett B, Assmann SF, et al. Regional variation in patients and outcomes in the Treatment of Preserved Cardiac Function Heart Failure with an Aldosterone Antagonist (TOPCAT) trial. Circulation 2015;131(1):34–42; with permission.)

associated with worse outcomes in patients with HFpEF.[45,46] Although natriuretic peptide levels are generally lower in patients with HFpEF compared with HFrEF, increased levels confer a prognosis in HFpEF that is as poor as that in HFrEF. In 687 patients from the Americas in the natriuretic peptide stratum of the TOPCAT study, spironolactone showed a significant benefit in the primary end point (HR, 0.64; 95% CI, 0.46–0.90; *P*<.01).[47] The patients with lower natriuretic peptide levels in this stratum benefited more than those with higher natriuretic peptide levels. Patients with the highest levels were older, had greater LV mass, worse LV diastolic dysfunction, and higher pulmonary pressure, all suggestive of more advanced structural heart disease.

RECOMMENDATIONS FOR ALDOSTERONE INHIBITION IN HEART FAILURE

Given the notable geographic disparities in the TOPCAT trial, it seems prudent to treat patients

with HFpEF who resemble those enrolled in North and South America with aldosterone antagonists. However, their use across all patients with HFpEF cannot be advocated, given the lack of clear benefit on mortality, hospitalization, or symptoms and the potential for harm in patients with renal dysfunction or prone to hyperkalemia. In the large clinical trials discussed earlier, patients were excluded with a creatinine level greater than 2.5 mg/dL, an estimated glomerular filtration rate less than 30 mL/min/1.73 m², or a serum potassium level of greater than 5.0 mmol/L before randomization. Aggregate data suggest that MRA provide a clear reduction in adverse cardiac events in patients with HFrEF, whereas there is an increased risk of harm from hyperkalemia and gynecomastia in HFpEF.[48] The 2017 ACC/AHA/Heart Failure Society of America Focused Update of the 2013 ACCF/AHA Guideline for the Management of Heart Failure provides a class IIb recommendation for the use of aldosterone receptor antagonists in HFpEF. Specifically, the guideline states, "in

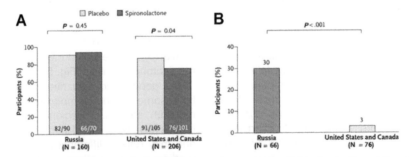

Fig. 5. Participants from the TOPCAT trial biorepository with samples available for testing at the 12-month study visit included 366 patients (206 patients from the United States or Canada and 160 patients from Russia). (*A*) The percentage of participants who reported that they were taking the assigned study drug; (*B*) the percentage of participants assigned to spironolactone who reported taking the drug but who did not have detectable canrenone concentrations at the visit. (*From* de Denus S, O'Meara E, Desai AS, et al. Spironolactone metabolites in TOPCAT - new insights into regional variation. N Engl J Med 2017;376(17):1690–2; with permission.)

appropriately selected patients with HFpEF (with EF $\geq$45%, elevated BNP levels or HF admission within 1 year, estimated glomerular filtration rate >30 mL/min, creatinine <2.5 mg/dL, potassium <5.0 mEq/L), aldosterone receptor antagonists might be considered to decrease hospitalizations."[49] Also, based on the results and subgroup analyses of the TOPCAT trial, clinicians may consider the use of these agents, especially in patients with HFpEF with increased BNP levels. Furthermore, careful monitoring of potassium level, renal function, and diuretic dosing should be performed to minimize the risk of hyperkalemia and worsening renal function.

SUMMARY

Given the expanding public burden of HFpEF, effective therapy is of critical importance. The β-blockers, such as nebivolol, may have potential benefit in reducing hospitalizations for HFpEF,[50] although there have been no large-scale studies evaluating mortality benefit or clinical outcomes only in patients with HFpEF. Phosphodiesterase-5 inhibition failed to improve exercise capacity or clinical status.[51] ARBs were shown to have a trend toward modest reduction in HF hospitalizations in only 1 trial, with neutral results for ACEIs and ARBs in other trials.[25–27] The only class I recommendations for HFpEF are for treating hypertension and diuretic therapy for volume overload.[49] The phenotypic heterogeneity among patients with HFpEF can account for the lack of clear benefit of any 1 therapy. Shah and colleagues[52] identified distinct groups based on clinical phenotypes: younger patients with moderate diastolic dysfunction and mildly increased BNP levels; obese patients with sleep disordered breathing and advanced diastolic dysfunction; and elderly patients with renal dysfunction, pulmonary hypertension, and right ventricular dysfunction. Outcomes were progressively worse across the last 2 groups. Using distinct phenotypic subtypes may allow effective targeted therapies. Despite the overall negative outcomes of the TOPCAT study, specific subsets of patients with HFpEF may benefit. Aldosterone antagonists remain a therapeutic option for HFpEF in carefully selected patients with evidence of volume overload or increased natriuretic peptide levels, with structural evidence of diastolic dysfunction, and without significant renal insufficiency.

REFERENCES

1. Benjamin EJ, Blaha MJ, Chiuve SE, et al. Heart disease and stroke statistics–2017 update: a report from the American Heart Association. Circulation 2017;135(10):e146–603.

2. Yancy CW, Jessup M, Bozkurt B, et al. 2013 ACCF/AHA guideline for the management of heart failure: a report of the American College of Cardiology Foundation/American Heart Association Task Force on Practice Guidelines. J Am Coll Cardiol 2013; 62(16):e147–239.

3. Redfield MM, Jacobsen SJ, Burnett JC Jr, et al. Burden of systolic and diastolic ventricular dysfunction in the community: appreciating the scope of the heart failure epidemic. JAMA 2003;289(2):194–202.

4. Bursi F, Weston SA, Redfield MM, et al. Systolic and diastolic heart failure in the community. JAMA 2006; 296(18):2209–16.

5. Deswal A. Diastolic dysfunction and diastolic heart failure: mechanisms and epidemiology. Curr Cardiol Rep 2005;7(3):178–83.

6. Aguilar D, Deswal A, Ramasubbu K, et al. Comparison of patients with heart failure and preserved left ventricular ejection fraction among those with versus without diabetes mellitus. Am J Cardiol 2010;105(3): 373–7.

7. Lewis GA, Schelbert EB, Williams SG, et al. Biological phenotypes of heart failure with preserved ejection fraction. J Am Coll Cardiol 2017;70(17): 2186–200.

8. Borbely A, Falcao-Pires I, van Heerebeek L, et al. Hypophosphorylation of the Stiff N2B titin isoform raises cardiomyocyte resting tension in failing human myocardium. Circ Res 2009;104(6):780–6.

9. van Heerebeek L, Borbely A, Niessen HW, et al. Myocardial structure and function differ in systolic and diastolic heart failure. Circulation 2006; 113(16):1966–73.

10. Zile MR, Baicu CF, Ikonomidis JS, et al. Myocardial stiffness in patients with heart failure and a preserved ejection fraction: contributions of collagen and titin. Circulation 2015;131(14):1247–59.

11. Adeniran I, MacIver DH, Hancox JC, et al. Abnormal calcium homeostasis in heart failure with preserved ejection fraction is related to both reduced contractile function and incomplete relaxation: an electro-mechanically detailed biophysical modeling study. Front Physiol 2015;6:78.

12. Paulus WJ, Tschope C. A novel paradigm for heart failure with preserved ejection fraction: comorbidities drive myocardial dysfunction and remodeling through coronary microvascular endothelial inflammation. J Am Coll Cardiol 2013;62(4):263–71.

13. Shah AM, Shah SJ, Anand IS, et al. Cardiac structure and function in heart failure with preserved ejection fraction: baseline findings from the echocardiographic study of the Treatment of Preserved Cardiac Function Heart Failure with an Aldosterone Antagonist trial. Circ Heart Fail 2014;7(1): 104–15.

14. Shah AM, Claggett B, Sweitzer NK, et al. Cardiac structure and function and prognosis in heart failure with preserved ejection fraction: findings from the echocardiographic study of the Treatment of Preserved Cardiac Function Heart Failure with an Aldosterone Antagonist (TOPCAT) trial. Circ Heart Fail 2014;7(5):740–51.

15. Shah AM, Claggett B, Sweitzer NK, et al. Prognostic importance of impaired systolic function in heart failure with preserved ejection fraction and the impact of spironolactone. Circulation 2015;132(5):402–14.

16. Pfeffer MA, Braunwald E. Treatment of heart failure with preserved ejection fraction: reflections on its treatment with an aldosterone antagonist. JAMA Cardiol 2016;1(1):7–8.

17. Struthers AD. The clinical implications of aldosterone escape in congestive heart failure. Eur J Heart Fail 2004;6(5):539–45.

18. Brilla CG, Matsubara LS, Weber KT. Anti-aldosterone treatment and the prevention of myocardial fibrosis in primary and secondary hyperaldosteronism. J Mol Cell Cardiol 1993;25(5):563–75.

19. Dzau VJ, Colucci WS, Hollenberg NK, et al. Relation of the renin-angiotensin-aldosterone system to clinical state in congestive heart failure. Circulation 1981;63(3):645–51.

20. Weber KT, Villarreal D. Aldosterone and antialdosterone therapy in congestive heart failure. Am J Cardiol 1993;71(3):3a–11a.

21. Pitt B, Zannad F, Remme WJ, et al. The effect of spironolactone on morbidity and mortality in patients with severe heart failure. Randomized Aldactone Evaluation Study investigators. N Engl J Med 1999;341(10):709–17.

22. Pitt B, Remme W, Zannad F, et al. Eplerenone, a selective aldosterone blocker, in patients with left ventricular dysfunction after myocardial infarction. N Engl J Med 2003;348(14):1309–21.

23. Zannad F, McMurray JJ, Krum H, et al. Eplerenone in patients with systolic heart failure and mild symptoms. N Engl J Med 2011;364(1):11–21.

24. Nair AP, Timoh T, Fuster V. Contemporary medical management of systolic heart failure. Circ J 2012;76(2):268–77.

25. Cleland JG, Tendera M, Adamus J, et al. The Perindopril in Elderly People with Chronic Heart Failure (PEP-CHF) study. Eur Heart J 2006;27(19):2338–45.

26. Yusuf S, Pfeffer MA, Swedberg K, et al. Effects of Candesartan in Patients with Chronic Heart Failure and Preserved Left-Ventricular Ejection Fraction: the CHARM-preserved trial. Lancet 2003;362(9386):777–81.

27. Massie BM, Carson PE, McMurray JJ, et al. Irbesartan in patients with heart failure and preserved ejection fraction. N Engl J Med 2008;359(23):2456–67.

28. Zannad F, Alla F, Dousset B, et al. Limitation of excessive extracellular matrix turnover may contribute to survival benefit of spironolactone therapy in patients with congestive heart failure: insights from the Randomized Aldactone Evaluation Study (RALES). RALES investigators. Circulation 2000;102(22):2700–6.

29. Mottram PM, Haluska B, Leano R, et al. Effect of aldosterone antagonism on myocardial dysfunction in hypertensive patients with diastolic heart failure. Circulation 2004;110(5):558–65.

30. Edelmann F, Holzendorf V, Wachter R, et al. Galectin-3 in patients with heart failure with preserved ejection fraction: results from the Aldo-DHF trial. Eur J Heart Fail 2015;17(2):214–23.

31. Edelmann F, Wachter R, Schmidt AG, et al. Effect of spironolactone on diastolic function and exercise capacity in patients with heart failure with preserved ejection fraction: the Aldo-DHF randomized controlled trial. JAMA 2013;309(8):781–91.

32. Deswal A, Richardson P, Bozkurt B, et al. Results of the Randomized Aldosterone Antagonism in Heart Failure with Preserved Ejection Fraction trial (RAAM-PEF). J Card Fail 2011;17(8):634–42.

33. Mak GJ, Ledwidge MT, Watson CJ, et al. Natural history of markers of collagen turnover in patients with early diastolic dysfunction and impact of eplerenone. J Am Coll Cardiol 2009;54(18):1674–82.

34. Kurrelmeyer KM, Ashton Y, Xu J, et al. Effects of spironolactone treatment in elderly women with heart failure and preserved left ventricular ejection fraction. J Card Fail 2014;20(8):560–8.

35. Pandey A, Garg S, Matulevicius SA, et al. Effect of mineralocorticoid receptor antagonists on cardiac structure and function in patients with diastolic dysfunction and heart failure with preserved ejection fraction: a meta-analysis and systematic review. J Am Heart Assoc 2015;4(10):e002137.

36. Kosmala W, Rojek A, Przewlocka-Kosmala M, et al. Effect of aldosterone antagonism on exercise tolerance in heart failure with preserved ejection fraction. J Am Coll Cardiol 2016;68(17):1823–34.

37. Pitt B, Pfeffer MA, Assmann SF, et al. Spironolactone for heart failure with preserved ejection fraction. N Engl J Med 2014;370(15):1383–92.

38. Pfeffer MA, Claggett B, Assmann SF, et al. Regional variation in patients and outcomes in the Treatment of Preserved Cardiac Function Heart Failure with an Aldosterone Antagonist (TOPCAT) trial. Circulation 2015;131(1):34–42.

39. Campbell RT, Jhund PS, Castagno D, et al. What have we learned about patients with heart failure and preserved ejection fraction from DIG-PEF, CHARM-preserved, and I-PRESERVE? J Am Coll Cardiol 2012;60(23):2349–56.

40. de Denus S, O'Meara E, Desai AS, et al. Spironolactone metabolites in TOPCAT - new insights into regional variation. N Engl J Med 2017;376(17):1690–2.

41. McMurray JJ, O'Connor C. Lessons from the TOP-CAT trial. N Engl J Med 2014;370(15):1453–4.

42. O'Connor CM, Fiuzat M, Swedberg K, et al. Influence of global region on outcomes in heart failure beta-blocker trials. J Am Coll Cardiol 2011;58(9): 915–22.

43. Mentz RJ, Kaski JC, Dan GA, et al. Implications of geographical variation on clinical outcomes of cardiovascular trials. Am Heart J 2012;164(3):303–12.

44. Blair JE, Zannad F, Konstam MA, et al. Continental differences in clinical characteristics, management, and outcomes in patients hospitalized with worsening heart failure results from the EVEREST (Efficacy of Vasopressin Antagonism in Heart Failure: Outcome Study with Tolvaptan) program. J Am Coll Cardiol 2008;52(20):1640–8.

45. van Veldhuisen DJ, Linssen GC, Jaarsma T, et al. B-type natriuretic peptide and prognosis in heart failure patients with preserved and reduced ejection fraction. J Am Coll Cardiol 2013;61(14):1498–506.

46. Khalid U, Wruck LM, Quibrera PM, et al. BNP and obesity in acute decompensated heart failure with preserved vs. reduced ejection fraction: the atherosclerosis risk in communities surveillance study. Int J Cardiol 2017;233:61–6.

47. Anand IS, Claggett B, Liu J, et al. Interaction between spironolactone and natriuretic peptides in patients with heart failure and preserved ejection fraction: from the TOPCAT trial. JACC Heart Fail 2017;5(4):241–52.

48. Berbenetz NM, Mrkobrada M. Mineralocorticoid receptor antagonists for heart failure: systematic review and meta-analysis. BMC Cardiovasc Disord 2016;16(1):246.

49. Yancy CW, Jessup M, Bozkurt B, et al. 2017 ACC/AHA/HFSA focused update of the 2013 ACCF/AHA guideline for the management of heart failure: a report of the American College of Cardiology/American Heart Association Task Force on Clinical Practice Guidelines and the Heart Failure Society of America. Circulation 2017;136(6):e137–61.

50. van Veldhuisen DJ, Cohen-Solal A, Bohm M, et al. Beta-blockade with nebivolol in elderly heart failure patients with impaired and preserved left ventricular ejection fraction: data from SENIORS (Study of Effects of Nebivolol Intervention on Outcomes and Rehospitalization in Seniors with Heart Failure). J Am Coll Cardiol 2009;53(23):2150–8.

51. Redfield MM, Chen HH, Borlaug BA, et al. Effect of phosphodiesterase-5 inhibition on exercise capacity and clinical status in heart failure with preserved ejection fraction: a randomized clinical trial. JAMA 2013;309(12):1268–77.

52. Shah SJ, Katz DH, Selvaraj S, et al. Phenomapping for novel classification of heart failure with preserved ejection fraction. Circulation 2015;131(3):269–79.

53. Kosmala W, Przewlocka-Kosmala M, Szczepanik-Osadnik H, et al. A randomized study of the beneficial effects of aldosterone antagonism on LV function, structure, and fibrosis markers in metabolic syndrome. JACC Cardiovasc Imaging 2011;4(12): 1239–49.

54. Shah AM, Claggett B, Sweitzer NK, et al. Prognostic importance of changes in cardiac structure and function in heart failure with preserved ejection fraction and the impact of spironolactone. Circ Heart Fail 2015;8(6):1052–8.

Intravenous Iron Therapy in Heart Failure

Natasha L. Altman, MD[a],*, Amit Patel, MD[b]

KEYWORDS

- Anemia • Intravenous (IV) iron • Iron deficiency • Heart failure • Peak oxygen consumption
- Ferrous carboxymaltose

KEY POINTS

- Iron deficiency is prevalent in heart failure and a marker of worse outcomes with respect to mortality, hospitalization, and quality of life.
- Repletion of iron with intravenous formulations, particularly ferrous carboxymaltose, has shown significant improvements in quality of life and rate of hospitalization in recent clinical trials.
- Repletion of iron with oral formulations has not resulted in significant improvements in outcomes, likely related to concerns with iron absorption in the gut.

INTRODUCTION

Anemia has long been acknowledged as a common comorbidity in patients with heart failure (HF) with reduced ejection fraction. There have been a number of studies that have shown that anemia is an independent predictor of mortality in patients with HF,[1–4] and anemia has been associated with reduced exercise capacity[5,6] and worse New York Heart Association (NYHA) class.[7] In addition, there is evidence that iron deficiency alone is related to poor functional capacity in patients with HF.[8] In particular, iron deficiency is more prevalent in the more advanced stages of HF (NYHA classes III and IV), in women, and in patients with higher levels of proinflammatory markers.

Recently, iron deficiency anemia has been evaluated as a potential target for therapeutic intervention in HF, with some notable results. Intravenous iron infusions have been found to significantly reduce HF hospitalizations and symptom burden in patients with HF in multiple recent studies. This article will focus on the evaluation and management of iron deficiency anemia, particularly in reference to management with intravenous (IV) iron repletion.

ANEMIA AND IRON DEFICIENCY IN HEART FAILURE

The World Health Organization defines anemia as a hemoglobin less than 13.0 g/dL in male individuals and hemoglobin less than 12.0 g/dL in nonpregnant female individuals, and is usually either due to red blood cell (RBC) destruction or inadequate RBC production. Of the multiple potential etiologies of anemia, iron deficiency is the most common in all patient groups and particularly in patients with HF.[9,10] Iron deficiency also may be present without clinical evidence of anemia.

THE PATHOPHYSIOLOGY OF IRON DEFICIENCY IN HEART FAILURE

The importance of iron in oxidative metabolism and other processes like fatty acid oxidation may explain why iron deficiency, even without anemia,

Disclosure Statement: The authors have nothing to disclose.
[a] Section of Advanced Heart Failure and Transplant, Division of Cardiology, Department of Medicine, University of Colorado Denver, 12631 East 17th Avenue, Aurora, CO 80045, USA; [b] Advanced Heart Failure and Cardiac Transplantation, St. Vincent Medical Group, 8333 Naab Road, Suite 400, Indianapolis, IN 46260, USA
* Corresponding author.
E-mail address: Natasha.altman@ucdenver.edu

Heart Failure Clin 14 (2018) 537–543
https://doi.org/10.1016/j.hfc.2018.06.003
1551-7136/18/© 2018 Elsevier Inc. All rights reserved.

can have consequences in the patient with HF[11,12] at the cellular level. The mitochondrial respiratory chain can be suppressed in states involving low cellular iron reserves, leading to reduced ATP production, and thus impairment in exercise capacity and increasing fatigue.[13,14]

The reduction in oxygen carrying capacity of blood reduces delivery of oxygen to organs, which, when coupled with reduced cardiac output in HF, results in a significant overall increase in relative oxygen extraction by tissues, requiring a higher cardiac output and more rapid circulatory time to keep up with demand.[15]

MECHANISMS OF IRON DEFICIENCY AND ANEMIA
The Role of Hepcidin

Regulation of iron absorption, storage, and distribution is a tightly controlled process in which hepcidin plays a central role. Hepcidin is a peptide hormone produced in the liver and released via the action of interleukin (IL)-6. It is considered the "master regulator" of systemic iron metabolism.[16] Hepcidin inhibits the protein ferroportin, which is found in the gastrointestinal tract, macrophages, and hepatocytes. Effectively, hepcidin functions to block duodenal iron absorption and recycling through the mononuclear phagocytic system,[16,17] thus inducing a "trapping" of iron within macrophages.[18] This results in decreased iron delivery to the bone marrow.

In HF, hepcidin is initially upregulated (likely related to the release of IL-6), resulting in the development of iron deficiency.[19] In the later stages of HF and with progression of disease, hepcidin is downregulated, possibly as an attempt to reverse prior iron deficiency.[19] In patients with chronic kidney disease (and in many cases cardiorenal syndrome), worsening glomerular filtration rate may also result in decreased hepcidin clearance in the kidneys,[20] further impacting iron deficiency. There is evidence that erythropoietin therapy in renal failure can suppress hepcidin levels,[20] but anemia resolves only after addition of iron therapy in iron-deficient individuals.

Diagnosing Iron Deficiency

The most well-accepted definition of iron deficiency is transferrin saturation (TSAT) <20% and ferritin less than 100 ng/mL.[18,21] Although both these indices are low in absolute iron deficiency, in states of functional iron deficiency whereby iron is sequestered within stores due to a proinflammatory state and elevated hepcidin levels, TSAT will remain low but ferritin levels may rise

above 100 ng/mL.[18] This reflects "anemia of chronic disease," which occurs frequently in HF.

Therapeutic Interventions

A number of randomized clinical trials have now been performed to better define the role of iron replacement therapy in HF. Starting with the Ferinject Assessment in Patients with Iron Deficiency and Chronic Heart Failure (FAIR-HF) trial,[22] we have seen improvements in functional capacity and possibly a reduction in HF hospitalizations. FAIR-HF was the first major randomized controlled trial to evaluate the effects of IV iron (ferric carboxymaltose) in patients with chronic HF and iron deficiency, regardless of evidence of anemia. Patients were NYHA class II-III with ejection fraction (EF) ≤45%, and randomized 2:1 to IV iron versus placebo. By 24 weeks, significant improvements in HF symptoms using NYHA class and the Patient Global Assessment (PGA) were found in patients treated with IV iron repletion. Six-minute walk test (6MWT), Kansas City Cardiomyopathy Questionnaire (KCCQ), and European Quality of Life–Five Dimensions (EQ-5D) scores also improved. The intervention showed benefit on "softer" endpoints, but more convincing evidence with regard to hospitalization and survival was needed.

In 2015, the CONFIRM-HF study[24] assessed the use of ferric carboxymaltose on the functional status of patients with EF ≤45% with signs/symptoms of HF (**Table 1** for inclusion/exclusion criteria). The primary endpoint of 6MWT was significantly improved, but importantly, this study showed a decrease in hospitalizations related to worsening HF in patients treated with IV iron versus placebo (**Fig. 1**). Although this was not a prespecified endpoint of the study, this result was notable. Serum ferritin, TSAT, and hemoglobin levels increased significantly ($P<.001$) between the groups by week 24, and there was a persistent effect up to week 52, without an increase in adverse events. This finding further extended the known effect of IV iron therapy up to 12 months with an objective measure of patient functionality using the 6MWT. In addition, subgroup analyses showed significant improvements specifically in patients with renal dysfunction and diabetes, with a larger treatment effect observed than most in these populations. This benefit deserves further study.

To further assess the effect of IV iron (ferric carboxymaltose [FCM]) on exercise capacity in patients with symptomatic chronic HF and iron deficiency, the EFFECT-HF[25] trial was undertaken. The investigators used cardiopulmonary stress testing as an objective measure of exercise

Table 1
Pivotal clinic trials of iron repletion in heart failure

Trial	Patient Criteria	Anemia Testing	Iron Formulation	Endpoints	Outcome	HF Hospitalization	Survival
FAIR-HF[22] (2009)	459 patients, LVEF ≤45%, NYHA II-III	Ferritin <100 ng/mL or Ferritin 100–299 ng/mL if TSAT <20%; Hg 95–135 g/L.	FCM (4 mL [200 mg iron] IV weekly × 3–7 wk until replete, then every 4 wk for maintenance) vs placebo (NS), randomized 2:1.	Primary: PGA, NYHA Class at wk 24. Secondary: 6MWT, KCCQ, EQ-5D.	Significant improvement in primary and secondary outcomes. Safety: No significant difference in AE.	Trend toward lower HF hospitalizations with IV iron (HR 0.53; 95% CI 0.25–1.09; $P = .08$)	No significant difference
IRON-HF[23] (2013)	23 patients, LVEF ≤40%, NYHA II-IV	Ferritin <500 ng/mL, TSAT <20% and Hg ≤12 g/dL and ≥9 g/dL.	Iron sucrose 200 mg IV weekly × 5 wk + oral placebo, vs FeSO4 200 mg po 3×/d × 8 wk + IV placebo, vs po and IV placebo.	Primary: Change in peak V_{O_2}.	Trial ended early due to lack of funding; insufficiently powered for determination of primary endpoint.		
CONFIRM-HF[24] (2015)	304 patients, LVEF <45%, NYHA II-III, BNP >100 pg/mL or NT-proBNP >400 pg/mL	Ferritin <100 ng/mL or Ferritin 100–300 ng/mL if TSAT <20%; Hg <15 g/dL.	FCM 10 mL or 20 mL (500 mg –2000 mg of iron) IV vs placebo (NS), randomized 1:1.	Primary: Increased 6MWT vs placebo. Secondary: NYHA class, PGA, KCCQ, Fatigue score, EQ-5D.	Significant improvements in primary and secondary endpoints.	Reduced in FCM group (HR 0.39; CI 0.19–0.82; $P = .009$)	No significant difference

(continued on next page)

Table 1
(continued)

Trial	Patient Criteria	Anemia Testing	Iron Formulation	Endpoints	Outcome	HF Hospitalization	Survival
EFFECT-HF[25] (2017)	172 patients with LVEF ≤45%, mild-moderate symptoms despite optimal HF medication, peak VO_2 10–20 mL/kg/min	Ferritin <100 ng/mL or Ferritin 100–300 ng/mL if TSAT <20%; Hg <15 g/dL.	FCM 10 mL or 20 mL (500 or 1000 mg iron) IV, follow-up dosing based on repeat iron levels at wk 6 and 12 vs standard of care, randomized 1:1.	Primary: Change in Peak VO_2 over 24 wk. Secondary: Hematologic indices, BNP/NT-proBNP, NYHA Class, PGA.	No significant difference in Peak VO_2. Significant improvement in NYHA Class, PGA.	No significant difference	Not calculable
IRONOUT-HF[26] (2017)	225 patients, LVEF ≤40%, NYHA II-IV	Ferritin 15–100 ng/mL or Ferritin 101–299 ng/mL if transferrin at <20%, Hg 9–15 g/dL (men) or 9–13.5 g/dL (women).	Oral iron polysaccharide 150 mg BID × 16 wk vs placebo, randomized 1:1.	Primary: Peak VO_2. Secondary: 6MWT, NT-proBNP, KCCQ.	No significant change in peak VO_2 or secondary endpoints; no significant change in hematologic indices.		

Abbreviations: 6MWT, 6-minute walk test; AE, adverse events; BID, twice a day; BNP, brain natriuretic peptide; CI, confidence interval; EQ-5D, European Quality of Life–Five Dimensions Score; FCM, ferric carboxymaltose; HF, heart failure; Hg, hemoglobin; HR, hazard ratio; IV, intravenous; KCCQ, Kansas City Cardiomyopathy Questionnaire; LVEF, left ventricular ejection fraction; NS, normal saline; NT-proBNP, N-terminal-pro-brain natriuretic peptide; NYHA, New York Heart Association; PGA, Patient Global Assessment; po, by mouth; TSAT, transferrin saturation.

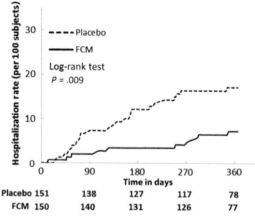

Fig. 1. Effect of IV iron on hospitalization rates from the CONFIRM-HF trial. Significant reduction in HF hospitalizations seen in patients treated with ferrous carboxy-maltose versus placebo. (*From* Ponikowski P, et al. Beneficial effects of long-term intravenous iron therapy with ferric carboxymaltose in patients with symptomatic heart failure and iron deficiency. Eur Heart J 2015;36(11):664; with permission.)

capacity on patients with symptomatic HF, EF ≤45% on optimal medical therapy, with documented iron deficiency. The primary endpoint was a change in peak Vo_2 from baseline to 24 weeks in patients randomized to standard HF therapy versus IV iron + standard therapy. The study design required the use of an imputation method for which patients who died had a peak Vo_2 of 0 at week 24, and a last observation carried forward imputation was used for subjects without assessment at week 24. Due to these imputations, the ultimate change in peak Vo_2 in patients treated with FCM could not be conclusively determined. Patients in this study did appear to derive benefit in terms of improved NYHA class and PGA.

Finally, Lewis and colleagues[26] assessed the effects of oral iron supplementation on exercise capacity in 225 patients with HF in the IRONOUT-HF study. There was no significant change in peak Vo_2 at 16 weeks between oral iron and placebo groups. There was also no significant difference between treatment groups in 6MWT or KCCQ score. The study concluded that high-dose oral iron supplementation did not cause an overall improvement in exercise capacity in patients with iron deficiency and HF. The investigators postulated that impact of hepcidin on iron absorption may be at play in patients who did not have improvements in TSAT and ferritin levels. It was noted, however, that changes in peak Vo_2 and N-terminal-pro-brain natriuretic peptide (NT-proBNP) did correlate with changes in TSAT.

Recommendations for Management of Iron Deficiency

There are a number of preparations approved by the Food and Drug Administration of IV iron available, including sodium ferric gluconate (Ferrlecit), iron sucrose (Venofer), ferumoxytol (Feraheme), and FCM (Injectafer).[27] Of these, FCM has been the agent most widely studied in clinical trials. Total cumulative doses for each can be based on the Ganzoni formula, a somewhat unwieldy but useful tool:

(Total iron deficit [mg] = Weight in kg × [Target Hb − Actual Hb in g/dL] × 2.4 + iron stores in mg)

or on recommended doses based on total iron deficits derived from the Ganzoni formula in clinical trials: 1500 mg for FCM and 1000 mg for the other agents.

Taken in total, results of recently published trials indicate that IV (and not oral) iron repletion improved functional capacity, HF symptoms, and may improve exercise capacity as measured by peak Vo_2. The lack of effect of oral iron on improvement in hematologic indices may be related to the effect of elevated hepcidin levels on gut absorption of iron.[21] **Fig. 2** provides an algorithm for management of iron deficiency based on current knowledge.

POTENTIAL ADVERSE EFFECTS OF INTRAVENOUS IRON

1. Anaphylaxis: Although older formulations of IV iron repletion (iron dextran) carried the risk of anaphylactic-type reactions, in more contemporary formulations this is no longer a concern.[28]
2. Tissue iron overload is now rare, but can occur at serum ferritin levels of more than 2000 ng/mL.[28]
3. Infections: The presence of iron in the circulation has been thought to support the growth of bacteria, and iron infusions in infected patients have been avoided for this reason. There has been no randomized controlled trial performed to date to substantiate this risk,[28] however, and some initial research has shown no impact on clinical outcomes in patients on dialysis admitted for infections who receive IV iron.[29]
4. Oxidative stress, although the long-term impact is unclear.[30]

FUTURE INVESTIGATIONS

Further study into the effect of iron repletion on HF hospitalizations and mortality is needed and

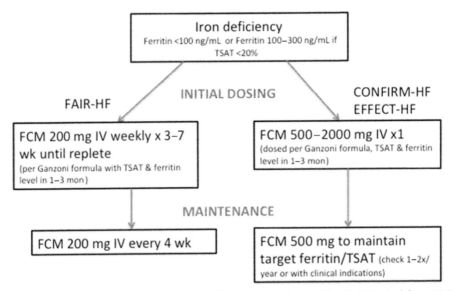

Fig. 2. Suggested algorithm for treatment of iron deficiency in patients with HF. (*Adapted from* McDonagh T, Macdougall IC. Iron therapy for the treatment of iron deficiency in chronic heart failure: intravenous or oral? Eur J Heart Fail 2015;17(3):259; with permission.)

currently in progress in 2 large trials: AFFIRM-AHF (Study to Compare Ferric Carboxymaltose With Placebo in Patients With Acute Heart Failure and Iron Deficiency; NCT02937454; evaluating the efficacy of IV iron repletion in 1100 patients after a hospitalization for acute HF) and FAIR-HF 2 NCT03036462, an randomized controlled trial to evaluate the effect of IV iron on rates of HF hospitalizations and cardiovascular death in 1200 patients with chronic HF.

SUMMARY

Iron deficiency anemia is a well-recognized co-morbidity in HF. Recent clinical trials have shown improvements in functional class and quality of life parameters in patients treated with IV iron formulations. Oral supplementation does not appear to be beneficial, likely related to poor absorption in the gastrointestinal tract. Given the initial positive results, further research is ongoing to determine the impact of IV iron supplementation on HF hospitalization and cardiovascular mortality.

REFERENCES

1. Berry C, Poppe KK, Gamble GD, et al. Prognostic significance of anaemia in patients with heart failure with preserved and reduced ejection fraction: results from the MAGGIC individual patient data meta-analysis. QJM 2016;109(6):377–82.
2. Sanchez-Torrijos J, Gudin-Uriel M, Nadal-Barange M, et al. Prognostic value of discharge hemoglobin level in patients hospitalized for acute heart failure. Rev Esp Cardiol 2006;59(12):1276–82 [in Spanish].
3. Szachniewicz J, Petruk-Kowalczyk J, Majda J, et al. Anaemia is an independent predictor of poor outcome in patients with chronic heart failure. Int J Cardiol 2003;90(2–3):303–8.
4. Groenveld HF, Januzzi JL, Damman K, et al. Anemia and mortality in heart failure patients a systematic review and meta-analysis. J Am Coll Cardiol 2008; 52(10):818–27.
5. Ebner N, Jankowska EA, Ponikowski P, et al. The impact of iron deficiency and anaemia on exercise capacity and outcomes in patients with chronic heart failure. Results from the Studies Investigating Co-morbidities Aggravating Heart Failure. Int J Cardiol 2016;205:6–12.
6. Kalra PR, Bolger AP, Francis DP, et al. Effect of anemia on exercise tolerance in chronic heart failure in men. Am J Cardiol 2003;91(7):888–91.
7. Silverberg DS, Wexler D, Blum M, et al. The use of subcutaneous erythropoietin and intravenous iron for the treatment of the anemia of severe, resistant congestive heart failure improves cardiac and renal function and functional cardiac class, and markedly reduces hospitalizations. J Am Coll Cardiol 2000; 35(7):1737–44.
8. Pozzo J, Fournier P, Delmas C, et al. Absolute iron deficiency without anaemia in patients with chronic systolic heart failure is associated with poorer functional capacity. Arch Cardiovasc Dis 2017;110(2): 99–105.
9. World Health Organization. Haemoglobin concentrations for the diagnosis of anaemia and assessment of severity. 2011. Available at: http://www.who.

int/iris/handle/10665/85839. Accessed June 29, 2018.

10. Cleland JG, Zhang J, Pellicori P, et al. Prevalence and outcomes of anemia and hematinic deficiencies in patients with chronic heart failure. JAMA Cardiol 2016;1(5):539–47.

11. Jankowska EA, Rozentryt P, Witkowska A, et al. Iron deficiency predicts impaired exercise capacity in patients with systolic chronic heart failure. J Card Fail 2011;17(11):899–906.

12. Haas JD, Brownlie T 4th. Iron deficiency and reduced work capacity: a critical review of the research to determine a causal relationship. J Nutr 2001;131(2S-2):676S–88S [discussion: 688S–90S].

13. Bayeva M, Gheorghiade M, Ardehali H. Mitochondria as a therapeutic target in heart failure. J Am Coll Cardiol 2013;61(6):599–610.

14. Guzman Mentesana G, Baez AL, Lo Presti MS, et al. Functional and structural alterations of cardiac and skeletal muscle mitochondria in heart failure patients. Arch Med Res 2014;45(3):237–46.

15. Duke M, Abelman W. The hemodynamic response to chronic anemia. Circulation 1969;39(4):503–15.

16. Singh B, Arora S, Agrawal P, et al. Hepcidin: a novel peptide hormone regulating iron metabolism. Clin Chim Acta 2011;412(11–12):823–30.

17. Nemeth E, Tuttle M, Powelson J, et al. Hepcidin regulates cellular iron efflux by binding to ferroportin and inducing its internalization. Science 2004; 306(5704):2090–3.

18. Silverberg DS, Iaina A, Schwartz D, et al. Intravenous iron in heart failure: beyond targeting anemia. Curr Heart Fail Rep 2011;8(1):14–21.

19. Jankowska EA, Malyszko J, Ardehali H, et al. Iron status in patients with chronic heart failure. Eur Heart J 2013;34(11):827–34.

20. Ashby DR, Gale DP, Busbridge M, et al. Plasma hepcidin levels are elevated but responsive to erythropoietin therapy in renal disease. Kidney Int 2009;75(9):976–81.

21. Macdougall IC. Evolution of IV iron compounds over the last century. J Ren Care 2009;35:8–13.

22. Anker SD, Comin Colet J, Filippatos G, et al. Ferric carboxymaltose in patients with heart failure and iron deficiency. N Engl J Med 2009;361:2436–48.

23. Beck-da-Silva L, Piardi D, Soder S, et al. IRON-HF study: a randomized trial to assess the effects of iron in heart failure patients with anemia. Int J Cardiol 2013;168(4):3439–42.

24. Ponikowski P, van Veldhuisen D, Comin-Colet J, et al. Beneficial effects of long-term intravenous iron therapy with ferric carboxymaltose in patients with symptomatic heart failure and iron deficiency. Eur Heart J 2015;36(11):657–68.

25. van Veldhuisen DJ, Ponikowski P, van der Meer P, et al. Effect of ferric carboxymaltose on exercise capacity in patients with chronic heart failure and iron deficiency. Circulation 2017;136(15):1374–83.

26. Lewis GD, Malhotra R, Hernandez AF, et al. Effect of oral iron repletion on exercise capacity in patients with heart failure with reduced ejection fraction and iron deficiency: the IRONOUT HF randomized clinical trial. JAMA 2017;317(19):1958–66.

27. Koch TA, Myers J, Goodnough LT. Intravenous iron therapy in patients with iron deficiency anemia: dosing considerations. Anemia 2015;2015:10.

28. Kovesdy CP, Kalantar-Zadeh K. Iron therapy in chronic kidney disease: current controversies. J Ren Care 2009;35:14–24.

29. Ishida JH, Marafino BJ, McCulloch CE, et al. Receipt of intravenous iron and clinical outcomes among hemodialysis patients hospitalized for infection. Clin J Am Soc Nephrol 2015;10(10):1799–805.

30. Agarwal R, Vasavada N, Sachs NG, et al. Oxidative stress and renal injury with intravenous iron in patients with chronic kidney disease. Kidney Int 2004;65(6):2279–89.

Management of Pulmonary Hypertension
Associated with Left Heart Disease

Veronica Franco, MD, MSPH

KEYWORDS

- Hypertension • Heart failure • Ejection fraction • Right ventricular • Pulmonary hypertension
- Pulmonary arterial hypertension

KEY POINTS

- Pulmonary hypertension (PH) due to left heart disease, or WHO group 2 PH, is the most frequent cause of PH.
- Long-standing PH results in right heart strain and failure, which further worsen symptoms and prognosis.
- The goal is to identify and treat the disease before onset of fixed pulmonary arterial hypertension and right heart failure.

INTRODUCTION

Pulmonary hypertension (PH) due to left heart disease, or WHO group 2 PH, is the most frequent cause of PH. It affects approximately 50% to 60% of patients with heart failure with preserved ejection fraction (HFpEF) as well as 60% of those with heart failure with reduced ejection fraction (HFrEF),[1,2] particularly advanced stages of disease, and contributes significantly to disease progression and unfavorable outcomes.

Elevated left-sided filling pressures secondary to diastolic or systolic dysfunction or valvular lesions (especially mitral valve disease) eventually result in postcapillary PH. Venous hypertension is back transmitted via capillaries to the pulmonary arterial system initially in a passive fashion resulting in passive pulmonary arterial hypertension.[3–5] During the passive phase, diuresing the patient is likely to result in complete normalization of pulmonary pressures. Over time, long-standing passive PH results in pulmonary arterial endothelial dysfunction, leading to elevated levels of endothelin 1 (ET-1), decreased nitric oxide level, and decrease in brain natriuretic peptide–mediated vasodilatation.[6,7] These biochemical changes result in active pulmonary arterial vasospasm, leading to further increase in pulmonary arterial pressures.

Eventually, pulmonary vascular remodeling is associated with fibrosis and decreased vascular compliance resulting in fixed elevation in pulmonary arterial pressures independent of the pressure changes in the left heart, no longer amenable to reversal with resolution of the underlying HF. Severity of PH is usually directly proportional to severity of underlying heart failure or valvular disease. Long-standing PH results in right heart strain and failure, which further worsen symptoms and prognosis. In view of the natural history of the disease, early diagnosis and management of volume overload is the key to favorable outcomes. The goal is to identify and treat the disease before onset of fixed pulmonary arterial hypertension and right heart failure.

Disclosure: Has served at advisory boards for Gilead, Bayer and United Therapeutics. The Ohio State University has received research funding from Actelion Pharmaceuticals, Arena, REATA, Bayer, Gilead and United Therapeutics.
Division of Cardiovascular Disease, Pulmonary Hypertension Program, Advanced Heart Failure, LVAD and Transplantation Program, The Ohio State University, DHLRI Suite 200, 473 West 12th Avenue, Columbus, OH 43210, USA
E-mail address: veronica.franco@osumc.edu

heartfailure.theclinics.com

HEMODYNAMIC DEFINITIONS

PH is defined hemodynamically by right heart catheterization, by a mean pulmonary arterial pressure (PAP) greater than or equal to 25 mm Hg at rest.[3] Pulmonary artery wedge pressure (PAWP) distinguishes precapillary ($\leq$15 mm Hg) and postcapillary (>15 mm Hg) PH in setting of normal or reduced left ventricular ejection fraction. As a consequence of these pressure cutoffs, the transpulmonary gradient (TPG = mean PAP − PAWP) has been used clinically for many years to distinguish between "passive" PH (TPG <12 mm Hg) and "reactive" PH (TPG $\geq$12 mm Hg).[3,8]

Patients with TPG greater than or equal to 12 mm Hg, also called to have "out of proportion" PH and assumed to have pulmonary pressures over that, can be explained by passive back transmission of elevated left heart pressures. However, the term "out of proportion" PH is challenging to interpret and could be unpredictable clinically. We should not assume that a high TPG represents superimposed pulmonary arterial hypertension because that is not always the clinical scenario.[9] For example, patients with HFrEF who were diagnosed with "reactive PH," unresponsive to vasodilator challenge, can completely normalize their pulmonary pressures solely by treatment of their left-sided HF with a left ventricular assist device (LVAD). The TPG depends flow rate and varies with stroke volume and cardiac output. The dependence of TPG on pulmonary vascular flow, resistance, and left heart filling pressures (PAWP) makes it a poor measure of pulmonary arterial vascular disease in the setting of left heart disease.[3,9]

The Fifth World Symposium in Pulmonary Hypertension from Nice, France took place in 2013. The use of the term "out of proportion" PH was discouraged.[5] Experts recommended the use of the diastolic pressure gradient (DPG = diastolic PAP − PAWP), rather than TPG, to better assess the development of pulmonary vascular disease in patients with left heart disease. Diastolic PAP is less sensitive to changes in pulmonary vascular flow rate (stroke volume/cardiac output), resistance, and PAWP.[4,9] It has been shown to be a less sensitive to pulmonary vascular distensibility. A study correlating PH with histology has demonstrated that DPG has a higher specificity to identify significant pulmonary vascular disease.[10]

The normal upper limit of DPG was assumed to be 5 mm Hg,[4] as derived from athletic young adults. The DPG was revisited by Gerges and colleagues[10] in a study of 2056 patients with HF. PH, defined by mean pulmonary arterial pressure (mPAP) greater than 25 mm Hg, was diagnosed in 1094 of these patients, a TPG greater than 12 mm Hg was diagnosed in 490, and a combination of TPG greater than 12 mm Hg and a DPG greater than 7 mm Hg in 179 (16%). Normal DPG values range from 1 to 3 mm Hg and remains less than 5 mm Hg in most patients with cardiac disease (excluding shunts).[9,11] Elevated DPG is a marker of pulmonary vascular remodeling. Studies correlating DPG with pulmonary vascular resistance (PVR) have shown that individuals with DPG less than 5 mm Hg are unlikely to have severe pulmonary vascular disease. A PAWP greater than 15 mm Hg with a DPG less than 7 mm Hg is more likely associated with isolated postcapillary PH, previously called "passive PH." Individuals with PAWP greater than 15 mm Hg with a DPG greater than or equal to 7 mm Hg have combined pre- and postcapillary PH, previously called "out of proportion PH" or "reactive PH"[3,10,12] (Table 1).

Elevated DPG has been shown to have prognostic value.[10] The survival of the patients with high TPG and DPG was very poor compared with that of patients with untreated pulmonary arterial hypertension. Some histopathologic examinations of the pulmonary small vessels in patients with both increased TPG and DPG have shown pulmonary vascular remodeling with medial hypertrophy, intimal thickening, and adventitial proliferation. From multivariate analysis, the DPG emerged as an independent predictor of survival, with a cutoff value of 7 mm Hg.[10] Patients with TPG greater than 12 mm Hg and diastolic pressure difference (DPD) greater than 7 mm Hg have a median survival of ~6.5 years. Patients with DPD less than

Table 1
Fifth World Symposium in Pulmonary Hypertension—classification of pulmonary hypertension due to left heart failure

PH-LHD	Mean PAP	PAWP	DPG	PVR
Isolated postcapillary PH	$\geq$25 mm Hg	>15 mm Hg	<7 mm Hg	$\leq$3 WU
Combined pre- and postcapillary PH	$\geq$25 mm Hg	>15 mm Hg	$\geq$7 mm Hg	>3 WU

Abbreviations: LHD, left heart disease; WU, Wood units.
Data from Refs.[3,5,10]

7 mm Hg have slightly better prognosis with median survival of ~8.4 years.

Another dynamic approach to the diagnosis of WHO group 2 PH is based on fluid or exercise challenge during catheterization to differentiate cases of pulmonary arterial hypertension from PH associated with HFpEF. These techniques are particularly important with patients with borderline PAWP (12–15 mm Hg) but several risk factors for HFpEF (ie, metabolic syndrome, hypertension, older patients, enlarged left atrium, etc.). "Fluid challenge" refers to the rapid intravenous fluid loading by the infusion of 0.5 to 1 L of saline over 5 to 10 min. Latent PH in left-sided disease is then diagnosed based on a PAWP increased to greater than 15 to 20 mm Hg. Robbins and colleagues[13] showed that a 0.5 L of saline fluid challenge may reclassify up the 22% of pulmonary arterial hypertension patients as HF-PH. However, the fluid challenge for the diagnosis of HF-PH is still in need of standardization.[1,14] A reanalysis of existing data in healthy subjects and accumulating clinical experience are drifting this cutoff value to 18 mm Hg, as recently demonstrated in 212 patients referred for PH, challenged with 7 mL/kg of saline given in 5–10 min.[15] There is too much disparity in amount of fluid, infusion rate, and cutoff pathologic values of PAWP and mPAP, and this is an area of growing research to differentiate between WHO group 1 and WHO group 2 PH.

Andersen and colleagues[16] showed that exercise elicits greater PAWP elevation compared with a fluid challenge with up to 20 mL/kg of saline in patients with HFpEF. Many questions remain in terms of exercise testing for diagnosis of PH, including appropriate mode of testing, the need for supine vs upright bicycle, evaluation of mean PAWP or end-of-expiration values, and diagnostic cutoffs for diagnosis. Hemodynamic measurements may be markedly affected by differences in ventilation and eventual dynamic hyperinflation. As of today, "fluid challenge" could help in the differential diagnosis between pre- and postcapillary PH; however, the test still needs standardization and better-defined clinical relevance. Further, the role of exercise testing in diagnosing PH in left heart disease has not been validated but can be used if fluid challenge is not feasible or contraindicated. Both tests should be interpreted with caution, particularly with "borderline" PAWP values.

The role of vasoreactive testing in diagnosis of PH suspected to be secondary to left heart disease is not well established. It has been shown to be of some benefit in evaluating patients for advanced heart failure therapies. When necessary, it is safest to use nitroprusside or nitric oxide as vasodilator agents as they are least likely to precipitate pulmonary edema and hemodynamic decompensations. Vasodilator testing with nitric oxide or epoprostenol is not recommended in patients with PAWP greater than 15 mm Hg to avoid risk of pulmonary edema and hemodynamic decompensation. It is best to avoid vasoreactive testing in PH secondary to fixed valvular disease for similar reasons.

MANAGEMENT OF PH ASSOCIATED TO LEFT HEART DISEASE
Management Goals

Identification of reversible abnormalities in LV filling as therapeutic targets is imperative in order to minimize PH. The lower the pulmonary pressures, the longer we will achieve preservation of right ventricular function, which is fundamental for good outcomes in HF. The first target should be to maintain euvolemia and keep a normal PAWP. Other important target therapies of WHO group 2 PH are the following: (a) treat the left heart by improving LV relaxation properties, (b) optimize volume status, (c) take care of comorbid conditions, and (d) be warned against the proper use of pulmonary vasodilators.[3,17] Finally, management of PH secondary to left heart disease should be geared toward appropriate interventions for the underlying left heart disease. HFpEF and HFrEF should be treated with optimal guideline-directed medical management.[18] Diuretics have been most helpful but the effect of neurohormonal antagonists on PH has not been systemically evaluated.

PH with HFrEF

Experts recommend a trial of nonspecific vasodilators, nitrates, and hydralazine to reduce pulmonary pressures as well as LV filling pressures. Patients with systolic dysfunction and PH can significantly improve and even normalize their pulmonary pressures in the catheterization suite with the use of nitroprusside, a very strong vasodilator. Usually, the pulmonary artery pressures decrease rapidly when the left heart is "unloaded," either pharmacologically or mechanically. This is the basis of "vasodilator challenges," which most commonly, as in the case of nitroprusside, nitroglycerin, and nesiritide, reduce PAWP, and typically pulmonary artery pressures decrease rapidly. A PVR greater than 5 Wood units is considered a relative contraindication for heart transplantation, and nitroprusside is the gold standard agent to evaluate vasoreactivity in heart transplant candidates.[19]

Patients with end-stage HFrEF and associated PH, not responding to medication, should be evaluated for advanced therapy with LVAD.[20–22] Mechanical LV support has been shown to dramatically improve pulmonary pressures and reduce right ventricular failure by unloading the LV. More importantly, benefit can be seen as early as 1 month, but it may take as long as 3 to 6 months to achieve maximum reversibility.[21,22] Therefore, in order to make full determination of reversibility after LVAD implantation, it is important to allow enough time for this therapy to have an effect.

PH with HFpEF

Elevated pulmonary pressure in patients with HFpEF is common and a cause of "diagnostic confusion," as commonly patients present with combined pre- and postcapillary PH hemodynamics. There are no good therapeutic pharmacologic strategies and this clinical group represents a challenge to date. Nonspecific vasodilators (nitrates and hydralazine) have shown to provide only a modest benefit of decrease in PVR and increase in cardiac output at the cost of significant hypotension.[23] In contrast to patients with HFrEF, in whom nitrate therapy can reduce pulmonary congestion and improve exercise capacity, the NEAT-HFpEF (Nitrate's Effect on Activity Tolerance in Heart Failure With Preserved Ejection Fraction) trial[24] randomized 110 patients with left ventricular ejection fraction greater than or equal to 50% on stable HF therapy, not including nitrates, and with activity limited by dyspnea, fatigue, or chest pain, to either isosorbide mononitrate or placebo and found no beneficial effects on activity levels, quality of life, exercise tolerance, or brain natriuretic peptide levels. Routine use of nitrates in patients with HFpEF is not recommended.[18]

PH with Valvular Disease and Others

Patients with severe aortic valvular disease, but most commonly, severe mitral stenosis or regurgitation, should be appropriately evaluated for valve repair or replacement to treat PH. Adequate treatment of the underlying valvular disease with improvement in left-sided pressures results in significant improvement in secondary PH especially if pulmonary arterial remodeling has not set in. Finally, it is imperative to screen early for comorbidities that could potentiate and worsen PH (eg, lung disease, obstructive sleep apnea, pulmonary thromboembolic disease, obesity, etc) and they should be treated aggressively in course of the disease.

Selective Pulmonary Vasodilators in Left Heart Disease

An established set of evidences suggest that even though pulmonary vasodilators are effective on hemodynamics, they have no clear beneficial effects in treating WHO group 2 PH and their use is complicated by side effects, such as systemic hypotension and fluid retention.[2,17,25] Further, acute pulmonary edema could be triggered by selective pulmonary vasodilators, as a result of increased blood return from the right ventricle to an noncompliant LV chamber, especially inhaled nitric oxide.[25] Pulmonary edema will worsen PH with a potential hemodynamic collapse from the resultant drop in cardiac output. At present time, none of the selective pulmonary vasodilators are recommended for the treatment of PH in left-sided disease.[3]

Endothelin 1 receptor blockers

ET-1 is one of the most potent endogenous vasoconstrictors and its pulmonary levels correlate with PVR.[26] Large-scale trials in patients with HF led to discouraging results. Treatment with bosentan increased the risk of worsening decompensated HF in the Endothelin Antagonist Bosentan for Lowering Cardiac Events in Heart Failure (ENABLE) study.[27] The use of bosentan caused a higher risk of HF during the first month of treatment, but lower risk of HF after 4 months of therapy, when compared with placebo.[28] The Endothelin A Receptor Antagonist Trial in Heart Failure (EARTH)[29] outcomes in patients with chronic HF were not improved by blockade of ET-1 with darusentan. Similarly, treatment with tezosentan, a short-acting intravenous ET-1 receptor antagonist, did not lower the incidence of death or worsening of HF in the Value of Endothelin Receptor Inhibition With Tezosentan in Acute Heart Failure Studies (VERITAS).[30] In the Heart Failure ET(A) Receptor Blockade Trial (HEAT),[31] cardiac index was improved by short-term administration of darusentan, whereas PAWP, PVR, or right atrial pressure did not change and trend toward increased death and early exacerbation of HF was reported.

Recently, the MELODY-1 trial was presented as an abstract.[32] This phase 2 study evaluated the safety and tolerability of macitentan in subjects with combined pre- and postcapillary PH due to HFpEF and showed that the macitentan-treated group was more likely to experience the composite endpoint of weight gain and need for intravenous diuretics or worsen functional class versus the placebo group at 12 weeks ($P = .34$). The main difference was driven by fluid retention. A follow-up, phase 2b trial with macitentan in patients with HFpEF (SERENADE; ClinicalTrials.gov Identifier: NCT03153111) is currently recruiting participants.

Prostacyclins

Trials that evaluated the benefit of prostanoids were negative for benefit with increased adverse reactions from the drugs and a trend for increased morbidity and mortality.[17,33,34] Acute administration of intravenous prostacyclin demonstrated a significant effect on PAWP and PVR, while cardiac index increased. However, these positive effects were paralleled by a decrease in systemic arterial pressure and resistance and some increase in plasma concentrations of epinephrine, norepinephrine, renin, and aldosterone.[33] The last large study on the use of prostanoids in patients with HFrEF, Flolan International Randomized Trial (FIRST),[34] was terminated early due to a strong trend toward negative survival rate. According to some insights, a positive inotropic effect of epoprostenol and some "steal effect" on the coronary circulation could have been responsible for the increased mortality.[17] Currently, there is also a study recruiting HFpEF subjects with PH and comparing oral treprostinil versus placebo to evaluate functional capacity as primary endpoint (SOUTHPAW; *ClinicalTrials.gov Identifier: NCT03037580*).

Guanylate cyclase stimulators

Riociguat has a dual mode of action; first it sensitizes the soluble guanylate cyclase (sGC) to endogenous nitric oxide (NO) and also directly stimulates sGC irrespective of NO.[35] A phase 2b study evaluated the acute hemodynamic response to a single riociguat administration in patients with HFpEF with PH.[36] It was well tolerated, without changes in PAWP or PVR, but increased stroke volume without significant change in the primary endpoint of mean PAP after 6 hours. The same group investigated the effects of riociguat in patients with HFrEF in a Phase 2b study (LEPHT).[37] Riociguat was well tolerated but again there was no change in the primary endpoint of mean PAP after 16 weeks. Two other studies done with another sGC, vericiguat, in patients with HFrEF and HFpEF, also failed to meet their primary endpoint of change in brain natriuretic values after 12 weeks of therapy.[38,39]

Phosphodiesterase type 5 inhibitors

This class of medications, particularly sildenafil, has been extensively evaluated in patients with HF.[5,17,40] There have been mixed outcomes in patients with left heart disease with or without PH; some single-center, small studies showed improvement in hemodynamics, exercise capacity, and symptoms; however, large randomized controlled trials did not have favorable clinical outcomes and the guidelines advised against the routine use of phosphodiesterase type 5 inhibitors in left heart disease.[3] Besides, these patients are on multiple guideline-directed medications to improve survival, which could lower blood

pressure; thus, hypotension is a limiting factor for the use of pulmonary vasodilators in subjects with left heart disease.

The RELAX study, the largest study to date, a randomized controlled trial that involved 216 participants with HFpEF, with or without PH, did not reveal improvement in the primary endpoint of functional capacity with sildenafil at 20 mg TID for 12 weeks, which was subsequently increased to 60 mg TID for another 12 weeks.[41] This study, however, did not evaluate hemodynamics or right ventricular function and nature of PH was not prespecified. Another large randomized controlled multicenter study, Sildenafil for Improving Outcomes after VAlvular Correction (SIOVAC),[42] also failed to show benefit in patients with persistent PH after correction of their valvular disease. It included 200 participants with mean PAP greater than or equal to 30 mm Hg, 1 year after their valve procedure and randomized to sildenafil, 40 mg TID, versus placebo for 6 months. Treatment with sildenafil was associated with worse outcomes. The acute administration of sildenafil lowered pulmonary pressures and increased cardiac output, whereas long-term administration induced both LV and right ventricle dilatation as compared with placebo, suggesting a possible negative inotropic effect of sildenafil in the setting of PH with left heart disease.

SUMMARY

The diagnosis of PH is associated with poor prognosis and significant morbidity and mortality. Group 2 PH is perhaps the most common as well as an underdiagnosed cause of PH. Management of PH in left heart disease is a widely prevalent poorly understood condition lacking evidence-based management approach. Current guidelines do not recommend treatment with selective pulmonary vasodilators ("specific pulmonary arterial hypertension drugs") in this patient population, but patients with combined pre- and postcapillary PH should be referred to specialized centers for individualized treatment decisions. Adequate management of underlying left heart disease remains the main stay of treatment.

REFERENCES

1. Guazzi M, Naeije R. Pulmonary hypertension in heart failure: pathophysiology, pathobiology and emerging clinical perspectives. J Am Coll Cardiol 2017;69:1719–34.
2. Guazzi M, Borlaug BA. Pulmonary hypertension due to left heart disease. Circulation 2012;126:975–90.
3. Galie N, Humbert M, Vachiery JL, et al. 2015 ESC/ERS guidelines for the diagnosis and treatment of

pulmonary hypertension: the joint task force for the diagnosis and treatment of pulmonary hypertension of the European Society of Cardiology (ESC) and the European Respiratory Society (ERS), endorsed by the International Society of Heart and Lung Transplantation (ISHLT) and association for European Pediatric and Congenital Cardiology. Eur Heart J 2016; 37:67–119.

4. Harvey RM, Enson Y, Ferrer MI. A reconsideration of the origins of pulmonary hypertension. Chest 1971; 59:82–94.

5. Vachiery JL, Adir Y, Barbera JA, et al. Pulmonary hypertension due to left heart disease. J Am Coll Cardiol 2013;62:D100–8.

6. Moraes DL, Colucci WS, Givertz MM. Secondary pulmonary hypertension in chronic heart failure: the role of the endothelium in pathophysiology and management. Circulation 2000;102:1718–23.

7. Guazzi M, Galie N. Pulmonary hypertension in left heart disease. Eur Respir Rev 2012;21:338–46.

8. Galie N, Hoeper M, Humbert M, et al. Guidelines on diagnosis and treatment of pulmonary hypertension: the Task Force on Diagnosis and Treatment of Pulmonary Hypertension of the European Society of Cardiology and of the European Respiratory Society. Eur Heart J 2009;30:2493–537.

9. Naeije R, Vachiery JL, Yerly P, et al. The transpulmonary pressure gradient for the diagnosis of pulmonary vascular disease. Eur Respir J 2013;41:217–23.

10. Gerges C, Gerges M, Lang MB, et al. Diastolic pulmonary vascular pressure gradient: a predictor of prognosis in "out-of-proportion" pulmonary hypertension. Chest 2013;143:758–66.

11. Rapp AH, Lange RA, Cigarroa JE, et al. Relation of pulmonary arterial diastolic and mean pulmonary arterial wedge pressures in patients with and without pulmonary hypertension. Am J Cardiol 2001;88:823–4.

12. Rosenkranz S, Gibbs JS, Wachter R, et al. Left ventricular heart failure and pulmonary hypertension. Eur Heart J 2016;37:942–54.

13. Robbins IM, Hemnes AR, Pugh ME, et al. High prevalence of occult pulmonary venous hypertension revealed by fluid challenge in pulmonary hypertension. Circ Heart Fail 2014;7:116–22.

14. Borlaug BA. Invasive assessment of pulmonary hypertension. Time for a more fluid approach? Circ Heart Fail 2014;7:2–4.

15. D'Alto M, Romeo E, Argiento P, et al. Clinical relevance of fluid challenge in patients evaluated for pulmonary hypertension. Chest 2017;151:119–26.

16. Andersen MJ, Olson TP, Melenovsky V, et al. Differential hemodynamic effects of exercise and volume expansion in people with and without heart failure. Circ Heart Fail 2015;8:41–8.

17. Guazzi M, Labate V. Group 2 PH: medical therapy. Prog Cardiovasc Dis 2016;59:71–7.

18. Yancy CW, Jessup M, Bozkurt B, et al. 2017 ACC/AHA/HFSA focused update of the 2013 ACCF/AHA guideline for the management of heart failure. a report of the American college of cardiology/american heart association task force on clinical practice guidelines and the heart failure society of America developed in collaboration with the American academy of family physicians, American college of chest physicians, and international society for heart and lung transplantation. Circulation 2017;136:e137–61.

19. Mehra MR, Kobashigawa J, Starling R, et al. Listing criteria for heart transplantation. J Heart Lung Transplant 2006;25:1024–42.

20. Mehra MR, Canter CE, Hannan MM, et al. The 2016 International Society for Heart Lung Transplantation listing criteria for heart transplantation: a 10-year update. J Heart Lung Transplant 2016;35:1–23.

21. Mikus E, Stepanenko A, Krabatsch T, et al. Reversibility of fixed pulmonary hypertension in left ventricular assist device support recipients. Eur J Cardiothorac Surg 2011;40:971–7.

22. Kutty RS, Parameshwar J, Lewis C, et al. Use of centrifugal left ventricular assist device as a bridge to candidacy in severe heart failure with secondary pulmonary hypertension. Eur J Cardiothorac Surg 2013;43:1237–42.

23. Schwartzenberg S, Redfield MM, From AM, et al. Effects of vasodilation in heart failure with preserved or reduced ejection fraction implications of distinct pathophysiologies on response to therapy. J Am Coll Cardiol 2012;59:442–51.

24. Redfield MM, Anstrom KJ, Levine JA, et al. Isosorbide mononitrate in heart failure with preserved ejection fraction. N Engl J Med 2015;373:2314–24.

25. Boilson BA, Schirgen JA, Borlaug BA. Caveal medicus! Pulmonary hypertension in the elderly: a word of caution. Eur J Heart Fail 2010;12:89–93.

26. Cody RJ, Haas GJ, Binkley PF, et al. Plasma endothelin correlates with the extent of pulmonary hypertension in patient with chronic congestive heart failure. Circulation 1992;85:504–9.

27. Kalra PR, Moon JC, Coats AJ. Do results of the ENABLE (endothelin antagonist bosentan for lowering cardiac events in heart failure) study spell the end for non-selective endothelin antagonism in heart failure? Int J Cardiol 2002;85:195–7.

28. Packer M, McMurray J, Massie BM, et al. Clinical effects of endothelin receptor antagonism with bosentan in patients with severe chronic heart failure: results of a pilot study. J Card Fail 2005;11:12–20.

29. Anand I, McMurray J, Cohn JN, et al. Long-term effects of darusentan on left-ventricular remodelling and clinical outcomes in the Endothelina Receptor Antagonist Trial in Heart Failure (EARTH): randomised, double-blind, placebo-controlled trial. Lancet 2004;364:347–54.

a preliminary study evaluating doxorubicin-mediated cardiomyopathy, moderate cardiotoxicity was described as a greater than or equal to 15% decrease in left ventricular ejection fraction (LVEF) to less than 45% on serial radionuclide angiocardiography.[4] According to the US Food and Drug Administration (FDA) package insert, doxorubicin-mediated cardiotoxicity is defined as either (1) greater than 20% absolute decline in LVEF or (2) greater than 10% decrease in LVEF to less than the lower limit of normal or absolute value of less than 45%.[5] The definition of trastuzumab-mediated cardiomyopathy, as determined by cardiac review and evaluation committee in trastuzumab trials, was either a greater than or equal to 10% decline in absence of symptoms or greater than or equal to 5% decrease in symptomatic patients to a final LVEF of less than 55%.[6,7] In the Herceptin Adjuvant (HERA) trial, LVEF decline by at least 10% from baseline to a value less than 50% was considered a significant LVEF decrease. New York Heart Association class III or IV symptoms with significant LVEF decrease was designated as symptomatic congestive HF.[8] The American Society of Echocardiography (ASE) defined CTRCD as greater than or equal to 10% decline in LVEF to a final value less than 53% confirmed on subsequent imaging performed 2 to 3 weeks after the initial measurement. If criteria for CTRCD were not met, greater than 15% relative decline in global longitudinal strain (GLS) compared with baseline strain was considered as subclinical left ventricular (LV) dysfunction. If there was less than 8% relative decline in GLS, LV dysfunction was unlikely.[9]

SELECTED CANCER THERAPEUTICS
Anthracyclines

Anthracyclines (eg, doxorubicin, daunorubicin, and epirubicin) are a group of chemotherapeutic agents that are very effective for the treatment of solid malignancies, lymphomas, and leukemias.[10] However, cardiotoxicity is a well-known dose-limiting adverse effect of anthracyclines that negatively affects their therapeutic efficacy.[11]

The exact pathophysiologic basis of anthracycline-related cardiotoxicity is not clear. According to one hypothesis, generation of reactive oxygen species and formation of iron complexes results in anthracycline-mediated cardiomyopathy. In cardiac myocytes, the quinone group of anthracyclines is reduced to a semiquinone form, which donates an electron to the oxygen molecule resulting in the production of superoxide ion, which in turn leads to the formation of hydrogen peroxide and reactive oxygen species. In the presence of reduced iron (Fe^{2+}), the oxidative potential of these compounds is greatly enhanced.[12] Anthracyclines can also form iron complexes that play a role in redox reactions in the cardiac myocytes.[12] These series of events result in lipid peroxidation, protein sulfhydryl oxidation, and injury to the mitochondrial DNA.[12,13] Dysfunction of oxidative phosphorylation and reduction of ATP production adds to the mitochondrial damage.[12,13] Anthracyclines bind to topoisomerase II, which negatively affects DNA repair and decreases protein production.[14] Inhibition of topoisomerase II-α in rapidly proliferating cancer cells results in tumoricidal effects. Inhibition of topoisomerase II-β in cardiomyocytes is probably responsible for cardiac damage.[15] According to a recently proposed theory, binding of anthracyclines to topoisomerase II-β induces breaks to double stranded DNA, causes alterations in transcriptome, damages the mitochondrial DNA, and results in the production of reactive oxygen species, all of which together may lead to cardiotoxicity (Fig. 1).[16]

The risk of HF exists at doses of doxorubicin less than 250 mg/m^2 and there is no clear dose threshold.[17] However, the risk of anthracycline-mediated cardiotoxicity is dose dependent. A pooled analysis of 3 studies revealed that the incidence of doxorubicin-induced symptomatic HF was 1.7%, 4.7%, 15.7%, and 48% at cumulative doses of 300 mg/m^2, 400 mg/m^2, 500 mg/m^2, and 650 mg/m^2 respectively.[18] Conventional cardiovascular risk factors, simultaneous or sequential treatment with other cardiotoxic therapies such as trastuzumab, and radiotherapy further increase the risk of cardiotoxicity.[19]

ALKYLATING AGENTS

Alkylating agents (eg, cyclophosphamide, ifosfamide, and melphalan) negatively affect DNA transcription, which in turn results in downregulation of protein production.[20] Cyclophosphamide is an integral part of combination chemotherapy used for treatment of leukemias, lymphomas, and solid tumors.[20] The incidence of symptomatic cardiomyopathy and fatal cardiotoxicity with cyclophosphamide has been estimated to be ~22% and 11% respectively.[21] Cardiotoxicity is dose dependent, with a dose ~180 to 200 mg/kg over a period of 48 to 96 hours associated with a significant risk. The dose based on body surface area is a good predictor of the cardiotoxicity, with a 25% risk of cardiomyopathy at 1.5 g/m^2/d or higher.[21] The exact mechanism underlying cyclophosphamide cardiotoxicity is not known. According to commonly accepted theory, injury to the endothelial layer causes leakage of potentially toxic

30. McMurray JJ, Teerlink JR, Cotter G, et al. Effects of tezosentan on symptoms and clinical outcomes in patients with acute heart failure: the veritas randomized controlled trials. JAMA 2007;298:2009–19.

31. Luscher TF, Enseleit F, Pacher R, et al. Hemodynamic and neurohumoral effects of selective endothelin A (ET(A)) receptor blockade in chronic heart failure: the Heart Failure Et(A) Receptor Blockade Trial (HEAT). Circulation 2002;106:2666–72.

32. Vachiery JL, Delcroix M, Al-Hiti H, et al. MELODY-1: a pilot study of macitentan in pulmonary hypertension due to left ventricular dysfunction. J Am Coll Cardiol 2017;69:1880 (presentation # 904-14).

33. Yui Y, Nakajima H, Kawai C, et al. Prostacyclin therapy in patients with congestive heart failure. Am J Cardiol 1982;50:320–4.

34. Califf RM, Adams KF, McKenna WJ, et al. A randomized controlled trial of epoprostenol therapy for severe congestive heart failure: the Flolan International Randomized Survival Trial (FIRST). Am Heart J 1997;134:44–54.

35. Grimminger F, Weimann G, Frey R, et al. First acute haemodynamic study of soluble guanylate cyclase stimulator riociguat in pulmonary hypertension. Eur Respir J 2009;33:785–92.

36. Bonderman D, Pretsch I, Steringer-Mascherbauer R, et al. Acute hemodynamic effects of riociguat in patients with pulmonary hypertension associated with diastolic heart failure (DILATE-1): a randomized, double-blind, placebo-controlled, single-dose study. Chest 2014;146:1274–85.

37. Bonderman D, Ghio S, Felix SB, et al. (LEPHT study group) Riociguat for patients with pulmonary hypertension caused by systolic left ventricular dysfunction: a phase IIb double-blind, randomized, placebo-controlled, dose-ranging hemodynamic study. Circulation 2013;128:502–11.

38. Gheorghiade M, Greene SJ, Butler J, et al. Effects of Vericiguat, a soluble guanylate cyclase stimulator, on natriuretic peptide levels in patients with worsening chronic heart failure and reduced ejection fraction (The SOCRATES-REDUCED randomized trial). JAMA 2015;314:2251–62.

39. Pieske B, Maggioni AP, CSP L, et al. Vericiguat in patients with worsening chronic heart failure and preserved ejection fraction: results of the SOluble guanylate Cyclase stimulatoR in heArT failurE patientS with PRESERVED EF (SOCRATES-PRESERVED) study. Eur Heart J 2017;38:1119–27.

40. Galie N, Manes A, Dardi F, et al. Aiming at the appropriate targete for the treatment of pulmonary hypertension due to left heart disease. Eur Heart J 2017;0:1–4.

41. Redfield MM, Chen HH, Borlaug BA, et al. Effect of phosphodiesterase-5 inhibition on exercise capacity and clinical status in heart failure with preserved ejection fraction: a randomized clinical trial. JAMA 2013;309:1268–77.

42. Bermejo J, Yotti R, Garcia-Orta R, et al. Sildenafil for improving outcomes in patients with corrected valvular heart disease and persistent pulmonary hypertension: a multicenter, double-blind, randomized clinical trial. Eur Heart J 2018;39(15):1255–64.

Management of Cancer Therapeutics–Related Cardiac Dysfunction

Ajay Vallakati, MD, MPH[a],*, Bhavana Konda, MD, MPH[b],
Daniel J. Lenihan, MD[c], Ragavendra R. Baliga, MD[a]

KEYWORDS

- Cancer therapy–mediated cardiotoxicity • Chemotherapy-induced cardiomyopathy
- Anthracyclines • HER2-targeted therapies • Trastuzumab • Radiotherapy-induced cardiotoxic
- β-Blockers • Renin-angiotensin inhibitors

KEY POINTS

- Cancer therapies are associated with different cardiac adverse effects. Cardiotoxicity is a known dose-limiting adverse effect of anthracyclines. Trastuzumab-related cardiomyopath dose independent and usually reversible.
- Vascular endothelial growth factor signaling pathway inhibitors include monoclonal antibodie bevacizumab), which block vascular endothelial growth factor, as well as small molecule inhib (eg, sunitinib, pazopanib, vandetanib). Apart from hypertension, these drugs can cause ventr dysfunction, heart failure, and myocardial ischemia.
- The goal of cardio-oncology is to ensure optimal cancer therapy while limiting adverse effect an emphasis on early recognition and treatment of cancer therapeutics–related ca dysfunction.
- Pre–cancer therapy evaluation begins with the assessment of cardiovascular disease burde risk stratification of each patient. Intra–cancer therapy evaluation involves close follow-up, toring, and treatment according to specific surveillance protocols and consensus guideline

INTRODUCTION

Improvements in the detection and treatment of cancer have resulted in a significant increase in the number of patients who are long-term survivors of cancers. In 2016, the estimated number of cancer survivors was more than 15.5 million.[1] However, cancer survivorship comes with long-term risk of adverse effects of cancer therapies. Complications caused by cancer therapies include cardiomyopathy, heart failure (HF), pericardial and valvular

disease, arrhythmias, vascular disease, heart disease, and hypertension.[2] This cusses the pathophysiology and m underlying cancer therapeutics–relate dysfunction (CTRCD) and presents an to the evaluation and treatment of these

DEFINITIONS

Different criteria have been used to def but no single definition is universally ac

Disclosure: The authors have nothing to disclose.
[a] Division of Cardiovascular Diseases, Department of Internal Medicine, The Ohio State Universit
10th, Avenue, Columbus, OH 43210, USA; [b] Division of Medical Oncology, Department of Interna
The Ohio State University, A440 Starling Loving Hall, 320 West 10th Avenue, Columbus, OH 4
[c] Division of Cardiovascular Diseases, Department of Internal Medicine, Washington University, S
63110, USA
* Corresponding author.
E-mail address: Ajay.Vallakati@osumc.edu

Heart Failure Clin 14 (2018) 553–567
https://doi.org/10.1016/j.hfc.2018.06.004
1551-7136/18/© 2018 Elsevier Inc. All rights reserved.

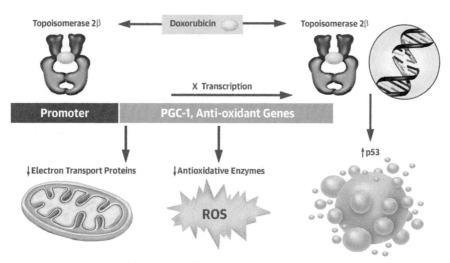

Fig. 1. One proposed mechanism of doxorubicin-induced cardiotoxicity. Doxorubicin binds to topoisomerase 2β and induces DNA double-strand break, resulting in p53 activation, which in turn causes death of cardiac myocytes. Doxorubicin-bound topoisomerase 2β interferes with the activity of promoters of antioxidative genes and peroxisome proliferator-activated receptor-γ coactivator 1 (PGC-1), which negatively affects the expression of antioxidative enzymes and electron transport chains. As a result, topoisomerase 2β hypothesis can explain the 3 classic features of doxorubicin-mediated cardiotoxicity: death of cardiac myocytes, production of reactive oxygen species (ROS), and mitochondrial dysfunction. (*From* Chang HM, Moudgil R, Scarabelli T, et al. Cardiovascular complications of cancer therapy: best practices in diagnosis, prevention, and management: part 1. J Am Coll Cardiol 2017;70(20):2540; with permission.)

metabolites into myocardium, which results in cardiac myocyte injury, interstitial edema, and hemorrhage. In addition, there is formation of intracapillary microthrombi leading to ischemic injury, which probably also contributes to cardiotoxicity.[21] High-dose ifosfamide (10–18 g/m^2) can cause severe but reversible LV dysfunction. The incidence of cardiomyopathy with high-dose ifosfamide has been estimated to be ~17%.[22]

HUMAN EPIDERMAL GROWTH FACTOR RECEPTOR 2–TARGETED CANCER THERAPIES

Human epidermal growth factor receptor 2 (HER2)–targeted agents (eg, trastuzumab, lapatinib, and pertuzumab) are used for the treatment of HER2-positive cancers, marked by the overexpression of the HER2 gene in malignant cells.[23] Trastuzumab is a monoclonal antibody against ErbB2, also known as HER2, a tyrosine kinase belonging to the epidermal growth factor receptor family.[24] Pertuzumab is a monoclonal antibody that binds to the dimerization domain of ErbB2 and blocks ligand-mediated ErbB2 activation.[24] Lapatinib inhibits ErbB1/2 tyrosine kinase activity.[24]

Trastuzumab-related cardiomyopathy is dose independent and usually reversible.[25] Concurrent treatment with doxorubicin and trastuzumab caused symptomatic HF in 16% of the patients

treated with this regimen.[24] Initiation of trastuzumab after the completion of anthracycline therapy decreased the rates of symptomatic HF to less than 5%, but the incidence of asymptomatic LV dysfunction/symptomatic HF was ~15%.[6,24]

Trastuzumab-mediated cardiomyopathy is likely related to HER2/HER4 blockade. Inhibition of the neuregulin ErbB pathway by trastuzumab interferes with cardiac homeostasis and contributes to myocardial dysfunction in response to stress.[26] ErbB4 ligand neuregulin (NRG)-1 binds to and activates Erb receptors in the heart,[24] which promotes cardiac homeostasis and restores cardiac function in a failing heart.[24,27] Molecular studies have shown that myocardial cells upregulate the production of neuregulin to facilitate cardiac repair in response to stress in HF.[28]

Risk factors for trastuzumab-mediated cardiotoxicity include age, diabetes, renal dysfunction, and underlying heart disease.[29] The risk of cardiotoxicity increases with concurrent anthracycline therapy.[7] Surprisingly, the risk is not increased beyond that associated with trastuzumab when other HER2-targeted therapies, such as pertuzumab and lapatinib, are used.[23]

TAXANES

Taxanes such as paclitaxel and docetaxel stabilize and prevent disassembly of microtubules and thereby inhibit cell multiplication.[30] The incidences of asymptomatic bradycardia, ventricular arrhythmias, supraventricular tachycardia including atrial fibrillation, and atrial flutter with paclitaxel are 30%, 0.26%, and 0.24% respectively.[21] Paclitaxel increases the risk of doxorubicin-mediated cardiotoxicity by interfering with the clearance of key metabolites of doxorubicin from the heart.[31] Incidence of HF when paclitaxel is combined with high-dose anthracycline chemotherapy is 20%. Limiting the dose of doxorubicin to less than 360 mg/m^2 and avoiding concomitant administration of paclitaxel and doxorubicin minimizes cardiotoxicity.[32] In contrast, adding paclitaxel to an epirubicin-based regimen does not increase the cardiotoxic metabolites.[32]

VASCULAR ENDOTHELIAL GROWTH FACTOR SIGNALING PATHWAY INHIBITORS

This class of drugs includes monoclonal antibodies (eg, bevacizumab), which block vascular endothelial growth factor (VEGF) as well as small molecule tyrosine kinase inhibitors (eg, sorafenib, sunitinib, pazopanib, vandetanib), which disrupt the downstream effects of vascular endothelial growth factor signaling pathway (VSP).[33,34] Hypertension is a well-known adverse effect of VSP inhibitors.[35] This class of drugs also causes LV dysfunction, HF, and myocardial ischemia.[36,37] Proposed mechanisms of cardiotoxicity include activation of myocardial proapoptotic kinases, microvascular dysfunction, and adenosine triphosphate depletion in the mitochondria and profound vasoconstriction resulting in LV remodeling.[37]

RADIATION THERAPY–INDUCED CARDIOTOXICITY

Radiation therapy refers to the treatment of cancer by exposure to x-rays, gamma rays, and high-energy charged particles. Exposure to radiation causes damage to DNA, which interferes with cell proliferation.[38] Malignant cells are susceptible to radiation therapy because of their high proliferation rate. Damage to the normal cells is determined by their inherent vulnerability and the dose of ionizing radiation.[38] There is a risk of damage to the heart caused by radiation exposure as a part of cancer treatment of Hodgkin's lymphoma and breast cancer.[39] A recent study revealed that almost half of the cancer survivors, who received mediastinal radiation between 1965 and 1995, developed cardiac diseases such as cardiomyopathy, valvular dysfunction, and coronary artery disease.[40] Radiation therapy can damage all layers of the heart, coronaries, valves, and electrical conduction

system.[41] This damage may manifest as long as 20 to 30 years after the initial exposure.[42] Injury to the pericardium results in increased capillary permeability, adhesions, and thickening causing pericardial effusions and acute and constrictive pericarditis. Improvements in radiation techniques have led to reduction in the incidence of radiation-induced acute pericarditis to ~2.5%.[39] Injury to the valves causes leaflet fibrosis, thickening, calcification, and valve retraction, which leads to valve insufficiency and stenosis.[43,44] Radiation causes microvascular injury leading to capillary rarefaction and accelerated atherosclerosis, which results in myocardial ischemia[44] and contributes to diffuse myocardial interstitial fibrosis and restrictive cardiomyopathy.[44,45]

EVALUATION OF CANCER THERAPY– MEDIATED CARDIOVASCULAR DYSFUNCTION

Cancer therapies are associated with different cardiovascular adverse effects. A multidisciplinary approach involving a cardio-oncology team with close communication between oncologist, primary care physician, and cardiologist is essential for providing optimal cancer therapy while limiting the risk of cardiovascular complications. Discussion of the entire spectrum of cardiovascular adverse effects is beyond the scope of this article. The risk factors, evaluation, prevention, and management of cardiovascular dysfunction before, during, and after cancer therapy are discussed.

RISK FACTORS

Risk factors can be arbitrarily divided into patient-related and cancer therapy–related categories. Conventional cardiovascular risk factors, such as hypertension, old age, female sex, diabetes mellitus, postmenopausal status, as well as previous coronary artery disease, LV dysfunction, or HF, represent patient-related risk factors.[46] Recent evidence suggests that genetic polymorphism may increase susceptibility to chemotherapy-mediated cardiac dysfunction.[47] Cancer therapy–related risk factors include high-dose chemotherapy, concomitant use of cardiotoxic chemotherapeutic agents, and the bolus form of chemotherapy.[48]

RISK PREDICTION

Different models have been proposed for risk prediction in patients receiving cancer therapy. Herrmann and colleagues[45] calculated cardiotoxicity risk score using patient-related and cancer therapy–related factors and recommended monitoring and management strategies based on the score. Dranitsaris and colleagues[49] proposed a risk prediction model in patients with breast cancer receiving doxorubicin. A composite score was calculated incorporating the following variables: age, administration of doxorubicin in conventional or pegylated form, age, weight, baseline anthracycline dose, number of chemotherapy cycles, and performance status.[49] The composite score was used to predict the risk of cardiac toxicity. For example, in patients with a composite score greater than or equal to 30 to less than 40, the risk of cardiac event after that chemotherapy cycle was 5.74%.[49] A risk prediction model for patients receiving trastuzumab was proposed by Ezaz and colleagues.[50] This model calculated 7-factor risk score based on age, adjuvant chemotherapy, the presence of comorbidities such as coronary artery disease, hypertension, atrial arrhythmias, diabetes mellitus, and renal dysfunction. The 7-factor risk score was used to predict 3-year risk of HF/cardiomyopathy.[50]

BIOMARKERS

The role of troponin in early detection and risk stratification of anthracycline-mediated cardiotoxicity is well known.[51] Increased troponin level, during or immediately after the completion of high-dose anthracycline therapy, predicted a high likelihood of future LV decline.[52] In contrast, troponin levels within normal limits after anthracycline therapy suggested low probability of LV dysfunction.[52] The European Society for Medical Oncology (ESMO) surveillance algorithm does not recommend an echocardiogram during anthracycline therapy if troponin levels are normal after each cycle of chemotherapy.[53] The ASE recommends baseline measurement of LVEF, GLS, and troponin levels in patients receiving anthracycline therapy.[9]

Increase in troponin levels with trastuzumab is mostly seen in patients who were previously treated with anthracyclines. Troponin peaks within the first 2 to 3 months and returns to normal in the next few months in most patients.[54–57] Cardinale and colleagues[54] showed that increased troponin level was associated with an increased risk of trastuzumab-mediated cardiomyopathy and lower likelihood of LV recovery. In contrast, Morris and colleagues[56] showed that increased troponin level is observed in two-thirds of the patients receiving trastuzumab and tyrosine kinase inhibitor lapatinib, but this did not predict the subsequent development of HF.

The role of natriuretic peptides for risk stratification and detection of CTRCD is unclear. A study by Lipshultz and colleagues[58] showed that increased levels of natriuretic peptides with doxorubicin are associated with subsequent cardiomyopathy. However, another study showed that natriuretic peptides did not predict subsequent cardiomyopathy.[57] Natriuretic peptides do not have a role in early detection of trastuzumab-mediated cardiotoxicity.[51] The utility of natriuretic peptides in patients receiving VEGF inhibitors is not clear. Asymptomatic increase in natriuretic peptide level was noted with VEGF inhibitors but it was not associated with subsequent cardiomyopathy.[59]

IMAGING MODALITIES

Preliminary studies using multigated acquisition (MUGA) scan revealed that LVEF decline during anthracycline therapy was a predictor of future symptomatic HF.[4,60] These findings supported the concept of surveillance imaging. Schwartz and colleagues[61] showed that the implementation of an LVEF surveillance protocol resulted in a lower incidence of HF in the patients receiving anthracycline therapy. This algorithm recommended a baseline LVEF measurement and serial imaging before each dose if LVEF was between 30% and 50%. In patients with no risk factors and baseline LVEF greater than 50%, subsequent LVEF measurement was recommended after a cumulative dose of 250 to 300 mg/m^2 and then at 450 mg/m^2 and each dose thereafter (**Fig. 2**).[61]

Accordingly, a baseline assessment of ventricular function before the initiation of cancer therapy is recommended to rule out structural heart disease.[9] Given its excellent reproducibility and widespread availability, MUGA scan was previously the primary tool for the evaluation of LV function.[62] However, the major concern with MUGA scan is exposure to radiation. Because one of the aims in clinical medicine is to minimize radiation exposure to as low as reasonably achievable, it is important to weigh the individual's risk versus benefit for every patient when considering this test.[9] MUGA scan has better reproducibility and lower interobserver variability, but echocardiogram is relatively inexpensive and allows comprehensive evaluation of LV structure and function.[9,62]

Two-dimensional (2D) echocardiogram is routinely used for surveillance imaging in patients with cancer.[9,63] Accurate measurement of LVEF is essential because cancer treatment may be affected by a change in cardiac function.[64] Poor image quality can prevent accurate estimation of LVEF. 2D echocardiogram is limited by its inability to detect small changes in LVEF.[63] The use of contrast, which enables precise demarcation of endocardial borders, is recommended in breast implant patients.[65] Three-dimensional echocardiogram is superior to 2D echocardiogram for

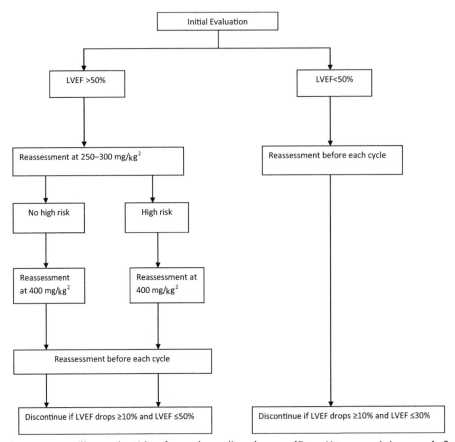

Fig. 2. Preliminary surveillance algorithm for anthracycline therapy. (*From* Herrmann J, Lerman A, Sandhu NP, et al. Evaluation and management of patients with heart disease and cancer: cardio-oncology. Mayo Clin Proc 2014;89(9):1296, with permission; and *Adapted from* Schwartz RG, McKenzie WB, Alexander J, et al. Congestive heart failure and left ventricular dysfunction complicating doxorubicin therapy. Seven-year experience using serial radionuclide angiocardiography. Am J Med 1987;82(6):1109–18, with permission.)

accurate measurement of ventricular function.[66] Recent study showed that three-dimensional echocardiogram was comparable with cardiac MRI for detection of subclinical cardiomyopathy.[67] However, this technology is expensive, not widely available, and requires initial training of the echocardiography staff, which has limited its widespread use.[9]

More recently, strain imaging by speckle tracking technology has been developed, which can detect subtle alterations in LV function.[57] An absolute value of GLS less than−17.5% before the initiation of anthracycline therapy was linked to 6-fold higher risk of cardiac events.[68] The reduction of systolic longitudinal strain to less than −19% at the end of breast cancer therapy predicted subsequent development of symptomatic HF.[57] A recent study showed that greater than 11% relative reduction of GLS in patients receiving trastuzumab was associated with future LVEF decline.[69] This technology is not widely

available and its application is further restricted by vendor variability in strain measurements.[2]

Cardiac magnetic resonance (CMR) is regarded as a gold standard for the evaluation of LV function.[2,70] CMR is a useful diagnostic tool because it can detect myocardial tissue changes such as edema, inflammation, and carring, which can help differentiate early and late cancer therapy–mediated cardiomyopathy.[71] CMR is also an effective prognostic tool because indexed LV mass measurement can serve as a valuable predictor of future cardiac events in patients with anthracycline-mediated cardiomyopathy.[72] Alterations in myocardial deformation parameters on cardiac MRI strain analysis can identify early CTRCD.[67] Because of its high sensitivity, application of CMR for assessment of LV function has resulted in an increase in the estimation of prevalence of chemotherapy-mediated cardiomyopathy.[2,70] Despite the advantages mentioned earlier, CMR is not a commonly used tool because it is expensive and not widely available, and because of patient-related factors such as claustrophobia.[2]

PRE–CANCER THERAPY AND INTRA–CANCER THERAPY CARDIOVASCULAR EVALUATION

Pre–cancer therapy evaluation includes obtaining complete history and performing comprehensive physical examination to determine the baseline cardiovascular risk. It is important to develop an institution-specific standard model for risk-based stratification of all patients. This stratification ensures systematic assessment of each patient, provides direction on treatment planning, and allows discussions between different providers. As a part of evaluation, clinicians should also consider the risk of cardiotoxicity and the potential therapeutic benefit of cancer treatment. An integrative approach proposed by Herrmann and colleagues[45] is presented in **Table 1**.

SURVEILLANCE PROTOCOL

Although there are different algorithms for surveillance imaging, there is no clear consensus on the frequency of imaging and discontinuation of anthracycline therapy. The American Society of Clinical Oncology (ASCO) recommends risk stratification of patients based on the dose of anthracycline, radiation therapy, cardiovascular risk factors, and administration of concomitant trastuzumab therapy. In patients with increased risk, baseline echocardiogram should be performed. Frequency of surveillance imaging should be based on each individual patient's risk factors,

---

Table 1
Framework of a risk assessment and management tool for cancer therapeutics–related cardiac dysfunction

(1) Risk Assessment	Tests: TTE with Strain, ECG, Troponin
Cancer therapy–related risk	*Patient-related risk factors*

High (risk score 4):
   Anthracyclines, cyclophosphamide, ifosfamide,
     clofarabine, Herceptin
 Intermediate (risk score 2):
   Docetaxel, pertuzumab, sunitinib, sorafenib
 Low (risk score 1):
   Bevacizumab, dasatinib, imatinib, lapatinib
 Rare (risk score 0):
   Eg, etoposide, rituximab, thalidomide
	• Cardiomyopathy or HF
	 • Coronary artery disease or equivalent
	 • Hypertension
	 • Diabetes mellitus
	 • Prior or concurrent anthracycline
	 • Age <15 or >65 y
	 • Female gender
	 • Heavy alcohol use
	 • Thyroid disease

Overall risk by CRS (risk categories by cancer therapy–related risk score plus number of patient-related risk factors: CRS>6, very high; 5–6, high; 3–4, intermediate; 1–2, low; 0, very low)

(2) Monitoring Recommendations

Very high cardiotoxicity risk: TTE with strain before every (other) cycle, end, 3–6 mo, and 1 y; optional ECG; troponins with TTE during cancer therapy
High cardiotoxicity risk: TTE with strain every 3 cycles, end, 3–6 mo, and 1 y after chemotherapy; optional ECG; troponins with TTE during cancer therapy
Intermediate cardiotoxicity risk: TTE with strain midterm, end, 3–6 mo, and 1 y after chemotherapy; optional ECG; troponins midterm of cancer therapy
Low cardiotoxicity risk: optional TTE with strain and/or ECG, troponin at the end of cancer therapy
Very low cardiotoxicity risk: none

(3) Management Recommendations

Very high cardiotoxicity risk: initiate ACEI/ARB, carvedilol, and/or spironolactone, starting at minimum dose, and start cancer therapy in 1 wk, uptitrate as tolerated
High cardiotoxicity risk: initiate ACEI/ARB, carvedilol, and/or statins
Intermediate cardiotoxicity risk: discuss risk and benefit of medications
Low cardiotoxicity risk: none, monitoring only
Very low cardiotoxicity risk: none, monitoring only

The model illustrates that risk stratification is based on patient- and medication-related risk factors. Screening and management strategies vary depending on the overall risk of cancer therapeutics–related cardiac dysfunction.
Abbreviations: ACEI, angiotensin-converting enzyme inhibitor; ARB, angiotensin receptor blocker; CRS, cardiotoxicity risk score; ECG, electrocardiogram; TTE, transthoracic echocardiogram.
Adapted from Herrmann J, Lerman A, Sandhu NP, et al. Evaluation and management of patients with heart disease and cancer: cardio-oncology. Mayo Clin Proc 2014;89(9):1295; with permission.

type of chemotherapy, and clinical judgment.[73] It is essential to develop an institution-specific surveillance protocol that is adjusted based on the patient's risk factors, baseline cardiac function, and type and dosing of cancer therapy.[74] The FDA recommends baseline LVEF measurement before initiation and surveillance LVEF measurement every 3 months during and at the completion of trastuzumab therapy and this should be followed by LVEF measurement every 6 months for 2 years after the completion of therapy (**Table 2**).[75]

ADJUSTMENTS TO CANCER THERAPY IN PATIENTS WITH LEFT VENTRICULAR DYSFUNCTION

The decision to adjust therapy protocols or withhold cancer therapy should be made taking into account the risk and potential benefits of continuing cancer therapy, which requires close collaboration between oncologists and cardiologists. Withholding cancer therapy should be the last resort. The FDA recommends discontinuation of anthracycline therapy in patients who develop HF.[76] The FDA recommends suspending trastuzumab therapy for at least 4 weeks for (1) greater than or equal to 16% LVEF decline from a baseline value, or (2) greater than or equal to 10% decline in LVEF to less than institution's lower cutoff limit.[75] Reinitiation of trastuzumab can be considered if LVEF on repeat measurement in 4 to 8 weeks is within normal limits and net decline from baseline is less than or equal to 15%.[75] Trastuzumab should not be readministered if LVEF does not improve within 8 weeks or therapy was withheld on more than 3 occasions for LVEF decline.[75] The ESMO surveillance algorithm suggests suspending trastuzumab therapy if (1) LVEF declines to 40% to 50% with a decrease of more than 10% from baseline or (2) LVEF decreases to less than 40%. Trastuzumab can be restarted if repeat LVEF in 3 weeks is greater than 40%.[53]

POST–CANCER THERAPY CARDIOVASCULAR EVALUATION

The National Comprehensive Cancer Network (NCCN) guidelines suggest comprehensive history and physical examination with assessment of HF risk factors in patients who have previously received anthracycline therapy.[77] Conventional cardiovascular risk factors, age greater than 65 years, family history of cardiomyopathy, high body mass index, low-normal baseline LV systolic function (ejection fraction 50%–54%), and exposure to high anthracycline dose

---

Table 2
Best practices for prevention, monitoring, and treatment of cardiomyopathy

Oncologist	Cardiologist
Identify high-risk patients (preexisting heart disease, diabetes, hyperlipidemia, young or old, female, plan for high-dose anthracycline therapy)	Modify cardiovascular risk factors (optimize cardiac medications, glucose control, diet, weight, exercise)
Order pretreatment imaging (if EF <50% or institution low normal, refer to cardiologist)	Repeat imaging studies (obtain high-quality EF, consider contrast, three-dimensional, strain). Order biomarkers (troponin and BNP)
Consider noncardiotoxic alternatives (consider noncardiotoxic alternatives in high-risk patients)	Advise on cardioprotection (interpret imaging and biomarker results and discuss with oncologist)
Adjust therapy protocols (for anthracycline, dose reduction, continuous infusion, liposomal doxorubicin, dexrazoxane; for anti-HER2, avoid concomitant treatment with anthracyclines)	Institute cardioprotective medications (start BB or ACEI if EF<50%, EF decrease >10%, abnormal GLS [>15% decrease])
Monitor during therapy (monitor with echocardiography at 3-mo intervals or symptom driven; if cardioprotective medications were given, monitor at 1-mo intervals).	
Withhold cardiotoxic therapy only as the last resort (for anthracycline, EF<45%; for anti-HER2 therapy, EF<40%).	
Monitor after completion of therapy (obtain posttherapy EF; repeat echocardiography in 6 mo or 1 y; if EF remains abnormal, follow ACC/AHA HF guidelines).	

Abbreviations: ACC, American College of Cardiology; AHA, American Heart Association; BB, β-blocker; BNP, brain natriuretic peptide; EF, ejection fraction.

Adapted from Chang HM, Moudgil R, Scarabelli T, et al. Cardiovascular complications of cancer therapy: best practices in diagnosis, prevention, and management: part 1. J Am Coll Cardiol 2017;70(20):2540; with permission.

(cumulative doxorubicin dose greater than or equal to 250 mg/m^2 or its equivalent) predispose cancer survivors to HF.[77] Therefore it is important to closely follow and treat modifiable cardiovascular risk factors in cancer survivors. The NCCN guidelines recommend 2D echocardiogram within 1 year of completion of anthracycline therapy in cancer survivors with greater than or equal to 1 risk factor.[77] Some centers suggest imaging at 6-month intervals in low-risk patients and 3-month intervals in high-risk patients for 1 year after completion of anthracycline chemotherapy.[45] The ASE does not support posttherapy surveillance imaging in patients with no risk factors with either (1) stable GLS during therapy and at 6 months posttherapy or (2) normal troponins during chemotherapy.[45] For the patients who received trastuzumab, the investigators recommend FDA guidelines that suggest LVEF measurement every 6 months for 2 years after the completion of therapy.[78]

MANAGEMENT OF CANCER THERAPEUTICS–RELATED CARDIAC DYSFUNCTION

Conventionally, HF is classified into stages A, B, C, and D. Stage C is symptomatic HF with structural heart disease such as LV systolic dysfunction.[79] The treatment of symptomatic CTRCD should be according to the pharmacologic strategies recommended in the American Heart Association (AHA)/American College of Cardiology (ACC) HF guidelines.[79] Stage D refers to the end-stage HF requiring advanced HF therapies such as inotropes, LV assist devices, and heart transplant. Readers are referred to the review by Mukku and colleagues[80] for the management of stage D CTRCD. Over the last decade, there has been renewed interest in the management of cancer therapy–related stage A HF, which refers to the patients who do not have structural heart disease or symptomatic HF but are at increased risk for HF. Different prevention strategies have been proposed for stage A HF secondary to cancer therapies.

  Primordial prevention: this novel approach to prevention refers to the initiation of cardioprotective medications after diagnosis of cancer and before starting chemotherapy.[3]
  Primary prevention: this refers to the initiation of medical therapy with cancer treatment in patients with increased risk of CTRCD,[3] which includes patients with multiple risk factors for cardiovascular disease or scheduled to receive high-risk chemotherapy; for example, cardiotoxic doses of anthracyclines.[81]
  Secondary prevention: this refers to the initiation of cardioprotective medications after the

development of cardiomyopathy, which may be a decline in LVEF, increased levels of cardiac biomarkers, or abnormalities in strain imaging.[3]

CARDIOPROTECTIVE STRATEGIES

The current data on the efficacy of various cardioprotective medications are discussed here.

Preclinical studies have shown that carvedilol protected against mitochondrial stress and histopathologic myocardial changes caused by doxorubicin. In contrast, atenolol did not inhibit the doxorubicin-mediated cardiotoxicity. This finding was attributed to the antioxidant properties of carvedilol.[82] The cardioprotective role of carvedilol in humans was shown in a randomized placebo-controlled trial that showed that prophylactic administration of carvedilol prevented detrimental changes in LV systolic and diastolic dimensions and attenuated a decline in LVEF.[83] In the Carvedilol Effect in Preventing Chemotherapy-Induced Cardiotoxicity (CECCY) trial, 200 patients with breast cancer scheduled to receive anthracycline-based chemotherapy were randomized to carvedilol and placebo arms. Carvedilol did not reduce the incidence of systolic dysfunction but decreased the rates of diastolic dysfunction and limited the increase in troponin levels during chemotherapy.[84] Nebivolol, a β$_1$ selective adrenergic receptor blocker, has vasodilating properties mediated by the nitric oxide pathway. Nebivolol reduced oxidative stress, decreased the production of cardiac biomarkers, and improved systolic and diastolic function in rat models treated with anthracyclines.[85] The efficacy of prophylactic nebivolol was shown in a prospective study involving 45 patients receiving anthracycline therapy. Initiation of nebivolol 1 week before and continuation during chemotherapy prevented an increase in natriuretic peptide levels and preserved LVEF.[86] Administration of bisoprolol during trastuzumab therapy attenuated LVEF decline but did not protect against cardiac remodeling.[87] In the patients who developed CTRCD defined as a decrease in GLS greater than 11%, the initiation of β-blockers reversed the ventricular dysfunction.[88] The beneficial effect noted with the aforementioned agents should not be extended to the entire β-blocker family. Concomitant use of metoprolol did not prevent doxorubicin-mediated LV decline in patients with hematologic malignancies.[89] Similar findings were observed in patients with breast cancer receiving adjuvant anthracycline therapy.[90] In mouse models, propranolol increased the Adriamycin-mediated cardiotoxicity.[91]

Experimental research has thrown light on the detrimental role of angiotensin II type a receptor in the pathogenesis of anthracycline-mediated cardiotoxicity.[92] Captopril and enalapril attenuated doxorubicin-mediated cardiotoxicity in rats.[93] The beneficial effects of renin-angiotensin-aldosterone antagonists have been attributed to their antioxidant and antifibrotic properties as well as downregulation of the inhibitory effect of angiotensin on the neuregulin/Erb system.[48,93] Studies in humans have shown benefit, albeit not consistently, with renin-angiotensin-aldosterone antagonists. In patients with positive troponins soon after chemotherapy, initiation of angiotensin-converting enzyme inhibitor protected against the development of anthracycline-mediated cardiomyopathy.[94] Prophylactic use of enalapril prevented a decline in LVEF in the patients receiving anthracycline therapy.[95] In contrast, enalapril did not decrease the rates of doxorubicin-mediated cardiotoxicity in patients with hematological malignancies.[89] Combined administration of enalapril and carvedilol attenuated anthracycline-mediated LV dysfunction and decreased the rates of the composite end point of death/HF.[96] In patients receiving trastuzumab therapy, perindopril reduced the decline in LVEF but did not prevent LV remodeling.[87]

The cardioprotective role of angiotensin receptor blockers (ARBs) has been shown, but not in all studies. Telmisartan protected against epirubicin-mediated inflammation and oxidative stress in the patients with cancer receiving this therapy. Importantly, telmisartan also prevented the development of subclinical cardiomyopathy.[97] Candesartan prevented a decline in LVEF in patients with breast cancer receiving adjuvant anthracycline-containing chemotherapy with or without radiation therapy and trastuzumab.[90] In contrast, in another study comparing candesartan with placebo in patients with breast cancer receiving trastuzumab therapy after an anthracycline-based regimen, there was no difference between the two groups in terms of LVEF decline and cardiac biomarkers.[98]

The cardioprotective role of aldosterone antagonists has been attributed to antifibrotic and antioxidant properties and inhibition of apoptosis.[99] Concurrent administration of spironolactone with anthracyclines in patients with breast cancer prevented a significant decline in LV systolic and diastolic function.[99]

Statins have been shown to possess pleotropic, antiinflammatory, antioxidative effects apart from cholesterol-lowering properties.[100] Prophylactic administration of atorvastatin in patients receiving anthracycline therapy prevented LVEF decline and negative ventricular remodeling.[100] A large observational study revealed that statins lowered the incidence of HF events in patients with breast cancer receiving anthracycline therapy.[101]

DEXRAZOXANE

Dexrazoxane is an intravenous metal chelating agent that is approved by the FDA for the prevention of anthracycline-mediated cardiomyopathy.[102] In addition to inhibition of the production of anthracycline-iron complexes and reactive oxygen species, dexrazoxane also prevents the formation of anthracycline–topoisomerase II DNA cleavage complexes.[103] The formation of topoisomerase II α-DNA complex in cancer cells is a proposed mechanism of action of anthracyclines.[14] This possibility generated concerns that dexrazoxane may compromise the antitumor efficacy of these agents. However, studies showed that dexrazoxane decreased the incidence of anthracycline-mediated cardiomyopathy without affecting the chemotherapeutic efficacy.[104,105] The ASCO supports the administration of dexrazoxane in adult patients with metastatic breast cancer who received a cumulative dose of 300 mg/m² of doxorubicin and were likely to benefit from continuation of anthracycline therapy.[106] There have been concerns that dexrazoxane use may result in hematological malignancies and secondary neoplasms in pediatric patients.[107] However, a subsequent Cochrane Review revealed that dexrazoxane use was not associated with increased risk of secondary neoplasms or decreased oncologic response. Although dexrazoxane reduced the HF risk caused by anthracyclines, there was no survival benefit.[108]

SUMMARY

Recent advances in cancer therapy have improved survival but are associated with different cardiac side effects. The goal of cardio-oncology is to ensure optimal cancer therapy while limiting adverse effects, with an emphasis on early recognition and treatment of cancer therapeutics–related cardiac dysfunction. Pre–cancer therapy evaluation begins with the assessment of cardiovascular disease burden and risk stratification of each patient. Intra–cancer therapy evaluation involves close follow-up, monitoring, and treatment according to specific surveillance protocols and consensus guidelines. Post–cancer therapy evaluation entails clinical assessment and imaging depending on the underlying cardiovascular burden and CTRCD noted during treatment. Close communication between the primary care physicians, cardiologists, and oncologists is essential to provide optimal care to these patients and thereby enhance cancer survivorship.

REFERENCES

1. Miller KD, Siegel RL, Lin CC, et al. Cancer treatment and survivorship statistics, 2016. CA Cancer J Clin 2016;66(4):271–89.
2. Bloom MW, Hamo CE, Cardinale D, et al. Cancer therapy-related cardiac dysfunction and heart failure: part 1: definitions, pathophysiology, risk factors, and imaging. Circ Heart Fail 2016;9(1):e002661.
3. Khouri MG, Douglas PS, Mackey JR, et al. Cancer therapy-induced cardiac toxicity in early breast cancer: addressing the unresolved issues. Circulation 2012;126(23):2749–63.
4. Alexander J, Dainiak N, Berger HJ, et al. Serial assessment of doxorubicin cardiotoxicity with quantitative radionuclide angiocardiography. N Engl J Med 1979;300(6):278–83.
5. Brabant SM, Eyraud D, Bertrand M, et al. Refractory hypotension after induction of anesthesia in a patient chronically treated with angiotensin receptor antagonists. Anesth Analg 1999;89(4):887–8.
6. Tan-Chiu E, Yothers G, Romond E, et al. Assessment of cardiac dysfunction in a randomized trial comparing doxorubicin and cyclophosphamide followed by paclitaxel, with or without trastuzumab as adjuvant therapy in node-positive, human epidermal growth factor receptor 2-overexpressing breast cancer: NSABP B-31. J Clin Oncol 2005;23(31):7811–9.
7. Seidman A, Hudis C, Pierri MK, et al. Cardiac dysfunction in the trastuzumab clinical trials experience. J Clin Oncol 2002;20(5):1215–21.
8. Suter TM, Procter M, van Veldhuisen DJ, et al. Trastuzumab-associated cardiac adverse effects in the Herceptin Adjuvant trial. J Clin Oncol 2007;25(25):3859–65.
9. Plana JC, Galderisi M, Barac A, et al. Expert consensus for multimodality imaging evaluation of adult patients during and after cancer therapy: a report from the American Society of Echocardiography and the European Association of Cardiovascular Imaging. J Am Soc Echocardiogr 2014;27(9):911–39.
10. Blum RH, Carter SK. Adriamycin. A new anticancer drug with significant clinical activity. Ann Intern Med 1974;80(2):249–59.
11. Shan K, Lincoff AM, Young JB. Anthracycline-induced cardiotoxicity. Ann Intern Med 1996;125(1):47–58.
12. Minotti G, Cairo G, Monti E. Role of iron in anthracycline cardiotoxicity: new tunes for an old song? FASEB J 1999;13(2):199–212.
13. Lebrecht D, Walker UA. Role of mtDNA lesions in anthracycline cardiotoxicity. Cardiovasc Toxicol 2007;7(2):108–13.
14. Tewey KM, Rowe TC, Yang L, et al. Adriamycin-induced DNA damage mediated by mammalian DNA topoisomerase II. Science 1984;226(4673):466–8.
15. Lyu YL, Kerrigan JE, Lin CP, et al. Topoisomerase II-beta mediated DNA double-strand breaks: implications in doxorubicin cardiotoxicity and prevention by dexrazoxane. Cancer Res 2007;67(18):8839–46.
16. Zhang S, Liu X, Bawa-Khalfe T, et al. Identification of the molecular basis of doxorubicin-induced cardiotoxicity. Nat Med 2012;18(11):1639–42.
17. Pein F, Sakiroglu O, Dahan M, et al. Cardiac abnormalities 15 years and more after Adriamycin therapy in 229 childhood survivors of a solid tumour at the Institut Gustave Roussy. Br J Cancer 2004;91(1):37–44.
18. Swain SM, Whaley FS, Ewer MS. Congestive heart failure in patients treated with doxorubicin: a retrospective analysis of three trials. Cancer 2003;97(11):2869–79.
19. Volkova M, Russell R 3rd. Anthracycline cardiotoxicity: prevalence, pathogenesis and treatment. Curr Cardiol Rev 2011;7(4):214–20.
20. Gershwin ME, Goetzl EJ, Steinberg AD. Cyclophosphamide: use in practice. Ann Intern Med 1974;80(4):531–40.
21. Pai VB, Nahata MC. Cardiotoxicity of chemotherapeutic agents: incidence, treatment and prevention. Drug Saf 2000;22(4):263–302.
22. Quezado ZM, Wilson WH, Cunnion RE, et al. High-dose ifosfamide is associated with severe, reversible cardiac dysfunction. Ann Intern Med 1993;118(1):31–6.
23. Sendur MA, Aksoy S, Altundag K. Cardiotoxicity of novel HER2-targeted therapies. Curr Med Res Opin 2013;29(8):1015–24.
24. De Keulenaer GW, Doggen K, Lemmens K. The vulnerability of the heart as a pluricellular paracrine organ: lessons from unexpected triggers of heart failure in targeted ErbB2 anticancer therapy. Circ Res 2010;106(1):35–46.
25. Ewer MS, Lippman SM. Type II chemotherapy-related cardiac dysfunction: time to recognize a new entity. J Clin Oncol 2005;23(13):2900–2.
26. Mercurio V, Pirozzi F, Lazzarini E, et al. Models of heart failure based on the cardiotoxicity of anti-cancer drugs. J Card Fail 2016;22(6):449–58.
27. Lemmens K, Doggen K, De Keulenaer GW. Role of neuregulin-1/ErbB signaling in cardiovascular physiology and disease: implications for therapy of heart failure. Circulation 2007;116(8):954–60.
28. Ky B, Kimmel SE, Safa RN, et al. Neuregulin-1 beta is associated with disease severity and adverse outcomes in chronic heart failure. Circulation 2009;120(4):310–7.
29. Onitilo AA, Engel JM, Stankowski RV. Cardiovascular toxicity associated with adjuvant trastuzumab therapy: prevalence, patient characteristics, and risk factors. Ther Adv Drug Saf 2014;5(4):154–66.

30. Field JJ, Kanakkanthara A, Miller JH. Microtubule-targeting agents are clinically successful due to both mitotic and interphase impairment of microtubule function. Bioorg Med Chem 2014;22(18):5050–9.

31. Colombo T, Parisi I, Zucchetti M, et al. Pharmacokinetic interactions of paclitaxel, docetaxel and their vehicles with doxorubicin. Ann Oncol 1999;10(4): 391–5.

32. Giordano SH, Booser DJ, Murray JL, et al. A detailed evaluation of cardiac toxicity: a phase II study of doxorubicin and one- or three-hour-infusion paclitaxel in patients with metastatic breast cancer. Clin Cancer Res 2002;8(11):3360–8.

33. Yang B, Papoian T. Tyrosine kinase inhibitor (TKI)-induced cardiotoxicity: approaches to narrow the gaps between preclinical safety evaluation and clinical outcome. J Appl Toxicol 2012;32(12):945–51.

34. Choueiri TK, Mayer EL, Je Y, et al. Congestive heart failure risk in patients with breast cancer treated with bevacizumab. J Clin Oncol 2011;29(6):632–8.

35. Maitland ML, Bakris GL, Black HR, et al. Initial assessment, surveillance, and management of blood pressure in patients receiving vascular endothelial growth factor signaling pathway inhibitors. J Natl Cancer Inst 2010;102(9):596–604.

36. Schmidinger M, Zielinski CC, Vogl UM, et al. Cardiac toxicity of sunitinib and sorafenib in patients with metastatic renal cell carcinoma. J Clin Oncol 2008;26(32):5204–12.

37. Steingart RM, Bakris GL, Chen HX, et al. Management of cardiac toxicity in patients receiving vascular endothelial growth factor signaling pathway inhibitors. Am Heart J 2012;163(2):156–63.

38. Groarke JD, Nguyen PL, Nohria A, et al. Cardiovascular complications of radiation therapy for thoracic malignancies: the role for non-invasive imaging for detection of cardiovascular disease. Eur Heart J 2014;35(10):612–23.

39. Jaworski C, Mariani JA, Wheeler G, et al. Cardiac complications of thoracic irradiation. J Am Coll Cardiol 2013;61(23):2319–28.

40. van Nimwegen FA, Schaapveld M, Janus CP, et al. Cardiovascular disease after Hodgkin lymphoma treatment: 40-year disease risk. JAMA Intern Med 2015;175(6):1007–17.

41. Filopei J, Frishman W. Radiation-induced heart disease. Cardiol Rev 2012;20(4):184–8.

42. Tukenova M, Guibout C, Oberlin O, et al. Role of cancer treatment in long-term overall and cardiovascular mortality after childhood cancer. J Clin Oncol 2010;28(8):1308–15.

43. van Leeuwen-Segarceanu EM, Bos WJ, Dorresteijn LD, et al. Screening Hodgkin lymphoma survivors for radiotherapy induced cardiovascular disease. Cancer Treat Rev 2011;37(5):391–403.

44. Lancellotti P, Nkomo VT, Badano LP, et al. Expert consensus for multi-modality imaging evaluation of cardiovascular complications of radiotherapy in adults: a report from the European Association of Cardiovascular Imaging and the American Society of Echocardiography. Eur Heart J Cardiovasc Imaging 2013;14(8):721–40.

45. Herrmann J, Lerman A, Sandhu NP, et al. Evaluation and management of patients with heart disease and cancer: cardio-oncology. Mayo Clin Proc 2014;89(9):1287–306.

46. Albini A, Pennesi G, Donatelli F, et al. Cardiotoxicity of anticancer drugs: the need for cardio-oncology and cardio-oncological prevention. J Natl Cancer Inst 2010;102(1):14–25.

47. Blanco JG, Sun CL, Landier W, et al. Anthracycline-related cardiomyopathy after childhood cancer: role of polymorphisms in carbonyl reductase genes–a report from the Children's Oncology Group. J Clin Oncol 2012;30(13):1415–21.

48. Valachis A, Nilsson C. Cardiac risk in the treatment of breast cancer: assessment and management. Breast Cancer (Dove Med Press) 2015;7:21–35.

49. Dranitsaris G, Rayson D, Vincent M, et al. The development of a predictive model to estimate cardiotoxic risk for patients with metastatic breast cancer receiving anthracyclines. Breast Cancer Res Treat 2008;107(3):443–50.

50. Ezaz G, Long JB, Gross CP, et al. Risk prediction model for heart failure and cardiomyopathy after adjuvant trastuzumab therapy for breast cancer. J Am Heart Assoc 2014;3(1):e000472.

51. Witteles RM. Biomarkers as predictors of cardiac toxicity from targeted cancer therapies. J Card Fail 2016;22(6):459–64.

52. Cardinale D, Sandri MT, Colombo A, et al. Prognostic value of troponin I in cardiac risk stratification of cancer patients undergoing high-dose chemotherapy. Circulation 2004;109(22):2749–54.

53. Curigliano G, Cardinale D, Suter T, et al. Cardiovascular toxicity induced by chemotherapy, targeted agents and radiotherapy: ESMO Clinical Practice Guidelines. Ann Oncol 2012;23(Suppl 7):vii155–66.

54. Cardinale D, Colombo A, Torrisi R, et al. Trastuzumab-induced cardiotoxicity: clinical and prognostic implications of troponin I evaluation. J Clin Oncol 2010;28(25):3910–6.

55. Ky B, Putt M, Sawaya H, et al. Early increases in multiple biomarkers predict subsequent cardiotoxicity in patients with breast cancer treated with doxorubicin, taxanes, and trastuzumab. J Am Coll Cardiol 2014;63(8):809–16.

56. Morris PG, Chen C, Steingart R, et al. Troponin I and C-reactive protein are commonly detected in patients with breast cancer treated with dose-dense chemotherapy incorporating trastuzumab and lapatinib. Clin Cancer Res 2011;17(10):3490–9.

57. Sawaya H, Sebag IA, Plana JC, et al. Assessment of echocardiography and biomarkers for the

extended prediction of cardiotoxicity in patients treated with anthracyclines, taxanes, and trastuzumab. Circ Cardiovasc Imaging 2012;5(5):596–603.

58. Lipshultz SE, Miller TL, Scully RE, et al. Changes in cardiac biomarkers during doxorubicin treatment of pediatric patients with high-risk acute lymphoblastic leukemia: associations with long-term echocardiographic outcomes. J Clin Oncol 2012;30(10):1042–9.

59. Hall PS, Harshman LC, Srinivas S, et al. The frequency and severity of cardiovascular toxicity from targeted therapy in advanced renal cell carcinoma patients. JACC Heart Fail 2013;1(1):72–8.

60. Choi BW, Berger HJ, Schwartz PE, et al. Serial radionuclide assessment of doxorubicin cardiotoxicity in cancer patients with abnormal baseline resting left ventricular performance. Am Heart J 1983;106(4 Pt 1):638–43.

61. Schwartz RG, McKenzie WB, Alexander J, et al. Congestive heart failure and left ventricular dysfunction complicating doxorubicin therapy. Seven-year experience using serial radionuclide angiocardiography. Am J Med 1987;82(6):1109–18.

62. Jiji RS, Kramer CM, Salerno M. Non-invasive imaging and monitoring cardiotoxicity of cancer therapeutic drugs. J Nucl Cardiol 2012;19(2):377–88.

63. Cheitlin MD, Armstrong WF, Aurigemma GP, et al. ACC/AHA/ASE 2003 guideline update for the clinical application of echocardiography: summary article: a report of the American College of Cardiology/American Heart Association Task Force on Practice Guidelines (ACC/AHA/ASE Committee to Update the 1997 Guidelines for the Clinical Application of Echocardiography). Circulation 2003;108(9):1146–62.

64. Kongbundansuk S, Hundley WG. Noninvasive imaging of cardiovascular injury related to the treatment of cancer. JACC Cardiovasc Imaging 2014;7(8):824–38.

65. Mulvagh SL, Rakowski H, Vannan MA, et al. American Society of Echocardiography consensus statement on the clinical applications of ultrasonic contrast agents in echocardiography. J Am Soc Echocardiogr 2008;21(11):1179–201 [quiz: 1281].

66. Thavendiranathan P, Grant AD, Negishi T, et al. Reproducibility of echocardiographic techniques for sequential assessment of left ventricular ejection fraction and volumes: application to patients undergoing cancer chemotherapy. J Am Coll Cardiol 2013;61(1):77–84.

67. Toro-Salazar OH, Ferranti J, Lorenzoni R, et al. Feasibility of echocardiographic techniques to detect subclinical cancer therapeutics-related cardiac dysfunction among high-dose patients when compared with cardiac magnetic resonance imaging. J Am Soc Echocardiogr 2016;29(2):119–31.

68. Ali MT, Yucel E, Bouras S, et al. Myocardial strain is associated with adverse clinical cardiac events in patients treated with anthracyclines. J Am Soc Echocardiogr 2016;29(6):522–7.e3.

69. Negishi K, Negishi T, Hare JL, et al. Independent and incremental value of deformation indices for prediction of trastuzumab-induced cardiotoxicity. J Am Soc Echocardiogr 2013;26(5):493–8.

70. Armstrong GT, Plana JC, Zhang N, et al. Screening adult survivors of childhood cancer for cardiomyopathy: comparison of echocardiography and cardiac magnetic resonance imaging. J Clin Oncol 2012;30(23):2876–84.

71. Thavendiranathan P, Wintersperger BJ, Flamm SD, et al. Cardiac MRI in the assessment of cardiac injury and toxicity from cancer chemotherapy: a systematic review. Circ Cardiovasc Imaging 2013;6(6):1080–91.

72. Neilan TG, Coelho-Filho OR, Pena-Herrera D, et al. Left ventricular mass in patients with a cardiomyopathy after treatment with anthracyclines. Am J Cardiol 2012;110(11):1679–86.

73. Armenian SH, Lacchetti C, Barac A, et al. Prevention and monitoring of cardiac dysfunction in survivors of adult cancers: American Society of Clinical Oncology clinical practice guideline. J Clin Oncol 2017;35(8):893–911.

74. Hamo CE, Bloom MW, Cardinale D, et al. Cancer therapy-related cardiac dysfunction and heart failure: part 2: prevention, treatment, guidelines, and future directions. Circ Heart Fail 2016;9(2):e002843.

75. Lindenauer PK, Pekow P, Wang K, et al. Lipid-lowering therapy and in-hospital mortality following major noncardiac surgery. JAMA 2004;291(17):2092–9.

76. Gupta PK, Gupta H, Sundaram A, et al. Development and validation of a risk calculator for prediction of cardiac risk after surgery. Circulation 2011;124(4):381–7.

77. Brabant SM, Bertrand M, Eyraud D, et al. The hemodynamic effects of anesthetic induction in vascular surgical patients chronically treated with angiotensin II receptor antagonists. Anesth Analg 1999;89(6):1388–92.

78. Coriat P, Richer C, Douraki T, et al. Influence of chronic angiotensin-converting enzyme inhibition on anesthetic induction. Anesthesiology 1994;81(2):299–307.

79. Yancy CW, Jessup M, Bozkurt B, et al. 2013 ACCF/AHA guideline for the management of heart failure: a report of the American College of Cardiology Foundation/American Heart Association Task Force on Practice Guidelines. J Am Coll Cardiol 2013;62(16):e147–239.

80. Mukku RB, Fonarow GC, Watson KE, et al. Heart failure therapies for end-stage chemotherapy-

induced cardiomyopathy. J Card Fail 2016;22(6): 439–48.

81. Finet JE. Management of heart failure in cancer patients and cancer survivors. Heart Fail Clin 2017; 13(2):253–88.

82. Oliveira PJ, Bjork JA, Santos MS, et al. Carvedilol-mediated antioxidant protection against doxorubicin-induced cardiac mitochondrial toxicity. Toxicol Appl Pharmacol 2004;200(2):159–68.

83. Kalay N, Basar E, Ozdogru I, et al. Protective effects of carvedilol against anthracycline-induced cardiomyopathy. J Am Coll Cardiol 2006;48(11): 2258–62.

84. Avila MS, Ayub-Ferreira SM, de Barros Wanderley MR Jr, et al. Carvedilol for prevention of chemotherapy-related cardiotoxicity: the CECCY trial. J Am Coll Cardiol 2018;71(20):2281–90.

85. de Nigris F, Rienzo M, Schiano C, et al. Prominent cardioprotective effects of third generation beta blocker nebivolol against anthracycline-induced cardiotoxicity using the model of isolated perfused rat heart. Eur J Cancer 2008;44(3):334–40.

86. Kaya MG, Ozkan M, Gunebakmaz O, et al. Protective effects of nebivolol against anthracycline-induced cardiomyopathy: a randomized control study. Int J Cardiol 2013;167(5):2306–10.

87. Pituskin E, Mackey JR, Koshman S, et al. Multidisciplinary Approach to Novel Therapies in Cardio-Oncology Research (MANTICORE 101-Breast): a randomized trial for the prevention of trastuzumab-associated cardiotoxicity. J Clin Oncol 2017;35(8): 870–7.

88. Negishi K, Negishi T, Haluska BA, et al. Use of speckle strain to assess left ventricular responses to cardiotoxic chemotherapy and cardioprotection. Eur Heart J Cardiovasc Imaging 2014;15(3):324–31.

89. Georgakopoulos P, Roussou P, Matsakas E, et al. Cardioprotective effect of metoprolol and enalapril in doxorubicin-treated lymphoma patients: a prospective, parallel-group, randomized, controlled study with 36-month follow-up. Am J Hematol Nov 2010;85(11):894–6.

90. Gulati G, Heck SL, Ree AH, et al. Prevention of cardiac dysfunction during adjuvant breast cancer therapy (PRADA): a 2 x 2 factorial, randomized, placebo-controlled, double-blind clinical trial of candesartan and metoprolol. Eur Heart J 2016; 37(21):1671–80.

91. Choe JY, Combs AB, Folkers K. Potentiation of the toxicity of Adriamycin by propranolol. Res Commun Chem Pathol Pharmacol 1978;21(3):577–80.

92. Toko H, Oka T, Zou Y, et al. Angiotensin II type 1a receptor mediates doxorubicin-induced cardiomyopathy. Hypertens Res 2002;25(4):597–603.

93. Abd El-Aziz MA, Othman AI, Amer M, et al. Potential protective role of angiotensin-converting enzyme inhibitors captopril and enalapril against Adriamycin-induced acute cardiac and hepatic toxicity in rats. J Appl Toxicol 2001;21(6):469–73.

94. Cardinale D, Colombo A, Sandri MT, et al. Prevention of high-dose chemotherapy-induced cardiotoxicity in high-risk patients by angiotensin-converting enzyme inhibition. Circulation 2006; 114(23):2474–81.

95. Janbabai G, Nabati M, Faghihinia M, et al. Effect of enalapril on preventing anthracycline-induced cardiomyopathy. Cardiovasc Toxicol 2017;17(2): 130–9.

96. Bosch X, Rovira M, Sitges M, et al. Enalapril and carvedilol for preventing chemotherapy-induced left ventricular systolic dysfunction in patients with malignant hemopathies: the OVERCOME trial (preventiOn of left Ventricular dysfunction with Enalapril and caRvedilol in patients submitted to intensive ChemOtherapy for the treatment of Malignant hEmopathies). J Am Coll Cardiol 2013; 61(23):2355–62.

97. Dessi M, Madeddu C, Piras A, et al. Long-term, up to 18 months, protective effects of the angiotensin II receptor blocker telmisartan on epirubin-induced inflammation and oxidative stress assessed by serial strain rate. Springerplus 2013; 2(1):198.

98. Boekhout AH, Gietema JA, Milojkovic Kerklaan B, et al. Angiotensin II-receptor inhibition with candesartan to prevent trastuzumab-related cardiotoxic effects in patients with early breast cancer: a randomized clinical trial. JAMA Oncol 2016;2(8): 1030–7.

99. Akpek M, Ozdogru I, Sahin O, et al. Protective effects of spironolactone against anthracycline-induced cardiomyopathy. Eur J Heart Fail 2015; 17(1):81–9.

100. Acar Z, Kale A, Turgut M, et al. Efficiency of atorvastatin in the protection of anthracycline-induced cardiomyopathy. J Am Coll Cardiol 2011;58(9): 988–9.

101. Seicean S, Seicean A, Plana JC, et al. Effect of statin therapy on the risk for incident heart failure in patients with breast cancer receiving anthracycline chemotherapy: an observational clinical cohort study. J Am Coll Cardiol 2012;60(23): 2384–90.

102. American Society of Anesthesiologists Task Force on Pulmonary Artery Catheterization. Practice guidelines for pulmonary artery catheterization: an updated report by the American Society of Anesthesiologists Task Force on Pulmonary Artery Catheterization. Anesthesiology 2003;99(4): 988–1014.

103. Hahn VS, Lenihan DJ, Ky B. Cancer therapy-induced cardiotoxicity: basic mechanisms and potential cardioprotective therapies. J Am Heart Assoc 2014;3(2):e000665.

104. Kalam K, Marwick TH. Role of cardioprotective therapy for prevention of cardiotoxicity with chemotherapy: a systematic review and meta-analysis. Eur J Cancer 2013;49(13):2900–9.

105. Marty M, Espie M, Llombart A, et al. Multicenter randomized phase III study of the cardioprotective effect of dexrazoxane (Cardioxane) in advanced/metastatic breast cancer patients treated with anthracycline-based chemotherapy. Ann Oncol 2006;17(4):614–22.

106. Hensley ML, Hagerty KL, Kewalramani T, et al. American Society of Clinical Oncology 2008 clinical practice guideline update: use of chemotherapy and radiation therapy protectants. J Clin Oncol 2009;27(1):127–45.

107. Tebbi CK, London WB, Friedman D, et al. Dexrazoxane-associated risk for acute myeloid leukemia/myelodysplastic syndrome and other secondary malignancies in pediatric Hodgkin's disease. J Clin Oncol 2007;25(5):493–500.

108. van Dalen EC, Caron HN, Dickinson HO, et al. Cardioprotective interventions for cancer patients receiving anthracyclines. Cochrane Database Syst Rev 2011;(6):CD003917.

Management of Heart Failure in Adult Congenital Heart Disease

Aarthi Sabanayagam, MD[a],*, Omer Cavus, MD[b],
Jordan Williams, BS[b], Elisa Bradley, MD[c]

KEYWORDS

- Congenital heart disease • Heart failure • Systemic ventricle dysfunction
- Single ventricle dysfunction • Fontan

KEY POINTS

- Children with congenital heart disease (CHD) are outnumbered by adults with CHD (ACHD).
- CHD–heart failure (HF) presentation differs based on anatomy and prior surgical repair.
- HF medical therapy is less well studied in CHD and needs to be considered in the context of CHD-related anatomy or physiology.
- The first step in evaluation of the adult CHD patient with HF is to examine the underlying anatomy for lesions with the possibility for intervention.
- Mechanical circulatory support and heart transplant in CHD is more complex secondary to anatomic limitations. These patients are at a disadvantage in the current allocation system.

INTRODUCTION

In the United States, children living with congenital heart disease (CHD) are outnumbered by adults with CHD (ACHD). Due to surgical and medical advances, it is now estimated that there are more than 1 million adults with CHD in the United States.[1,2] Advances in surgical technique, transcatheter intervention, imaging modalities, and focus on high-quality multidisciplinary care teams has contributed to improved CHD survival. Recent studies have shown that the median age of patients with severe CHF has increased from 11 years in 1985 to 17 years in 2000, and the overall age at death increased from 37 years in 2002 to 57 years in 2007.[3] Improved survival to adult age and late adulthood translates to a population with both cardiac and extracardiac disease, and specialized care needs. In particular, heart failure (HF) is common in the adult patient with CHD. Adults with CHD experience more hospitalizations, episodes of decompensation, and ultimately have higher mortality than non-CHD cohorts.[4–6] Therefore, it is critical to understand the heterogenetic nature of HF in ACHD population, assessment and management across the spectrum of CHD, and treatment options, as well as current gaps in treatments available to this unique group.

THE DISTINCT NATURE OF HEART FAILURE IN ADULT CONGENITAL HEART DISEASE

As CHD patients live to older age, the population becomes even more diverse because it includes

Disclosures: The authors have nothing to disclose.
[a] Division of Cardiology, The Ohio State University, Nationwide Children's Hospital, Davis Heart and Lung Research Institute, 473 West 12th Avenue Suite 200, Columbus, OH 43210, USA; [b] Department of Physiology and Cell Biology, Davis Heart and Lung Research Institute, The Ohio State University, 473 West 12th Avenue Suite 200, Columbus, OH 43210, USA; [c] Department of Physiology and Cell Biology, The Ohio State University, Nationwide Children's Hospital, Davis Heart and Lung Research Institute, 473 West 12th Avenue Suite 200, Columbus, OH 43210, USA
* Corresponding author.
E-mail address: Aarthi.sabanayagam@osumc.edu

Heart Failure Clin 14 (2018) 569–577
https://doi.org/10.1016/j.hfc.2018.06.005
1551-7136/18/© 2018 Elsevier Inc. All rights reserved.

patients who survived several percutaneous and surgical procedures in childhood, and adults who presented and were diagnosed later in life. Residual anatomic and hemodynamic lesions accompanied by acquired heart disease lead to an increasingly complex group of patients with varied presentation. HF, along with arrhythmia, sudden death, and late vascular complications are the most common late cardiac presentations in adults.[7]

Bolger and colleagues[8] described CHD as the original HF syndrome as "...characterized by a triad comprising cardiac abnormality, exercise limitation, and neurohormonal activation." The Heart Failure Society of America guidelines' define HF as "...a syndrome characterized by either or both pulmonary and systemic venous congestion or inadequate peripheral oxygen delivery, at rest of during stress caused by cardiac dysfunction."[9,10] In the CHD population, it is often difficult to stratify patients into common categories such as left-sided failure or right-sided failure. Standard functional class categorization is also difficult because it based on the premise that patients do not have structural abnormalities at baseline. For instance, the 2005 American College of Cardiology and American Heart Association guidelines recommend HF be divided into 4 subtypes: A, at risk for HF; B, structural heart disease without signs or symptoms; C, structural heart disease with previous or current symptoms; and D, refractory heart disease requiring advanced therapies.[11] One may wonder how CHD patients fit into this classification, which, despite updating in 2013, still did not account for the CHD patient with an underlying congenital cardiac defect. Guideline-level documents such as this are often not particularly helpful in the management of CHD patients because they amass data in the acquired HF population, which is often significantly different if not less well-studied than CHD patients.[9,12,13]

From an epidemiologic perspective, CHD patients do not fare as well as patients with HF from acquired forms of heart disease. Hospitalization rates in CHD patients with HF are higher (214 admissions/1000 adults) and the mean length of stay is longer (11.5 days in complex CHD vs 8 days in the acquired HF cohort).[14] The underlying anatomic defect and prior surgical interventions have been identified as independent risk factors for HF admission in CHD. When admitted for HF, CHD patients have a 5-fold higher risk of in-hospital mortality; death at 1 and 3 years post-HF admission was exceptionally high at 24% and 35%, respectively.[15]

Predictors of death due to HF include endocarditis, supraventricular tachycardia, ventricular tachyarrhythmia, conduction disturbances, pulmonary arterial hypertension, and myocardial infarction (hazard ratio 2–5; $P<.05$).[7] In 2 different European cohorts, HF has been shown to be the most common cause of mortality with the average age of death reported between 47 to 50 years of age.[7,16] As the CHD population continues to age, both outpatient and inpatient care for HF will continue to become among the most important aspects of managing these patients.[17–19]

ANATOMY DICTATES HEART FAILURE PHENOTYPE

HF in CHD is a broad topic that is often difficult to understand. It is easy to see why this may be the case, given the broad spectrum of CHD. Clinically, CHD is subdivided into categories based on the complexity of the structural lesions. Defects are classified as simple CHD, moderately complex CHD, or severely complex CHD. Published guidelines in the treatment of ACHD have indicated follow-up intervals for continued care based on the severity of underlying CHD[20] (**Table 1**). Prior interventions, including cardiac surgery, also play a role in the development of HF and late CVD risk; therefore, they are crucial to consider in caring for the ACHD patient. Given the heterogenous nature of CHD and palliative or surgical repair, the cause and presentation of HF in CHD is diverse. Some common themes in describing HF in this population include the side of the HF (subpulmonic ventricular vs subsystemic ventricular dysfunction),[21] cyanotic versus acyanotic HF, single ventricular failure, and pressure versus volume-mediated HF, among others.

ETIOLOGIC FACTORS OF CONGENITAL HEART DISEASE–HEART FAILURE

The mechanisms leading to HF in CHD are numerous and variable. Some potential causes include abnormal pressure or volume-loading of either the morphologic right ventricle (RV) or left ventricle, myocardial ischemia from either a supply demand mismatch or coronaries anomalies, ventricular hypertrophy, and constriction from prior sternotomy. Myocardial architecture must be considered in patients with CHD. Data suggest embryologic development of the right ventricular myocardium may be different from the left ventricle and more susceptible to dysfunction in lesions where the RV is the systemic ventricle.[9,22] Perfusion also seems to also be important as evidenced by the high prevalence of RV systolic function following

Table 1
Complexity of adult congenital heart disease

Simple CHD	Moderate CHD	Severely Complex CHD

• Native disease
  ○ Isolated congenital aortic valve disease
  ○ Isolated congenital MV disease
  ○ Small ASD
  ○ Isolated small VSD
  ○ Mild PS
  ○ Small PDA
• Repaired conditions (without residua)
  ○ Ligated or occluded PDA
  ○ Repaired VSD
  ○ Repaired secundum or sinus venosus
  ○ ASD
	• Aorto-left ventricular fistulas
	• Anomalous pulmonary venous drainage
	• AVSD (partial or complete)
	• CoA
	• Ebstein anomaly
	• Infundibular RVOTO of significance
	• Ostium primum ASD
	• PDA, not closed
	• Pulmonary valve regurgitation (moderate to severe)
	• Pulmonary valve stenosis (moderate to severe)
	• Sinus of Valsalva fistula or aneurysm
	• Sinus venosus ASD
	• Subvalvular AS or supra-AS
	• Tetralogy of Fallot
	• VSD with absent valves, AI, CoA, mitral disease, RVOTO, straddling TV or MV, sub-AS
		• Conduits
		• Cyanotic CHD (all forms)
		• Double-outlet ventricle
		• Eisenmenger syndrome
		• Fontan procedure
		• Mitral atresia
		• Single ventricle
		• Pulmonary atresia (all forms)
		• Transposition of the great arteries
		• Tricuspid atresia
		• Truncus arteriosus, hemitruncus
		• Abnormalities of atrioventricular or ventriculoarterial connection NOS (ie, crisscross heart, isomerism, heterotaxy, ventricular inversion)

Abbreviations: AI, aortic insufficiency; AS, aortic stenosis; ASD, atrial septal defect; AVSD, atrioventricular septal defect; CoA, coarctation of the aorta; MV, mitral valve; NOS, not otherwise specified; PDA, patent ductus arteriosus; PS, pulmonic stenosis; RVOTO, right ventricular outflow tract obstruction; TV, tricuspid valve; VSD, ventricular septal defect.

Modified from Connelly MS, Webb GD, Somerville J, et al. Canadian consensus conference on adult congenital heart disease, 1996. Can J Cardiol 1998;14:395–452; with permission.

the atrial switch operation in complete transposition.[23,24] Reduced right ventricular myocardial microvascular density of the septal wall is seen in complete transposition and in RV hypertrophy in tetralogy of Fallot patients. This seems to be related to a reduced myocardial perfusion reserve and impaired right ventricular systolic function.[25] It is likely that myocardial perfusion defects are a sensitive predictor of systemic ventricular impairment.[26] Similar to acquired heart disease, activation of natriuretic peptides, the sympathoadrenergic system, and the endothelin and renin angiotensin aldosterone system have been implicated to play an important role in CHD-HF.[27] Fibrosis and aberrant remodeling are also important deleterious processes important to HF in CHD.[28–30]

CLINICAL PRESENTATION AND EVALUATION

Presentation of HF in CHD can vary depending on anatomic and physiologic factors related to underlying anatomy and prior repair. Systolic function may not necessarily be the primary cause of HF in these patients. Typical HF symptoms, such as exertional dyspnea, fatigue, exercise intolerance, and signs of volume overload,

although present may not always be dramatic. A comprehensive history and examination is critical in evaluation of this population. Special testing often involves imaging, such as transthoracic echocardiogram or cardiac MRI–computed tomography, to provide information about anatomic detail and function. Cardiopulmonary stress testing is an invaluable tool to assess functional capacity and other vital information, such as chronotropic competence and oxygenation level with exercise. Patients with CHD exhibit lower than normal oxygen consumption per unit time (Vo_2) in comparison with age-matched healthy cohorts[31,32] and, given that New York Heart Association status is not accurate in CHD, trends in peak Vo_2 and functional capacity are valuable. A rhythm monitor is also very important in CHD because arrhythmia and requirement for pacemaker are more common than in other forms of acquired heart disease.

MANAGEMENT OF HEART FAILURE IN CONGENITAL HEART DISEASE

In acquired HF, medical treatment is the cornerstone of management; however, the same therapy is not well-studied in CHD patients. Treatment typically focuses on correcting structural abnormalities and potentially reversing abnormalities. The management of arrhythmia is also critically important in the ACHD patient because it occurs in 15% of CHD patients and more than doubles the risk of HF.[33] Common late anatomic, physiologic, or arrhythmogenic problems, as well as available interventions in select moderate and severely complex ACHD patients, are reviewed in **Table 2**.

Medical Therapy

Traditional HF medications are not well-studied in the ACHD population (**Table 3**). Even with the lack of substantial data, there may be a role for these treatments because some of the mechanisms for HF overlap.[34] In general, one must consider all the indications for cardiac medications in these patients because there are often multiple reasons to use medications such as beta-blockers, diuretics, and angiotensin-converting enzyme inhibitors. Typically,

Table 2
Common procedural and surgical interventions in moderate-severe adult congenital heart disease–heart failure patients

	Late (Adult) Anatomic or Physiologic Problem	Intervention
Tetralogy of Fallot	• PI • RV enlargement and dysfunction due to PI • RVOT obstruction, specifically if a conduit is present • High risk of VT and SCD	• Transcatheter pulmonary valve replacement • Balloon pulmonary valvuloplasty • Surgical pulmonary valve replacement or conduit replacement • EPS, VT ablation, ICD placement
DTGA with atrial switch	• Baffle leak and/or stenosis in up to 25%[37,38] • Baffle leak can impact ventricular volume and lead to volume-related HF, systemic desaturation, and paradoxic emboli • Atrial scarring leads to increased IART, and other atrial arrhythmias[39] • High risk of atrial arrhythmia degenerating to VT and SCD[40,41] • High risk of chronotropic incompetence and need for pacemaker[42–44]	• Transcatheter baffle intervention (stent placement or occlusion of leak) • EPS with or without RFA, pacemaker, ICD placement
CCTGA	• Tricuspid regurgitation may occur due to a dysplastic TV • Increased risks of heart block and need for pacemaker[20,45]	• Surgical pulmonary valve replacement • Surgical TV repair or replacement • EPS, pacemaker placement
Ebstein anomaly	• Tricuspid regurgitation • RV enlargement and dysfunction • Atrial arrhythmias • Heart block • ASD often present	• Surgical TV repair or replacement • EPS, pacemaker placement • Transcatheter ASD closure
Fontan palliation	• Fontan failure is common later in life • Up to 40% diagnosed with HF[46] • Residual fenestration or collateral formation → ↑ Fontan pressures → ↑shunt → worsening hypoxia • Hemoptysis due to collateral formation • Fontan pathway leak • Branch pulmonary artery stenosis • High risk for atrial arrhythmias and heart block • Extracardiac disease: PLE, FALD, renal dysfunction, hematologic	• Transcatheter fenestration closure • Transcatheter collateral coiling • Transcatheter baffle puncture • Transcatheter pulmonary artery angioplasty and stenting • Surgical Fontan conversion • EPS with or without RFA, pacemaker placement

Abbreviations: CCTGA, congenitally corrected transposition of the great arteries; DTGA, dextro-transposition of the great arteries; EPS, electrophysiology study; FALD, Fontan-associated liver disease; IART, intra-atrial reentrant tachycardia; ICD, implantable cardiac defibrillator; PI, pulmonic insufficiency; PLE, protein-losing enteropathy; RFA, radiofrequency ablation; SCD, sudden cardiac death; Side arrows, leads to; upward arrow, increased; VT, ventricular tachycardia.

patients with significant HF and ACHD are followed by both congenital heart specialists and HF specialists. This allows each team to provide expertise on the nature of CHD and recommended HF therapies, respectively. A reasonable approach to the clinical evaluation of some common ACHD-HF phenotypes is outlined in **Fig. 1** with potential treatment considerations and strategies.

Table 3
Heart failure medication use in congenital heart disease patients

Diagnosis	Medications (Reference)	Important Findings
TGA, systemic RV	Beta blockers: Giardini et al,[47] 2007; Shaddy et al,[48] 2007; Doughan et al,[49] 2007; Bouallal et al,[50] 2010; Khairy et al,[41] 2017	• Positive RV remodeling[47] vs neutral or possible worsening function,[48] improved exercise duration,[47] improved NYHA functional class[49,50] and QOL,[50] protective against appropriate shocks[41]
	ACE inhibitors: Therrien et al,[51] 2008; Hechter et al,[52] 2001; Robinson et al,[53] 2001; Tutarel et al,[54] 2012	• No effect on RVEF, RVEDV and RVESV,[51] no improvement in exercise performance[52,53] • Decreases NT-pro (BNP) levels[54]
	Angiotensin receptor blockers: Van der Bom et al,[55] 2013; Dore et al,[56] 2005; Lester et al,[57] 2001	• No effect on RVEF, QOL,[55] and exercise capacity[55,56] • During active treatment, systolic BP and degree of TR decreased and duration of exercise increased[57]
	Aldosterone receptor blockers: Dos et al,[58] 2013	• Improvement of an altered baseline CTB profile suggesting reduction in myocardial fibrosis[58]
Tetralogy of Fallot, subpulmonic RV	Beta blockers: Norozi et al,[59] 2007	• No effect on peak V_{O_2} or ventricular function in patients with BNP >100 pg/mL and peak V_{O_2} <25 mL/kg/min[59]
	ACE inhibitors: Babu-Narayan et al,[60] 2012	• No improvement in RVEF[60]
	Angiotensin receptor blockers: Bokma et al (REDEFINE),[61] 2018	• No significant effect on RVEF, and secondary outcomes such as LVEF, peak aerobic exercise capacity, and NT-pro (BNP)[61]
Single ventricle circulation	Beta blockers: Ishibashi et al,[62] 2011	• Cardiothoracic ratio improved, dosage of furosemide reduced, and ejection fraction improved[62]
	ACE inhibitors: Hsu et al,[63] 2010; Kouatli et al,[64] 1997	• In infants, no improvement in somatic growth, ventricular function or HF severity; incidence of death and transplantation did not differ between groups[63] • No change in exercise capacity diastolic function, resting cardiac index, and SVR[64]
	Aldosterone receptor blockers: Mahle et al,[65] 2009	• Did not improve endothelial function or alter most serum cytokine levels[65]
	Phosphodiesterase inhibitors: Goldberg et al,[66] 2011 Endothelin receptor blockers: Hebert et al (TEMPO),[67] 2014; Schuuring et al,[68] 2013	• Increase in peak V_{O_2} and improved exercise time and functional class[67] • No effect on peak V_{O_2}, NT-pro (BNP) level, and mental QOL[68] • Improved ventilator efficiency during peak and submaximal exercise but no effect on peak V_{O_2}[66]

Abbreviations: ACE, angiotensin converting enzyme; APPROPRIATE, Ace Inhibitors for Potential Prevention of the Deleterious Effects of Pulmonary Regurgitation in Adults with Repaired Tetralogy of Fallot; BNP, brain natriuretic peptide; CTB, collagen turnover biomarker; LVEF, left ventricular ejection fraction; NT-pro (BNP), N-terminal pro (brain natriuretic peptide); NYHA, New York Heart Association; QOL, quality of life; RVEDV, right ventricular end diastolic volume; RVEF, right ventricular ejection fraction; RVESV, right ventricular systolic; SVR, systemic vascular resistance; TGA, transposition of the great arteries (here includes DTGA with atrial switch and CCTGA); TR, tricuspid regurgitation.

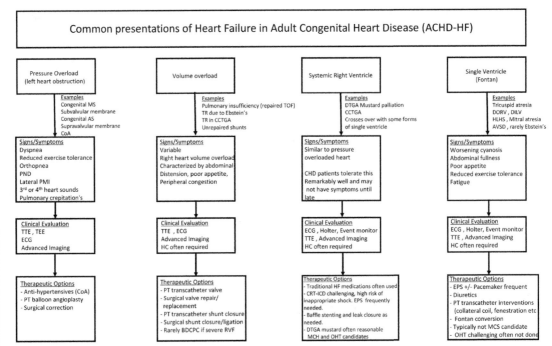

Fig. 1. Approach to managing HF in ACHD. Common presentations of ACHD-HF are outlined inclusive of example CHD lesions, signs, or symptoms; reasonable clinical evaluation or special testing; and potential therapeutic options. +/−, with or without; AS, aortic stenosis; AVSD, atrioventricular septal defect; BDCPC, bidirectional cavopulmonary connection; CCTGA, congenitally corrected transposition of the great arteries; CoA, coarctation of the aorta; CRT-ICD, cardiac resynchronization therapy–implantable cardiac defibrillator; CoA, coarctation of the aorta; CRT-ICD, cardiac resynchronization therapy–implantable cardiac defibrillator; DILV, double inlet left ventricle; DORV, double-outlet RV; DTGA, dextrotransposition of the great arteries; ECG, electrocardiogram; EPS, electrophysiology study; HC, hemodynamic catheterization; HLHS, hypoplastic left heart syndrome; MCS, mechanical circulatory support; MS, mitral stenosis; OHT, orthotopic heart transplant; PMI, point of maximum impulse; PND, paroxysmal nocturnal dyspnea; PT, percutaneous; RVF, RV failure; TEE, transesophageal echocardiogram; TOF, tetralogy of Fallot; TR, tricuspid regurgitation; TTE, transthoracic echocardiogram.

Mechanical Circulatory Support and Cardiac Transplantation

Advanced therapies for HF, which include the use of mechanical circulatory support (MCS), total artificial heart, and organ transplantation, are challenging in the CHD population owing to prior surgical repair, repeat sternotomy, nontraditional anatomy, elevated panel reactive antibodies, bleeding risk, hypercoagulability, and extracardiac disease secondary to CHD. Several studies have shown that up-front mortality is higher in the CHD population; however, long-term outcomes (>1 year posttransplant) are favorable.[35,36] The current organ allocation system is predicated on the sickest patients receiving listing preference. Unfortunately for many CHD patients, their anatomy may not be suitable for traditional measures for HF decompensation. In particular, this is true of the patient with a single functioning ventricle or Fontan that may have preserved systolic function but presents with congestive right-sided failure symptoms. There are only a handful of centers that have the resources and multidisciplinary teams required to care for these unique patients when MCS and transplant are considered.

SUMMARY

As the CHD population continues to age, managing late HF will continue to be an important part of long-term care. Important first steps in evaluating these patients are to consider prior anatomy and procedures, and to identify potentially reversible or treatable lesions. Device therapy, MCS, and transplant have a limited role in this population, and require evaluation by an experienced and specialized team.

REFERENCES

1. Marelli AJ, Mackie AS, Ionescu-Ittu R, et al. Congenital heart disease in the general population: changing prevalence and age distribution. Circulation 2007;115:163–72.

2. Hoffman JI, Kaplan S, Liberthson RR. Prevalence of congenital heart disease. Am Heart J 2004;147: 425–39.

3. van der Bom T, Zomer AC, Zwinderman AH, et al. The changing epidemiology of congenital heart disease. Nat Rev Cardiol 2011;8:50–60.

4. Wren C, O'Sullivan JJ. Survival with congenital heart disease and need for follow up in adult life. Heart 2001;85:438–43.

5. Harrison DA, Connelly M, Harris L, et al. Sudden cardiac death in the adult with congenital heart disease. Can J Cardiol 1996;12:1161–3.

6. Oechslin EN, Harrison DA, Connelly MS, et al. Mode of death in adults with congenital heart disease. Am J Cardiol 2000;86:1111–6.

7. Verheugt CL, Uiterwaal CS, van der Velde ET, et al. Mortality in adult congenital heart disease. Eur Heart J 2010;31:1220–9.

8. Bolger AP, Coats AJ, Gatzoulis MA. Congenital heart disease: the original heart failure syndrome. Eur Heart J 2003;24:970–6.

9. Stout KK, Broberg CS, Book WM, et al, American Heart Association Council on Clinical Cardiology CoFG, Translational B, council on cardiovascular R and imaging. Chronic heart failure in congenital heart disease: a scientific statement from the American Heart Association. Circulation 2016;133: 770–801.

10. Heart Failure Society of America. Executive summary: HFSA 2006 Comprehensive heart failure practice guideline. J Card Fail 2006;12:10–38.

11. Hunt SA, American College of Cardiology, American Heart Association Task Force on Practice Guidelines. ACC/AHA 2005 guideline update for the diagnosis and management of chronic heart failure in the adult: a report of the American College of Cardiology/American Heart Association Task Force on Practice Guidelines (Writing Committee to Update the 2001 Guidelines for the Evaluation and Management of Heart Failure). J Am Coll Cardiol 2005;46: e1–82.

12. Yancy CW, Jessup M, Bozkurt B, et al. 2013 ACCF/AHA guideline for the management of heart failure: executive summary: a report of the American College of Cardiology Foundation/American Heart Association Task Force on practice guidelines. Circulation 2013;128:1810–52.

13. Acker MA, Pagani FD, Stough WG, et al. Statement regarding the pre and post market assessment of durable, implantable ventricular assist devices in the United States: executive summary. Circ Heart Fail 2013;6:145–50.

14. Mackie AS, Pilote L, Ionescu-Ittu R, et al. Health care resource utilization in adults with congenital heart disease. Am J Cardiol 2007;99:839–43.

15. Zomer AC, Vaartjes I, van der Velde ET, et al. Heart failure admissions in adults with congenital heart disease; risk factors and prognosis. Int J Cardiol 2013;168:2487–93.

16. Diller GP, Kempny A, Alonso-Gonzalez R, et al. Survival prospects and circumstances of death in contemporary adult congenital heart disease patients under follow-up at a large tertiary centre. Circulation 2015;132:2118–25.

17. Opotowsky AR, Siddiqi OK, Webb GD. Trends in hospitalizations for adults with congenital heart disease in the U.S. J Am Coll Cardiol 2009;54:460–7.

18. Briston DA, Bradley EA, Sabanayagam A, et al. Health Care costs for adults with congenital heart disease in the United States 2002 to 2012. Am J Cardiol 2016;118:590–6.

19. Bhatt AB, Foster E, Kuehl K, et al. Association Council on Clinical C. Congenital heart disease in the older adult: a scientific statement from the American Heart Association. Circulation 2015;131:1884–931.

20. Warnes CA, Williams RG, Bashore TM, et al. ACC/AHA 2008 Guidelines for the management of adults with congenital heart disease: a report of the American College of Cardiology/American Heart Association Task Force on Practice Guidelines (writing committee to develop guidelines on the management of adults with congenital heart disease). Circulation 2008;118:e714–833.

21. Konstam MA, Kiernan MS, Bernstein D, et al. Evaluation and management of right-sided heart failure: a scientific statement from the American Heart Association. Circulation 2018;137:e578–622.

22. Black BL. Transcriptional pathways in second heart field development. Semin Cell Dev Biol 2007;18: 67–76.

23. Puley G, Siu S, Connelly M, et al. Arrhythmia and survival in patients >18 years of age after the mustard procedure for complete transposition of the great arteries. Am J Cardiol 1999;83:1080–4.

24. Kirjavainen M, Happonen JM, Louhimo I. Late results of Senning operation. J Thorac Cardiovasc Surg 1999;117:488–95.

25. Rutz T, de Marchi SF, Schwerzmann M, et al. Right ventricular absolute myocardial blood flow in complex congenital heart disease. Heart 2010;96: 1056–62.

26. Lubiszewska B, Gosiewska E, Hoffman P, et al. Myocardial perfusion and function of the systemic right ventricle in patients after atrial switch procedure for complete transposition: long-term follow-up. J Am Coll Cardiol 2000;36:1365–70.

27. Bolger AP, Sharma R, Li W, et al. Neurohormonal activation and the chronic heart failure syndrome in adults with congenital heart disease. Circulation 2002;106:92–9.

28. Babu-Narayan SV, Goktekin O, Moon JC, et al. Late gadolinium enhancement cardiovascular magnetic resonance of the systemic right ventricle in adults with previous atrial redirection surgery for

transposition of the great arteries. Circulation 2005; 111:2091–8.

29. Broberg CS, Prasad SK, Carr C, et al. Myocardial fibrosis in Eisenmenger syndrome: a descriptive cohort study exploring associations of late gadolinium enhancement with clinical status and survival. J Cardiovasc Magn Reson 2014;16:32.

30. Rathod RH, Prakash A, Powell AJ, et al. Myocardial fibrosis identified by cardiac magnetic resonance late gadolinium enhancement is associated with adverse ventricular mechanics and ventricular tachycardia late after Fontan operation. J Am Coll Cardiol 2010;55:1721–8.

31. Fredriksen PM, Veldtman G, Hechter S, et al. Aerobic capacity in adults with various congenital heart diseases. Am J Cardiol 2001;87:310–4.

32. Diller GP, Dimopoulos K, Okonko D, et al. Exercise intolerance in adult congenital heart disease: comparative severity, correlates, and prognostic implication. Circulation 2005;112:828–35.

33. Bouchardy J, Therrien J, Pilote L, et al. Atrial arrhythmias in adults with congenital heart disease. Circulation 2009;120:1679–86.

34. McMurray JJ, Adamopoulos S, Anker SD, et al, Avrupa Kardiyoloji Derneği (ESC) Akut ve Kronik Kalp Yetersizliği Tani ve Tedavisi 2012 Görev Grubu, ESC Kalp Yetersizliği Birliğinin İşbirliğiyle hazirlanmiştir, Heart Failure Association. ESC Guidelines for the diagnosis and treatment of acute and chronic heart failure 2012. Turk Kardiyol Dern Ars 2012; 40(Suppl 3):77–137 [in Turkish].

35. Davies RR, Russo MJ, Yang J, et al. Listing and transplanting adults with congenital heart disease. Circulation 2011;123:759–67.

36. Bradley EA, Pinyoluksana KO, Moore-Clingenpeel M, et al. Isolated heart transplant and combined heart-liver transplant in adult congenital heart disease patients: insights from the united network of organ sharing. Int J Cardiol 2017;228:790–5.

37. Park SC, Neches WH, Mathews RA, et al. Hemodynamic function after the Mustard operation for transposition of the great arteries. Am J Cardiol 1983;51: 1514–9.

38. Bradley EA, Cai A, Cheatham SL, et al. Mustard baffle obstruction and leak - how successful are percutaneous interventions in adults? Prog Pediatr Cardiol 2015;39:157–63.

39. Bradley EA, Zaidi AN, Morrison J, et al. Effectiveness of early invasive therapy for atrial tachycardia in adult atrial-baffle survivors. Tex Heart Inst J 2017;44:16–21.

40. Khairy P. Sudden cardiac death in transposition of the great arteries with a Mustard or Senning baffle: the myocardial ischemia hypothesis. Curr Opin Cardiol 2017;32:101–7.

41. Khairy P, Harris L, Landzberg MJ, et al. Sudden death and defibrillators in transposition of the great

arteries with intra-atrial baffles: a multicenter study. Circ Arrhythm Electrophysiol 2008;1:250–7.

42. Diller GP, Dimopoulos K, Okonko D, et al. Heart rate response during exercise predicts survival in adults with congenital heart disease. J Am Coll Cardiol 2006;48:1250–6.

43. Diller GP, Okonko DO, Uebing A, et al. Impaired heart rate response to exercise in adult patients with a systemic right ventricle or univentricular circulation: prevalence, relation to exercise, and potential therapeutic implications. Int J Cardiol 2009;134:59–66.

44. Kaltman JR, Ro PS, Zimmerman F, et al. Managed ventricular pacing in pediatric patients and patients with congenital heart disease. Am J Cardiol 2008; 102:875–8.

45. Huhta JC, Maloney JD, Ritter DG, et al. Complete atrioventricular block in patients with atrioventricular discordance. Circulation 1983;67:1374–7.

46. Piran S, Veldtman G, Siu S, et al. Heart failure and ventricular dysfunction in patients with single or systemic right ventricles. Circulation 2002;105: 1189–94.

47. Giardini A, Lovato L, Donti A, et al. A pilot study on the effects of carvedilol on right ventricular remodelling and exercise tolerance in patients with systemic right ventricle. Int J Cardiol 2007;114: 241–6.

48. Shaddy RE, Boucek MM, Hsu DT, et al. Carvedilol for children and adolescents with heart failure: a randomized controlled trial. JAMA 2007;298:1171–9.

49. Doughan AR, McConnell ME, Book WM. Effect of beta blockers (carvedilol or metoprolol XL) in patients with transposition of great arteries and dysfunction of the systemic right ventricle. Am J Cardiol 2007;99:704–6.

50. Bouallal R, Godart F, Francart C, et al. Interest of beta-blockers in patients with right ventricular systemic dysfunction. Cardiol Young 2010;20:615–9.

51. Therrien J, Provost Y, Harrison J, et al. Effect of angiotensin receptor blockade on systemic right ventricular function and size: a small, randomized, placebo-controlled study. Int J Cardiol 2008;129: 187–92.

52. Hechter SJ, Fredriksen PM, Liu P, et al. Angiotensin-converting enzyme inhibitors in adults after the Mustard procedure. Am J Cardiol 2001;87: 660–3. a11.

53. Robinson B, Heise CT, Moore JW, et al. Afterload reduction therapy in patients following intraatrial baffle operation for transposition of the great arteries. Pediatr Cardiol 2002;23:618–23.

54. Tutarel O, Meyer GP, Bertram H, et al. Safety and efficiency of chronic ACE inhibition in symptomatic heart failure patients with a systemic right ventricle. Int J Cardiol 2012;154:14–6.

55. van der Bom T, Winter MM, Bouma BJ, et al. Effect of valsartan on systemic right ventricular function: a

double-blind, randomized, placebo-controlled pilot trial. Circulation 2013;127:322–30.

56. Dore A, Houde C, Chan KL, et al. Angiotensin receptor blockade and exercise capacity in adults with systemic right ventricles: a multicenter, randomized, placebo-controlled clinical trial. Circulation 2005; 112:2411–6.

57. Lester SJ, McElhinney DB, Viloria E, et al. Effects of losartan in patients with a systemically functioning morphologic right ventricle after atrial repair of transposition of the great arteries. Am J Cardiol 2001;88: 1314–6.

58. Dos L, Pujadas S, Estruch M, et al. Eplerenone in systemic right ventricle: double blind randomized clinical trial. The evedes study. Int J Cardiol 2013; 168:5167–73.

59. Norozi K, Bahlmann J, Raab B, et al. A prospective, randomized, double-blind, placebo controlled trial of beta-blockade in patients who have undergone surgical correction of tetralogy of Fallot. Cardiol Young 2007;17:372–9.

60. Babu-Narayan SV, Uebing A, Davlouros PA, et al. Randomised trial of ramipril in repaired tetralogy of Fallot and pulmonary regurgitation: the APPROPRIATE study (Ace inhibitors for Potential PRevention of the deleterious effects of Pulmonary Regurgitation in Adults with repaired TEtralogy of Fallot). Int J Cardiol 2012;154:299–305.

61. Bokma JP, Winter MM, van Dijk AP, et al. Effect of losartan on RV dysfunction: results from the double-blind, randomized REDEFINE trial in adults with repaired tetralogy of Fallot. Circulation 2018; 137(14):1463–71.

62. Ishibashi N, Park IS, Waragai T, et al. Effect of carvedilol on heart failure in patients with a functionally univentricular heart. Circ J 2011;75:1394–9.

63. Hsu DT, Zak V, Mahony L, et al. Enalapril in infants with single ventricle: results of a multicenter randomized trial. Circulation 2010;122:333–40.

64. Kouatli AA, Garcia JA, Zellers TM, et al. Enalapril does not enhance exercise capacity in patients after Fontan procedure. Circulation 1997;96:1507–12.

65. Mahle WT, Wang A, Quyyumi AA, et al. Impact of spironolactone on endothelial function in patients with single ventricle heart. Congenit Heart Dis 2009;4:12–6.

66. Goldberg DJ, French B, McBride MG, et al. Impact of oral sildenafil on exercise performance in children and young adults after the fontan operation: a randomized, double-blind, placebo-controlled, crossover trial. Circulation 2011;123:1185–93.

67. Hebert A, Mikkelsen UR, Thilen U, et al. Bosentan improves exercise capacity in adolescents and adults after Fontan operation: the TEMPO (treatment with Endothelin receptor antagonist in fontan patients, a randomized, placebo-controlled, double-blind study measuring peak oxygen consumption) study. Circulation 2014;130:2021–30.

68. Schuuring MJ, Vis JC, van Dijk AP, et al. Impact of bosentan on exercise capacity in adults after the Fontan procedure: a randomized controlled trial. Eur J Heart Fail 2013;15:690–8.

Short-Term Circulatory and Right Ventricle Support in Cardiogenic Shock
Extracorporeal Membrane Oxygenation, Tandem Heart, CentriMag, and Impella

Ibrahim Sultan, MD[a,b,*], Arman Kilic, MD[c], Ahmet Kilic, MD[c]

KEYWORDS

- Right ventricular failure • Heart failure • Cardiac surgery • Mechanical circulatory support

KEY POINTS

- Right ventricular (RV) failure can lead to significant in-hospital mortality.
- Some patients with acute RV dysfunction may require mechanical circulatory support.
- Mechanical circulatory support in the short term can rest and recover the right ventricle.

INTRODUCTION

Severe right ventricular (RV) failure is seen in 4% to 5% of patients following cardiac surgery. A lesser degree of RV dysfunction can be seen in up to 20% of patients. Severe RV failure is a significant cause of morbidity and mortality, with an in-hospital mortality rate of up to 70% to 75%.[1–3] Medical management is employed and is successful for most of these patients. However, a small percentage of patients will continue to have persistent RV failure, for which mechanical support is used for management.

Despite the clinical impact of RV failure, the right ventricle has generally been considered a mere bystander, a victim of pathologic processes affecting the cardiovascular system. Consequently, most mechanical circulatory devices have been discovered and utilized for the right ventricle, prior to their implementation for the right ventricle. As such, not all mechanical circulatory devices can be used for the right ventricle but some have been used quite successfully.

PATHOPHYSIOLOGY

Unlike the left ventricle, the right ventricle has the distinct advantage of pumping blood into a low-compliance pulmonary vasculature. This allows the right ventricle to maintain low systolic pressure, and any change in the afterload can cause RV dysfunction to a variable degree. Acute RV failure can be a consequence of impaired pump function, acute pulmonary hypertensive crises, or right-sided valvular pathology. Impaired pump function can be a consequence of an RV infarct or inadequate myocardial protection when seen

Disclosure: The authors have nothing to disclose.

[a] Division of Cardiac Surgery, Department of Cardiothoracic Surgery, University of Pittsburgh and Heart and Vascular Institute, University of Pittsburgh Medical Center, 5200 Centre Avenue, Pittsburgh, PA 15206, USA; [b] Cardiothoracic Surgery, University of Pittsburgh, 5200 Centre Avenue, Suite 715, Pittsburgh, PA 15213, USA; [c] Division of Cardiac Surgery, Department of Surgery, Johns Hopkins Hospital, 600 N Wolfe Street, Baltimore, MD 21234, USA

* Corresponding author. Cardiothoracic Surgery, University of Pittsburgh, 5200 Centre Avenue, Suite 715, Pittsburgh, PA 15213.

E-mail address: sultani@upmc.edu

Heart Failure Clin 14 (2018) 579–583
https://doi.org/10.1016/j.hfc.2018.06.014
1551-7136/18/© 2018 Elsevier Inc. All rights reserved.

in the postcardiotomy setting. Acute pulmonary hypertensive crises can be a consequence of a large pulmonary embolus, hypoxia or as a consequence of an LV dysfunction causing increased filling pressures. All of these factors can increase the work load on the right ventricle, thereby causing dysfunction.

MEDICAL MANAGEMENT OF RIGHT VENTRICULAR FAILURE

A pulmonary artery catheter, right heart catheterization, or an echocardiogram can all provide means for the diagnosis of acute RV failure. Gated computed tomography CT angiograms can also do the same with reproducibility. The medical management of acute RV dysfunction is directed toward treating the reversible cause. This may include thrombolysis or embolectomy in the setting of a pulmonary embolus, percutaneous coronary intervention (PCI) in the setting of an RV infarct or aggressive diuresis in the setting of a dilated dysfunctional right ventricle. Treating hypoxia in a patient with respiratory distress may also help alleviate increasing pulmonary artery pressures, thus helping with RV afterload. Filling pressure can help guide subsequent management after initial therapy. Patients may benefit from atrial pacing, particularly if bradycardic, as the atrial kick in patients with RV dysfunction can be beneficial. The details of each therapeutic measure are beyond the scope of this article.

MECHANICAL SUPPORT FOR RIGHT VENTRICULAR FAILURE

Mechanical circulatory support (MCS) for the RV can be instrumental in stabilizing patients with cardiogenic shock while allowing the right ventricle to recover. Both percutaneous and open surgical options are available, which allow the heart failure team to choose the appropriate therapy for each patient depending on cause of RV dysfunction and associated comorbidities.[4–6]

PERCUTANEOUS MECHANICAL CIRCULATORY SUPPORT DEVICES
Extracorporeal Membrane Oxygenation

Extracorporeal membrane oxygenation (ECMO) is one of the most widely used mechanical circulatory support (MCS) options because of ease of availability for patients with acute RV failure. ECMO can be initiated both percutaneously and via open surgical access. ECMO is typically employed in patients with biventricular failure. A venous or drainage cannula is placed in the right atrium, most commonly via the femoral vein, and

an arterial cannula is placed via the femoral artery in absence of peripheral arterial disease. Because of the large size cannulas (18–20 French) that are placed in the common femoral artery, this may cause distal leg ischemia, and a distal perfusion cannula is typically placed in the superficial femoral artery or the posterior tibial artery. The axillary artery can also be used for in-flow in patients with peripheral arterial disease. ECMO is not a direct therapy targeted for the right ventricle, but rather best suited in the setting of biventricular function. ECMO decreases RV preload by draining the right atrium and passing blood through an oxygenator before circulating through the arterial system. This can further increase left ventricular (LV) afterload, and in cases of significantly impaired LV function, can increase LV end diastolic and pulmonary artery (PA) pressures. This can be addressed with an intra-aortic balloon pump (IABP), a decompressive vent across the left ventricle via the right superior pulmonary vein, or an Impella (Abiomed, Danvers, Massachusetts) device that can be placed via the femoral artery across the aortic valve. The LV vent would be connected to the ECMO circuit and be part of the venous drainage, in which the Impella would be independent; both methods have their advantages and disadvantages.[6–8]

Intra-aortic Balloon Pump

IABPs are most commonly employed in the setting of LV failure as a result of a myocardial infarction or in the acute setting of cardiomyopathy. IABPs mainly serve 2 purposes in this setting. During diastole, IABP inflation causes increased pressure and thus flow in the sinuses of Valsalva, increasing coronary perfusion. During systole, the deflated pump creates a low pressure system in the descending thoracic aorta, which then allows for increasing LV ejection, increasing mean arterial pressure while reducing LV afterload. In the setting of acute RV failure, IABP may be helpful by unloading the LV and eventually reducing right-sided filling pressures. Additionally, it can be helpful by increasing right coronary perfusion. Both these effects on the right ventricle are indirect and may not be solely helpful in ameliorating acute RV failure. Studies have shown that IABP has a limited effect in RV failure and has not been consistent in improving measured cardiac output. The advantage of using an IABP is that this can be placed via a small-bore femoral arterial sheath (6 French) or without a sheath if so desired. When placed appropriately, the vascular access complication rate can be negligible.

Impella

The Impella device was initially used and approved for patients with LV dysfunction or for patients undergoing high-risk PCI or cardiac procedure without the use of cardiopulmonary bypass. The Impella RP used exclusively for right heart support can be inserted percutaneously via the femoral vein. It is a 3-dimensional based microaxial pump that recently won premarket approval by the US Food and Drug Administration for RV support. The Impella RP is a 23F pump head mounted on an 11 French catheter. The pump head consists of an electric motor, axial blood pump, and outflow cannula. This can be placed percutaneously via the femoral vein under live echocardiographic and fluoroscopic guidance. Via the femoral vein, the pump is advanced into the inferior vena cava (IVC)/right atrial junction, after which it can be carefully advanced via the tricuspid valve into the right ventricle and via the pulmonic valve into the main pulmonary artery. This allows the inflow to be in the IVC while the flexible nitinol pump is advanced into the pulmonary artery. The Impella RP can be used up to 14 days and can provide flow up to 5 L/min. Initial studies on the Impella RP indicated significant increase in cardiac output and decrease in central venous pressure following placement of the device. The effect was tempered but continued to be better than baseline once the device was removed. Once placed via the femoral vein, the vascular complication rate is negligible. However, some patients may experience lower extremity swelling if the femoral vein is narrowed significantly after removal of the device. Prior to the availability of the Impella RP, the Impella RD was utilized for RV support. Installation of the Imeplla RD requires a sternotomy with direct cannulation of the right atrium and the pulmonary artery. This requires general anesthesia and carries with it increased risk of bleeding and infection in a patient who is already in cardiogenic shock. Cheung and colleagues examined their results in patients who underwent Impella RD and RP implantation for acute RV failure. Their results replicated what was seen before in patients undergoing short-term RV support: 30-day survival of 72% and 1-year survival of 50%.[9,10]

Tandem Heart

The Tandem Heart (TH) (Tandem Life, Pittsburgh, Pennsylvania) is a centrifugal pump that is a direct RV assist device (RVAD) such as the Impella (**Fig. 1**). Two venous cannulas are

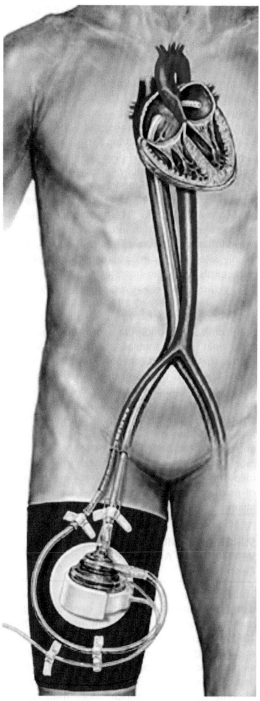

Fig. 1. Tandem heart pump. (*Courtesy of* CardiacAssist Inc. dba TandemLife; with permission.)

placed: one for drainage from the right atrium which drains blood into the extracorporeal system followed by another venous cannula that works as an outflow cannula in to the pulmonary artery. The inflow cannula is typically placed via the left femoral vein into the right atrium. The outflow cannula is placed via the right femoral vein and advanced into the pulmonary artery. In tall patients, in whom the cannula may not be long enough to reach the pulmonary artery from the femoral vein, it can be placed via the internal jugular vein thereby utilizing a shorter course. Like the Impella, the TH does not have an in-built oxygenator. However, one can be spliced in as can be done with most extracorporeal circuits. The major disadvantage to femoral venous cannulation with the TH, like the Impella, is the inability to successfully ambulate patients, particularly if RVAD support is utilized for more than 7 to 10 days. Kapur and colleagues[7,9,10] studied the use of the TH where most of the patients were postcardiotomy or postacute myocardial infarction. The population being mainly skewed toward postcardiotomy patients may explain the in-hospital mortality rate of 57% in the series. However, changes in hemodynamics were observed after implantation of the TH in these patients. An alternative to this is the Protek Duo, which can be placed via the jugular vein. The cannulas are 29 French or 31 French in size and have dual channels. The inflow channels are placed in the SVC and the right atrium, and the blood is drained into the extracorporeal centrifugal pump, after which it is pumped into the pulmonary artery. Flow up to 4 L/min can be obtained with both the TH and the Protek Duo. The use of Protek Duo has most commonly been reported in RV failure following LVAD implantation and in the setting of pulmonary hypertensive crises leading to RV failure.[10,11]

SURGICALLY IMPLANTED RIGHT VENTRICULAR ASSIST DEVICE
CentriMag

The CentriMag (Thoratec, Pleasanton, CA) is an extracorporeal RVAD with a centrifugal pump and a motor. The pump can generate up to 10 L/min of continuous flow (**Fig. 2**). Bhama and colleagues[3] reported their initial experience with the CentriMag pump in patients with an LV assist device (LVAD), heart transplant or postcardiotomy cardiogenic shock. More than half the patients were weaned off successfully. Cannulation is performed via sternotomy or thoracotomy. The right atrium and the pulmonary artery are cannulated for drainage and outflow. Because large and short cannulas can be used, the ability to achieve higher flows is seen. This is an advantage seen in all patients with surgically implanted RVADs that most percutaneous devices cannot offer at this stage. This advantage, however,

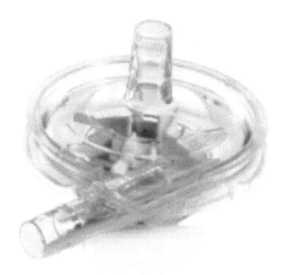

Fig. 2. Centrimag pump. (*Courtesy of* Thoratec Corporation, Pleasanton, CA; with permission.)

can be countered by the higher risk of bleeding and infection as a result of sternotomy or thoracotomy.[12–15]

ANTICOAGULATION

It is prudent to anticoagulate all RVADs. This is typically done as a loading dose with heparin at the time of insertion followed by a heparin drip that can be managed by the local nurse-managed protocol. It is imperative to have frequent activated clotting time (ACT) or partial thromboplastin time (PTT) checks when initiating RVAD support, after which they can be liberalized once the levels are therapeutic and stable. With surgical implantation, it is typical to not use any anticoagulation for up to 6 hours after implantation because of bleeding risks after initiating RVAD support. It is, however, critical to maintain support of at least 3 to 4 L/min in order to avoid any stasis and discourage development of thrombus in the circuit and the oxygenator, if one is being used. The standard PTT target is approximately 1.5 to 1.9 times the laboratory normal levels. Excessive bleeding may be seen after RVAD implantation, which is typically a consequence of coagulopathy. Patients are more likely to need blood products such as platelets and cryoprecipitate as a consequence of bleeding rather than heparin in the immediate postoperative setting. Because of multiple exposures to intravenous heparin, patients are at risk for developing heparin-induced thrombocytopenia. Any suspicion should promptly lead to discontinuation of heparin and use of bivalrudin or argatroban, with eventual transition to warfarin.

WEANING FROM RIGHT VENTRICULAR SUPPORT

Most patients in whom RV support has been instituted are on multiple inotropes and vasopressors. It is important to ensure that hemodynamics have normalized and the inotropic requirement has improved significantly prior to RVAD wean. Weaning trials can be performed and hemodynamics observed carefully, as flow on the RVAD is gradually decreased. Live echocardiography is employed to visualize the right ventricle while weaning the RVAD over several hours. If there is no significant change in filling pressures, cardiac index, and the function of the right ventricle on echocardiography, the RVAD can be removed surgically or percutaneously. Heparin is reversed with protamine, and careful medical management is continued to help nurse the right ventricle.[16,17]

SUMMARY

Severe RV dysfunction can be managed with RVADs in the short term with reasonable success. Choosing the right patient for RVAD implantation may help in ensuring success in the short term with a successful wean and long-term RV recovery.

REFERENCES

1. Abnousi F, Yong CM, Fearon W, et al. The evolution of temporary percutaneous mechanical circulatory support devices: a review of the options and evidence in cardiogenic shock. Curr Cardiol Rep 2015;17(6):40.
2. Aissaoui N, Morshuis M, Schoenbrodt M, et al. Temporary right ventricular mechanical circulatory support for the management of right ventricular failure in critically ill patients. J Thorac Cardiovasc Surg 2013;146(1):186–91.
3. Bhama JK, Kormos RL, Toyoda Y, et al. Clinical experience using the Levitronix CentriMag system for temporary right ventricular mechanical circulatory support. J Heart Lung Transplant 2009;28(9):971–6.
4. Cheung AW, White CW, Davis MK, et al. Short-term mechanical circulatory support for recovery from acute right ventricular failure: clinical outcomes. J Heart Lung Transplant 2014;33(8):794–9.
5. Gilotra NA, Stevens GR. Temporary mechanical circulatory support: a review of the options, indications, and outcomes. Clin Med Insights Cardiol 2014;8(Suppl 1):75–85.
6. Kapur NK, Esposito ML, Bader Y, et al. Mechanical circulatory support devices for acute right ventricular failure. Circulation 2017;136(3):314–26.
7. Kapur NK, Paruchuri V, Jagannathan A, et al. Mechanical circulatory support for right ventricular failure. JACC Heart Fail 2013;1(2):127–34.
8. Sultan I, Habertheuer A, Wallen T, et al. The role of extracorporeal membrane oxygenator therapy in the setting of type A aortic dissection. J Card Surg 2017;32(12):822–5.
9. Kapur NK, Paruchuri V, Korabathina R, et al. Effects of a percutaneous mechanical circulatory support device for medically refractory right ventricular failure. J Heart Lung Transplant 2011;30(12):1360–7.
10. Mulaikal TA, Bell LH, Li B, et al. Isolated right ventricular mechanical support: outcomes and prognosis. ASAIO J 2018;64(2):e20–7.
11. Ravichandran AK, Baran DA, Stelling K, et al. Outcomes with the tandem protek duo dual-lumen percutaneous right ventricular assist device. ASAIO J 2018;64(4):570–2.
12. Saffarzadeh A, Bonde P. Options for temporary mechanical circulatory support. J Thorac Dis 2015;7(12):2102–11.
13. Soliman OI, Akin S, Muslem R, et al. Derivation and validation of a novel right-sided heart failure model after implantation of continuous flow left ventricular assist devices:the EUROMACS (European Registry for Patients with Mechanical Circulatory Support) right-sided heart failure risk score. Circulation 2018;137(9):891–906.
14. Yoshioka D, Takayama H, Garan RA, et al. Contemporary outcome of unplanned right ventricular assist device for severe right heart failure after continuous-flow left ventricular assist device insertion. Interact Cardiovasc Thorac Surg 2017;24(6):828–34.
15. Kilic A, Sultan I, Yuh DD, et al. Ventricular assist device implantation in the elderly: nationwide outcomes in the United States. J Card Surg 2013;28(2):183–9.
16. Keebler ME, Haddad EV, Choi CW, et al. Venoarterial extracorporeal membrane oxygenation in cardiogenic shock. JACC Heart Fail 2018;6(6):503–16.
17. Konstam MA, Kiernan MS, Bernstein D, et al. Evaluation and management of right-sided heart failure: a scientific statement from the American Heart Association. Circulation 2018;137(20):e578–622.

Mitral Valve Surgery for Congestive Heart Failure

Juan A. Crestanello, MD

KEYWORDS

- Mitral valve disease • Mitral valve repair • Congestive heart failure • Mitral regurgitation
- Transcatheter device

KEY POINTS

- Mitral valve disease is a common cause of congestive heart failure. It can be categorized from the functional standpoint in mitral regurgitation, mitral stenosis, or mixed lesions.
- Every year approximately 22,500 patients undergo surgery for mitral valve disease. More than 95% of the mitral repairs and 75% of the replacements are performed to correct mitral regurgitation.
- An increased number of patients with mitral regurgitation who are considered either inoperable or at high risk for surgery are treated with transcatheter devices. More than 5000 patients received a transcatheter mitral procedure in 2016.
- Transcatheter mitral valve procedures is an evolving treatment modality that will likely expand the number of mitral valve procedures performed.
- Mitral valve disease can be categorized from the functional standpoint in regurgitant lesions, stenosis, or both.

INTRODUCTION

Mitral valve disease is a common cause of congestive heart failure.[1,2] It can be categorized from the functional standpoint in mitral regurgitation, mitral stenosis, or mixed lesions.

Every year approximately 22,500 patients undergo surgery for mitral valve disease.[3] More than 95% of the mitral repairs and 75% of the replacements are performed to correct mitral regurgitation. In addition, an increased number of patients with mitral regurgitation who are considered either inoperable or at high risk for surgery are treated with transcatheter devices.[3] More than 5000 patients received a transcatheter mitral procedure in 2016 (Society of Thoracic Surgery [STS]/American College of Cardiology [ACC] Transcatheter Valve Therapy Registry, personal communication, 2017). This is an evolving treatment modality that will likely expand the number of mitral valve procedures performed.

MITRAL REGURGITATION

Mitral valve regurgitation can be categorized based on its etiology as either primary (organic) or secondary (functional). This discussion is limited to chronic mitral regurgitation.

PRIMARY OR ORGANIC MITRAL VALVE REGURGITATION

In primary mitral valve disease, the regurgitation occurs as a consequence of a structural defect on the valvular apparatus (leaflets, chordae, or papillary muscles).[2] The most common etiology for primary mitral regurgitation is mitral valve prolapse secondary to either myxomatous degeneration or fibro-elastic deficiency[4] (Fig. 1). Other less common etiologies include rheumatic heart disease, infective endocarditis, connective tissue disorders, radiation, and congenital heart disease.

Disclosure: The author has nothing to disclose.
Senior Associate Consultant, Department of Cardiovascular Surgery, Mayo Clinic, 200 First Street Southwest, Rochester, MN 55905, USA
E-mail address: crestanello.juan@mayo.edu

Heart Failure Clin 14 (2018) 585–600
https://doi.org/10.1016/j.hfc.2018.06.006
1551-7136/18/© 2018 Elsevier Inc. All rights reserved.

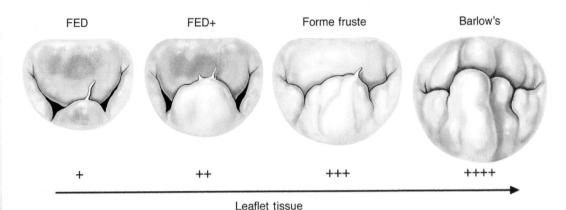

FED   FED+   Forme fruste   Barlow's

+   ++   +++   ++++

Leaflet tissue

Fig. 1. Degenerative mitral valve disease ranges from fibroelastic deficiency (FED) to full myxomatous valve disease (Barlow disease). In FED, there is a deficiency of collagen with thin and almost transparent leaflets and 1 or more ruptured chordae. In myxomatous valve disease, the leaflets are diffusely thickened, redundant, with excess tissue with elongation or rupture of 1 or several chordae tendinea leading to leaflet prolapse or flail. +, increased amount of leaflet tissue. (*From* Adams DH, Rosenhek R, Falk V. Degenerative mitral valve regurgitation: best practice revolution. Eur Heart J 2010;31(16):1959; with permission.)

SECONDARY OR FUNCTIONAL MITRAL VALVE REGURGITATION

Secondary or functional mitral regurgitation is a ventricular disease in which there are no abnormalities of the mitral valve leaflet or subvalvular apparatus. The mitral regurgitation is secondary to remodeling and global or regional dysfunction of the left ventricle. Remodeling of the left ventricle leads to apical and lateral papillary muscle displacement with leaflet tethering that prevents coaptation and leads to mitral regurgitation (**Fig. 2**).[5–7] Annular dilatation plays a small role as a mechanism for the mitral regurgitation. Ischemic and nonischemic cardiomyopathy are the most common causes of functional mitral regurgitation.[8]

The presence of functional mitral regurgitation after a myocardial infarction and in patients with heart failure is a marker of poor prognosis.[9–12] It is associated with increased mortality, increased severity of heart failure symptoms, and increased rate of readmissions to the hospital. The severity of the regurgitation also affects the prognosis. Patients with mild to moderate functional (effective regurgitant orifice [ERO] 1–19 mm^2) had a 5-year survival of 49%, whereas patients with severe functional mitral regurgitation (ERO $\geq$20 mm^2) had a 5-year survival of 29%.[9–11] In functional mitral regurgitation, lesser regurgitant volumes have significantly more impact in prognosis than in patients with primary mitral regurgitation.

The pattern of annular dilation, leaflet tethering, and the direction of the mitral regurgitant jet differ with the etiology and severity of functional mitral regurgitation[13–16] (see **Fig. 2**). In ischemic cardiomyopathy, the initial ventricular remodeling occurs in the posterior-medial papillary muscle. Thus, the posterior-medial portion of the posterior leaflet (P3) is tethered and lower than the anterior, leading to a posteriorly directed mitral regurgitation jet (see **Fig. 2**, parts 1 and 2). This pattern is called "asymmetric tethering." Ischemia of the anterior wall of the left ventricle leads to functional mitral regurgitation in more advanced stages of ventricular remodeling than in patients with inferior infarction (more spherical ventricles with more tenting and lower left ventricular ejection fraction [LVEF]). Both papillary muscles are displaced laterally and apically, and therefore, both leaflets are tethered. The regurgitant jet is central. This pattern is called "symmetric tethering" (see **Fig. 2**, parts 3 and 4). Ventricular remodeling in nonischemic cardiomyopathy is also "symmetric," involving both papillary muscles and leading to a central regurgitation jet[13–16] (see **Fig. 2**, parts 3 and 4).

Because functional mitral regurgitation is a ventricular problem, reestablishing the competency of the mitral valve is not curative. In addition, there is no conclusive evidence that correcting functional mitral regurgitation improves survival.[17,18]

TREATMENT OF PRIMARY OR ORGANIC MITRAL VALVE REGURGITATION

The surgical treatment of organic mitral regurgitation is well established. Mitral valve repair is the preferred treatment for patients with mitral valve

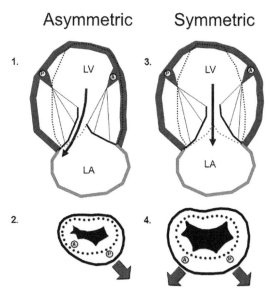

Asymmetric   ## Symmetric

Fig. 2. Secondary or functional mitral valve regurgitation. LV remodeling with displacement of the papillary muscles leads to leaflet tethering and mitral regurgitation. The most common type is asymmetric (1, 2) with displacement of the inferior wall and postero-medial papillary muscle (P) with tethering of the posterior leaflet, dilatation of the postero-medial annulus, and posteriorly directed regurgitant jet. Symmetric tethering is seen in advanced ischemic cardiomyopathy or in nonischemic cardiomyopathy (3, 4). Both papillary muscles are involved and the jet is central. A, anterolateral papillary muscle; LA, left atrium. Dotted lines represent the normal status of the LV, the mitral leaflet in systole, and the mitral valve annulus. Blue arrow demonstrates the direction of the mitral regurgitation jet. *Red arrows* demonstrate the pattern of dilatation of the mitral annulus.

prolapse. Mitral valve repair can be achieved by several techniques, including leaflet resection, plication, neochordae insertion, and chord transposition reinforced with either a partial or complete annuloplasty ring.[19–21]

Mitral valve repair in organic mitral regurgitation is associated with a very low operative mortality and excellent long-term results.[19–21] Mitral valve repair cures primary mitral regurgitation and restores survival to the expected survival of a gender-matched and age-matched population[22,23] (**Fig. 3**). Compared with replacement, mitral valve repair is associated with lower operative mortality, improved left ventricular function, and improved long-term survival.[24] The long-term survival benefit of valve repair is seen in posterior and bileaflet prolapse, whereas the survival benefit in the less common isolated anterior leaflet prolapse repair is less clear[24] (**Fig. 4**). Mitral valve repair is a durable procedure. It is at least as durable as mitral valve replacement with a mechanical valve and far exceeds the durability of a biological valve. The annualized risk of reoperation varies by the leaflet subset: for posterior leaflet repair the risk is 0.5% per year, for bileaflet repair the risk is 0.9% per year, and for anterior leaflet repair the risk is 1.6% per year. All of them compare very favorably to the risk of reoperation with a mechanical valve: 0.66% per year (**Fig. 5**).[24]

The functional results are also good with freedom from +2 mitral regurgitation greater than 90% at 8 years (**Fig. 6**).[25,26]

Mitral valve replacement for organic mitral regurgitation is reserved for patients with complex sessions that cannot be reliably repaired and

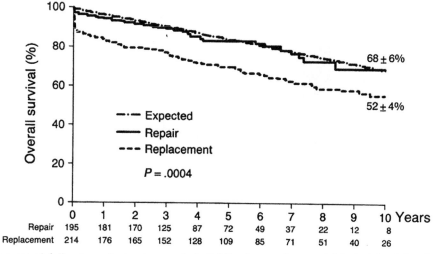

Fig. 3. Late survival following mitral valve repair (*solid lines*) or replacement (*dashed lines*) for degenerative mitral valve disease compared with expected survival (*dotted lines*). (*From* Enriquez-Sarano M, Schaff HV, Orszulak TA, et al. Valve repair improves the outcome of surgery for mitral regurgitation. A multivariate analysis. Circulation 1995;91(4):1023; with permission.)

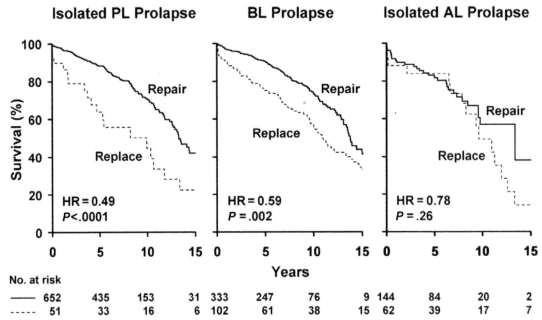

Fig. 4. Late survival among patients having mitral valve repair versus replacement for anterior (AL), posterior (PL), or bileaflet prolapse (BL). Solid line: valve repair; dashed line: valve replacement. HR, hazard ratio for survival of replacement group compared with repair group. (*From* Suri RM, Schaff HV, Dearani JA, et al. Survival advantage and improved durability of mitral repair for leaflet prolapse subsets in the current era. Ann Thorac Surg 2006;82(3):822; with permission.)

for failed repairs. Regardless of the reason, it is essential to maintain the mitral to left ventricular (LV) continuity by completely preserving the subvalvular apparatus that better preserves LV function, dimensions, and survival.[27,28]

Indications for mitral valve surgery in organic mitral regurgitation are well established in the American Heart Association (AHA)/ACC guidelines.[18] Severe mitral regurgitation is defined as (1) central jet of mitral regurgitation that occupies more than 40% of the left atrium or holosystolic eccentric jet mitral regurgitation, (2) vena contracta $\geq$0.7 cm, (3) regurgitant volume $\geq$60 mL, (4) regurgitant fraction $\geq$50%, (5) ERO $\geq$0.40 cm^2, (6) angiographic grade +3 to 4.[18]

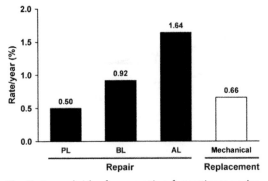

Fig. 5. Annual risk of reoperation for patients undergoing surgical correction of organic mitral regurgitation. Posterior leaflet repair (PL) has the lowest risk of reoperation, followed by mechanical valve replacement, bileaflet repair (BL), and anterior leaflet repair (AL). (*From* Suri RM, Schaff HV, Dearani JA, et al. Survival advantage and improved durability of mitral repair for leaflet prolapse subsets in the current era. Ann Thorac Surg 2006;82(3):825; with permission.)

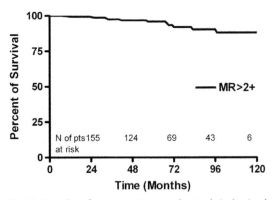

Fig. 6. Freedom from recurrent moderate (>2+) mitral regurgitation after mitral valve repair for organic mitral regurgitation due to degenerative disease. Semin Thorac Cardiovasc Surg 2007;19:118; with permission.)

For patients with severe mitral regurgitation, mitral surgery is indicated when they became symptomatic (New York Heart Association [NYHA] functional class $\geq$2), or for asymptomatic patients when they develop LV dysfunction (LVEF $\leq$60%), LV dilation (LV end-systolic diameter $\geq$40 mm) atrial fibrillation, or pulmonary hypertension (systolic pulmonary artery pressure >50 mm Hg).[18] Mitral valve repair is also reasonable in asymptomatic patients with preserved ventricular function and dimensions when a successful and durable repair can be achieved with greater than 95% certainty and with an operative mortality less than 1% or when there has been a progressive increase in LV size or decrease in ejection fraction (EF) on serial imaging studies.[18] Concomitant mitral valve repair should be consider in patients with moderate or severe organic mitral regurgitation who are undergoing cardiac surgery for other indications.[18] Mitral valve repair in patients with less than severe mitral regurgitation is an area of ongoing research.[29]

TREATMENT OF SECONDARY OR FUNCTIONAL MITRAL VALVE REGURGITATION
Medical Management for Functional Mitral Valve Regurgitation

The severity of functional mitral regurgitation and clinical presentation are dynamic and are significantly influenced by the ventricular loading conditions. Optimizing the preload and afterload with guideline-directed medical therapy, including diuretics, beta blockers, angiotensin-converting enzyme inhibitors or angiotensin receptor blockers, aldosterone antagonist, and cardiac resynchronization therapy (if indicated) is essential before deciding on surgical intervention.[5,6,17,18] Medical optimization decreases mitral regurgitation, pulmonary congestion, fluid overload, and myocardial ischemia.[5,6,17,18] Cardiac resynchronization therapy with biventricular pacing is indicated in patients with wall motion abnormalities and left bundle branch block resulting in improved LV function and wall motion abnormalities, increasing mitral closing force reducing or eliminating mitral regurgitation. The benefit of cardiac resynchronization therapy is more pronounced in patients with nonischemic cardiomyopathy.[5,6,17,18] It is reasonable to consider placing an epicardial pacing lead on the lateral wall of the LV in all patients at the time of mitral valve surgery.

Surgery for Functional Mitral Valve Regurgitation

The ideal goals of treatment in functional mitral regurgitation would be to restore competency of

the valve and to stop or reverse the LV remodeling and dysfunction. Addressing the ventricular problem is as important as restoring the competency of the mitral valve. Although we have effective treatments to address the mitral regurgitation, an effective and predictable treatment for the LV remodeling and dysfunction is not yet available. Coronary revascularization to the ischemic myocardium should be undertaken when technically feasible. Although coronary revascularization with coronary artery bypass grafting (CABG) restores blood supply to the ischemic myocardium, improves long-term survival compared with medical therapy alone, and improves LV function, and reverse remodels the LV, the effect on mitral regurgitation is uncertain.[30–33] In many cases, revascularization alone improves moderate and mild mitral regurgitation.[33] However, there are no well-established predictors that allow for the identification of those patents in advance. Because of our inability to address the ventricular problem, it has never been demonstrated that reducing or eliminating mitral regurgitation alters the natural history of the underlying LV disease or that it improves survival.[17,18]

Mitral Valve Repair for Functional Mitral Valve Regurgitation

Mitral valve repair with a restrictive annuloplasty has been the treatment of choice to address functional mitral regurgitation for many years.[34–36] Mitral annuloplasty restores leaflet coaptation by reducing the anteroposterior distance and the valve area. The annuloplasty should be performed with a complete and rigid ring at least 1 or 2 sizes smaller than the size necessary to improve leaflet coaptation.[17,34–36] If the LV remodeling continues, further displacement of the papillary muscles will lead to further teetering and recurrent mitral regurgitation. The rate of mitral regurgitation recurrence after mitral valve repair with a restrictive annuloplasty is a very large rate (**Fig. 7**) with 10% to 20% rates of persistent mitral regurgitation early after operation and with 50% to 70% rates of recurrent mitral regurgitation at 5 years[5,37]

Multiple annuloplasty rings have been designed to address the changes in annular shape associated with functional mitral regurgitation. However, there are no studies that prove their superiority.[38] Other adjuvant techniques, like division of secondary chordae,[39] placement of edge-to-edge stitches,[40,41] and reposition of papillary muscles,[42,43] have been advocated to improve coaptation and decrease the rate of recurrence. Long-term results and precise indications for those techniques are lacking.

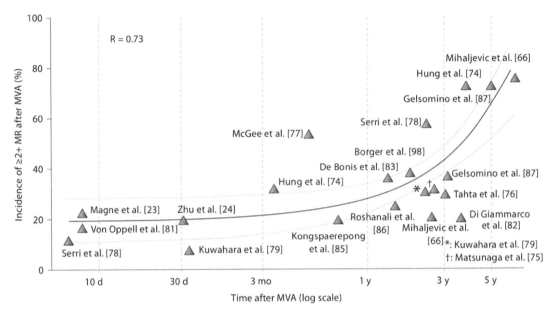

Fig. 7. Recurrence of greater than +2 mitral regurgitation after mitral valve annuloplasty (MVA) for ischemic mitral regurgitation. MR, mitral regurgitation. (*From* Magne J, Sénéchal M, Dumesnil JG, et al. Ischemic mitral regurgitation: a complex multifaceted disease. Cardiology 2009;112(4):244–59; with permission.)

Mitral Valve Replacement for Functional Mitral Valve Regurgitation

Mitral valve replacement provides a more durable correction of mitral regurgitation.[44] To prevent further deterioration of LV function, mitral valve replacement should be performed with preservation of the subvalvular apparatus of both the anterior and posterior leaflet.[27,28] Preservation of the subvalvular apparatus reduces LV systolic size and improves LV function compared with partial or no preservation.[27,28] Mitral valve replacement has been perceived for many years as detrimental to the short-term and long-term outcomes of patients with functional mitral regurgitation. Perceived disadvantages were longer operative times, increased operative mortality and morbidity, and worsened ventricular function secondary to the elimination of the continuity between the mitral annulus and the LV wall with the consequent decreased long-term survival. Many of these concerns were not supported by prospective randomized trials but by observational retrospective studies and metanalysis.[23,45,46] They were also encouraged by the demonstrated superiority of mitral valve repair over replacement for organic mitral regurgitation.[24] Other concerns associated with mitral valve repair were the need for anticoagulation to prevent thromboembolic complications, risk of endocarditis, and the durability of the valve prosthesis. In terms of durability, the median survival of patients with ischemic

cardiomyopathy ranges from 6 to 7 years and more than 60% of the patients dead at 10 years.[30] Therefore, it is unlikely that these patients outlive a mitral bioprosthesis.

Repair or Replacement for Severe Functional Mitral Valve Regurgitation

The current ACC/AHA and the European guidelines recommend mitral valve surgery for symptomatic patients with severe ischemic mitral regurgitation who do not respond to medical therapy.[18,47] However, they do not specify how to select repair over replacement or whether one is superior to the other. There was no clear conclusive evidence in the literature that proved the superiority of one over the other until the Cardiothoracic Surgical Trials Network (CTSN) trial. The CTSN conducted a prospective randomized trial that examined mitral valve repair versus replacement for severe ischemic mitral regurgitation.[44] This is a landmark study that has changed the way we approach ischemic mitral regurgitation. The study randomized 251 patients with severe ischemic mitral regurgitation, LVEF of 40% and dilated LV (LV end-systolic volume index >60 mL/m²) to mitral valve repair with a complete undersized ring or to chordal sparing valve replacement. The study showed that operative mortality was similar in repair and in replacement (4.0% in replacement vs 1.6% in repair $P = .26$). The 1-year and 2-year mortality, LV function, and degree of ventricular remodeling was similar among the groups (**Fig. 8**).[44,48] However, the proportion of patients with recurrence of moderate to severe mitral regurgitation at 2 years was 12 times higher on the repair group (59% vs 3.9%, P<.001) as well as the rate of heart-failure–related adverse events and readmissions for heart failure.[44] Factors associated with the recurrence of moderate or severe mitral regurgitation in the repair group were (1) less reverse remodeling after surgery and (2) the presence of preoperative basal aneurysm or dyskinesis.[37,44] This study did not identify any other preoperative criteria that would predict the recurrence of mitral regurgitation and help discriminate between mitral valve replacement (MVR) and repair in patients with severe mitral regurgitation. Previous studies have identified severe tethering or significant LV dilatation (LV end diastolic size >6.5 cm) as predictors of recurrent mitral regurgitation.[5,8,17] Several retrospective studies had confirmed the findings that the nature of mitral valve surgery (repair or replacement) had no influence on long-term survival in ischemic mitral regurgitation.[45,49]

Management of Functional Mitral Valve Regurgitation in the Patient Who Needs Coronary Artery Bypass Surgery

The most common situation that the surgeon or cardiologist encounters is patients with coronary artery disease who need CABG and have functional mitral regurgitation. The severity of the mitral regurgitation and the decision to address it at the time of the surgery should be made with data obtained from the preoperative transthoracic echocardiogram.[8,17] The intraoperative transesophageal echocardiogram performed under general anesthesia downgrades the severity of the mitral

regurgitation given the reduction in afterload induced by general anesthesia. Because ischemic mitral regurgitation is functional and depends on the loading conditions, a trial of guideline-directed optimal medical therapy should be attempted and the mitral regurgitation severity reevaluated before surgery. This medical therapy usually positively affects mitral regurgitation severity.[8,17]

The decision to perform concomitant mitral valve surgery during the CABG procedure rests on several factors, including the severity of the mitral regurgitation, the surgical risk, and the experience of the surgeon.

The addition of a mitral valve procedure to CABG is associated with increased operative mortality. Even though trial data showed that in centers of excellence, CABG with mitral valve repair or replacement can be performed with low operative mortality,[48] the mortality in the real world is much higher. The STS database shows that although the unadjusted operative mortality for CABG is a little more than 2%, the addition of mitral valve repair increases the mortality to 5% and the addition of MVR increases the mortality to 9.5%.[3] In addition, the experience of the surgeon counts. The median number of mitral valve procedures performed annually by surgeons in the United States is only 5 (range 1–166), and the probability of repairing the mitral valve increases with the number of mitral valve procedures performed by the surgeon and is associated with improved freedom from reoperation and long-term survival.[50,51]

The most important factor in deciding whether to address or not the mitral valve is the mitral regurgitation severity determined by the preoperative transthoracic echocardiogram.

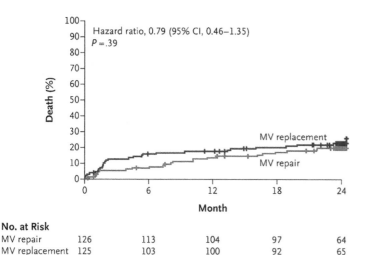

Fig. 8. Long-term survival of mitral valve repair versus replacement for severe ischemic mitral valve regurgitation: 2-year results of the CTSN trial. CI, confidence interval; MV, mitral valve. (*From* Goldstein D, Moskowitz AJ, Gelijns AC, et al. Two-year outcomes of surgical treatment of severe ischemic mitral regurgitation. N Engl J Med 2016;374(4):344–53; with permission.)

No. at Risk					
MV repair	126	113	104	97	64
MV replacement	125	103	100	92	65

Although patients with severe mitral regurgitation will benefit from a mitral valve procedure to alleviate their symptoms and the benefit of the additional procedure will justify the risk, patients with mild mitral regurgitation should undergo CABG alone.

The management of patients with moderate mitral regurgitation is still controversial. Several questions arise in this group of patients: Is the risk of adding a mitral valve procedure justified? Are there clinical benefits associated with mitral valve repair? Does adding mitral valve repair improve symptoms, survival, and freedom from mitral regurgitation compared with CABG alone? Is there a role for MVR in this group? Does mitral valve repair prevent progression of mitral regurgitation and LV remodeling? Several of these questions were addressed in another landmark trial from the CTSN that was recently published.[52,53] In this trial, 301 patients with moderate ischemic mitral regurgitation were randomly assigned to CABG and mitral valve repair or CABG alone. Preoperatively, the mean LVEF was 40% and the LV end-systolic volume index was 55 mL/m². Mitral valve repair was performed with a complete annuloplasty ring and prolonged operative time and length of hospital stay. Mitral valve repair did not increase operative mortality but was associated with an increased rate of neurologic events and supraventricular arrhythmias. At 2 years, the prevalence of moderate or severe mitral regurgitation was higher in the CABG-alone group than in the combined-procedure group (32.3% vs 11.2%, P<.001); only 2% of patients in the CABG-alone group and none in the combined-procedure group had severe mitral regurgitation. CABG alone or with mitral valve repair resulted in reverse remodeling of the LV and in improved LV function. Mitral

valve repair did not lead to significant differences in heart failure symptoms, degree of LV reverse remodeling, changes in LV function, or survival at 2 years (**Fig. 9**). Patients without mitral regurgitation recurrence had large reverse remodeling and more improvement in the inferior posterior lateral wall motion. Patients with combined CABG-mitral valve repair had improved exercise tolerance.[52,53]

THE GUIDELINES: HOW TO APPROACH THE PATIENT WITH FUNCTIONAL MITRAL VALVE REGURGITATION

So how do we make sense of these data? There are several guidelines that address the indications for surgery in functional mitral regurgitation. They include the 2014 AHA/ACC guidelines and the European Society of Cardiology/European Association for Cardio-Thoracic Surgery guidelines[18,47] and the recently published American Association for Thoracic Surgery (AATS) guidelines.[17] The AATS guidelines provide the most comprehensive recommendations that take into account the results of the most recent clinical trials. All guidelines recommendations are summarized in **Table 1**.

Severe Mitral Regurgitation

Severe mitral regurgitation will not improve with coronary revascularization alone. Therefore patients with severe mitral regurgitation undergoing CABG should have their mitral valve repaired or replaced. For patients with (1) severe ischemic mitral regurgitation with no targets for revascularization (or when revascularization is not indicated) or (2) severe nonischemic functional mitral regurgitation who remain symptomatic despite guideline-directed medical therapy, isolated mitral valve surgery can be considered. Isolated mitral valve

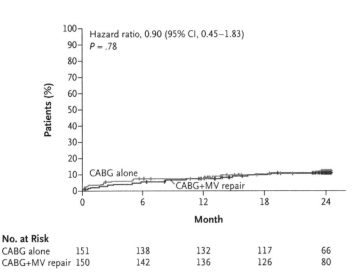

Fig. 9. Rate of death among patients undergoing either CABG or CABG plus mitral valve (MV) repair for moderate ischemic mitral regurgitation: 2-year results of the CTSN trial. CI, confidence interval. (*From* Michler RE, Smith PK, Parides MK, et al. Two-year outcomes of surgical treatment of moderate ischemic mitral regurgitation. N Engl J Med 2016;374(20):1932–41; with permission.)

No. at Risk					
CABG alone	151	138	132	117	66
CABG+MV repair	150	142	136	126	80

Table 1
Summary of the European Society of Cardiology (ESC)/European Association for Cardio-Thoracic Surgery (EACTS), American Heart Association (AHA)/American College of Cardiology (ACC), and American Association for Thoracic Surgery (AATS) guidelines for the management of patients with functional mitral regurgitation

Severity of Mitral Regurgitation	Type of Surgery Considered	2012 ESC/EACTS Guidelines (47)	2014 AHA/ACC Guidelines (18)	2017 AATS Guidelines (17)
Mild	CABG ± mitral valve surgery or isolated mitral valve surgery	There are no data to support surgical correction of mild mitral regurgitation.	Not addressed (*)	Not addressed (*)
Moderate	CABG ± mitral valve surgery	Surgery should be considered in patients with moderate MR undergoing CABG. *Class IIb, Level of Evidence C*	*Mitral valve repair may be considered for patients with chronic moderate secondary MR (stage B) who are undergoing other cardiac surgery Class IIb, Level of Evidence C*	In patients with moderate ischemic mitral regurgitation undergoing CABG, mitral valve repair with an undersized complete rigid annuloplasty ring may be considered *Class IIb, Level of Evidence B*
	Isolated mitral valve surgery	Not addressed	Not addressed	Not addressed

(continued on next page)

Table 1
(continued)

Severity of Mitral Regurgitation	Type of Surgery Considered	2012 ESC/EACTS Guidelines (47)	2014 AHA/ACC Guidelines (18)	2017 AATS Guidelines (17)
Severe	CABG ± mitral valve surgery	Surgery is indicated in patients with severe MR undergoing CABG, and LVEF >30%. *Class I, Level of Evidence C* Surgery should be considered in symptomatic patients with severe MR, LVEF <30% option for revascularization and evidence of viability *Class IIa, Level of Evidence C*	Mitral valve surgery is reasonable for patients with chronic severe secondary MR (stages C and D) who are undergoing CABG or AVR *Class IIa, Level of Evidence C*	*Mitral valve replacement* is reasonable in patients with severe ischemic mitral regurgitation who remain symptomatic despite guideline-directed medial and cardiac device therapy, and who have a basal aneurysm/dyskinesis, significant leaflet tethering, and/or severe LV dilatation (end diastolic diameter >6.5 cm) *Class IIa, Level of Evidence B* *Mitral valve repair* with an undersized complete rigid annuloplasty ring may be considered in patient with severe IMR who remain symptomatic despite guideline-directed medical and cardiac device therapy and who do not have a basal aneurysm/dyskinesis, significant leaflet tethering, or severe LV enlargement *Class IIb, Level of Evidence B*
	Isolated mitral valve surgery	Surgery may be considered in patients with severe MR, LVEF >30%, who remain symptomatic despite optimal medical management (including CRT if indicated) and have low comorbidity, when revascularization is not indicated. *Class IIb, Level of Evidence C*	Mitral valve surgery may be considered for severely symptomatic patients (NYHA class III/IV) with chronic severe secondary MR (stage D) *Class IIb, Level of Evidence B*	Not addressed

| Repair vs. replacement | Not addressed | Not addressed | *Mitral valve replacement* for ischemic mitral regurgitation is performed with complete preservation of both anterior and posterior leaflet
Class I, Level of Evidence B
Mitral valve repair for ischemic mitral regurgitation is performed with small, undersized complete rigid annuloplasty ring
Class IIa, Level of Evidence B |

(*) It is not indicated.

Abbreviations: AVR, aortic valve replacement; CABG, coronary artery bypass surgery; CRT, cardiac resynchronization therapy; IMR, ischemic mitral regurgitation; LV, left ventricle; LVEF, left ventricular ejection fraction; MR, mitral regurgitation; NYHA, New York Heart Association.

Data from Refs. [17,18,47]

surgery should be considered cautiously on patients with very low LVEF (<30%), no targets for revascularization, or no viability because their operative risk is very high and the benefits may be limited. Those patients should be considered for mechanical circulatory support or heart transplantation.[54] In terms of the type of mitral valve surgery, the decision to repair or replace remains controversial given the high rate of recurrence with repair (32% at 1 year and 59% at 2 years). It appears that the patients at higher risk of mitral regurgitation recurrence are those who have larger degree of LV remodeling as evidenced by significant leaflet tethering, severe LV dilatation (LV end diastolic diameter >6.5 cm), aneurysm, or dyskinesis of the basal inferior wall, or no targets for revascularization on that region. Those patients would benefit from replacement rather than repair. In addition, the experience of the surgeon and the presence of technical issues that would require the performance of more complex, prolonged, or less reliable repairs should also weigh into replacing the valve. Even though the 2-year results of the CTSN trial did not show any difference in survival or LV function or remodeling between mitral valve repair or replacement in spite of the high rate of mitral regurgitation recurrence, the study showed a higher rate of heart failure events and readmissions.[44,48] The lack of significant demonstrable clinical adverse effect of recurrent or persistent mitral regurgitation at 2 years is likely the result of the short follow-up. It is reasonable to expect that the persistence or recurrence of mitral regurgitation will have adverse long-term consequences that may manifest beyond 2 years.

Moderate Mitral Regurgitation

For patients with moderate ischemic mitral regurgitation undergoing CABG, the addition of mitral valve repair is associated with an increased rate of perioperative stroke and supraventricular arrhythmias with no significant differences in heart failure symptoms, degree of LV reverse remodeling, LV function, or survival at 2 years.[52,53] The AATS guidelines recommend the consideration of mitral valve repair on these patients (see **Table 1**) but it does not provide conclusive recommendations on when to perform it.[17] The investigators also recommend the consideration of other clinical aspects that, although unsupported by evidence, make clinical sense: (1) Is the patient complaining mostly of heart failure symptoms, dyspnea rather than angina? Are the left-sided filling pressures elevated or the left atrium dilated? If the answer is yes to any of these questions, the addition of an annuloplasty may be

reasonable. (2) To how much additional risk would this patient be subjected? Risk considerations include, for example, technical issues, left atrial size, presence of calcification of the mitral annulus, length of the surgical procedure, frailty, or need to convert to an on-pump approach. (c) The viability and presence of targets for bypass in the inferior wall is also important to consider. If the inferior wall is ischemic but viable with good revascularization targets, it is possible that the mitral regurgitation will improve after CABG alone.

There are no data to support mitral valve replacement in patients with moderate mitral regurgitation undergoing CABG. There are also no data to support the performance of isolated mitral valve surgery in these patients.

Mild Mitral Regurgitation

There are no data to support the surgical correction of mild mitral regurgitation.

MANAGEMENT OF FUNCTIONAL MITRAL VALVE REGURGITATION IN NONISCHEMIC CARDIOMYOPATHY

The treatment of functional mitral regurgitation in nonischemic cardiomyopathy follows the same principles and guidelines as in ischemic cardiomyopathy: both the mitral valve and ventricular remodeling should be addressed.[55] Surgery is indicated in patients with severe mitral regurgitation with persistent symptoms in spite of optimal medical therapy.[17,18] The uncertainties in terms of mitral valve repair versus replacement are similar to those in ischemic mitral regurgitation. However, restrictive mitral valve annuloplasty appears more effective in resolving mitral regurgitation than ischemic cardiomyopathy.[56–58] The rate of mitral regurgitation recurrence and survival are also better. Patients with very low EF, severely remodeled ventricles, and severe leaflet tethering also should be considered for chordal sparing valve replacement rather than repair.

The addition of ventricular restraint devices (CorCap; Acorn Cardiovascular Inc, St Paul, MN) to mitral valve repair has been associated with greater LV reverse remodeling and lower rate of mitral regurgitation recurrence.[59]

TRANSCATHETER MITRAL VALVE PROCEDURES

Transcatheter procedures to address mitral regurgitation can be grouped in annuloplasty procedures, leaflet procedures, chordal procedures, and mitral valve replacement.

Many of these procedures are in early stages of development or in clinical trials, but promise to revolutionize the treatment of mitral valve disease and expand the treatment to patients who are not candidates for open surgical procedures.[60,61]

The most studied device has been the MitraClip (Abbott Vascular; Santa Clara, CA), which creates an edge-to-edge repair similar to the Alfieri stitch. It has been approved by the Food and Drug Administration (FDA) for organic mitral regurgitation in symptomatic patients who are not surgical candidates and is being studied for functional mitral regurgitation. MitraClip is also approved in Europe for functional mitral regurgitation. The EVEREST II (Endovascular Valve Edge-to-Edge Repair) trial randomized patients with either organic (73%) or functional (27%) mitral regurgitation to mitral valve repair (n = 95) or MitraClip (n = 184). At 4 years, there was no difference in survival, or in the degree of improvement in LV dimensions, or in NYHA functional class between surgery and MitraClip. Both groups showed significant improvement in mitral regurgitation. However, at 4 years, the proportion of patients with grade +3 or +4 mitral regurgitation was higher in the MitraClip group (20.6% vs 9.1%). Patients who received the MitraClip required surgery for valve dysfunction more often (24.8% vs 5.5%, $P<.001$). Interestingly in the functional subgroup, +3 or +4 mitral regurgitation recurrence was more common in the surgical arm.[62,63] The results of this trial supported the FDA approval of MitraClip for the treatment of organic mitral regurgitation. The COAPT trial (Clinical Outcomes Assessment of the MitraClip Percutaneous Therapy for Extremely High-Surgical-Risk Patients) trial randomized nonsurgical candidates with functional $\geq$ +3 mitral regurgitation to (1) optimal medical therapy and MitraClip procedure, or (2) optimal medical therapy alone. The primary effectiveness endpoint of the trial was survival and heart failure hospitalizations.

MITRAL VALVE STENOSIS

Mitral stenosis is commonly associated with rheumatic heart disease and senile calcific stenosis. The incidence of rheumatic heart disease has decreased in the developed world but continues to increase in third-world countries, in immigrant populations, and in underserved areas.[1] There is also senile calcific mitral stenosis characterized by calcification of the leaflets extending into the annulus without fusion of the commissures. This is increasingly prevalent in the elderly.[18]

Severe mitral stenosis leads to congestive heart failure by increasing left atrial pressure and pulmonary venous pressure. It is usually associated with atrial fibrillation that exacerbates the hemodynamic impairment and symptoms. Rheumatic and calcific mitral stenosis can be associated with variable degrees of mitral regurgitation.[18]

The indications for intervention in mitral stenosis are well stabilized in the AHA/ACC Guidelines. Percutaneous mitral balloon commissurotomy is the preferred treatment for symptomatic patents with severe rheumatic mitral stenosis, favorable anatomy, and no contraindications.[18] Percutaneous mitral balloon commissurotomy is not an option for patients with senile calcific stenosis. Mitral valve replacement is indicated in symptomatic patients with severe mitral stenosis who have failed or who are not candidates for percutaneous mitral balloon commissurotomy. Several centers outside the United States have developed extensive experience with mitral valve repair for rheumatic mitral valve disease achieving excellent long-term results.[64] Mitral annular calcification possesses a formidable technical challenge during mitral valve surgery and is associated with atrioventricular dissociation and perivalvular leak. The excision or exclusion of the left atrial appendage and the management of atrial fibrillation during mitral valve surgery is important to decrease the risk of thromboembolic complications.

SUMMARY

Mitral valve diseases are common causes of congestive heart failure. Chronic primary and secondary (functional) mitral valve regurgitation are the most common reasons. Valve repair for primary mitral regurgitation cures mitral valve disease, whereas in functional regurgitation, mitral valve repair is associated with high failure rates secondary to persistent/progressive ventricular dysfunction and remodeling. Most patients can be managed with strict adherence to the valve guidelines. Mitral valve replacement has an increased role in the management of functional mitral regurgitation. Surgery for mitral valve disease is indicated in symptomatic patients with severe valve disease and in asymptotic patients before irreversible ventricular damage occurs.

REFERENCES

1. Benjamin EJ, Blaha MJ, Chiuve SE, et al, American Heart Association Statistics Committee and Stroke Statistics Subcommittee. Heart disease and stroke statistics-2017 update: a report from the American Heart Association. Circulation 2017; 135(10):e146–603 [Erratum appears in Circulation

2017;135(10):e646; Erratum appears in Circulation 2017;136(10):e196].

2. Nkomo VT, Gardin JM, Skelton TN, et al. Burden of valvular heart diseases: a population- based study. Lancet 2006;368:1005–11.

3. Harvest 1- Executive summary adult cardiac surgery database. 2017. Available at: https://www.sts.org/sites/default/files/documents/ACSD2017Harvest3_ExecutiveSummary.pdf Accessed November 30, 2017.

4. Adams DH, Rosenhek R, Falk V. Degenerative mitral valve regurgitation: best practice revolution [review]. Eur Heart J 2010;31(16):1958–66.

5. Magne J, Sénéchal M, Dumesnil JG, et al. Ischemic mitral regurgitation: a complex multifaceted disease. Cardiology 2009;112(4):244–59.

6. Lancellotti P, Marwick T, Pierard LA. How to manage ischaemic mitral regurgitation. Heart 2008;94(11):1497–502.

7. Levine RA, Hung J, Otsuji Y, et al. Mechanistic insights into functional mitral regurgitation. Curr Cardiol Rep 2002;4(2):125–9.

8. Crestanello JA. Surgical approach to mitral regurgitation in chronic heart failure: when is it an option? [review]. Curr Heart Fail Rep 2012;9(1):40–50.

9. Grigioni F, Detaint D, Avierinos JF, et al. Contribution of ischemic mitral regurgitation to congestive heart failure after myocardial infarction. J Am Coll Cardiol 2005;45(2):260–7.

10. Grigioni F, Enriquez-Sarano M, Zehr KJ, et al. Ischemic mitral regurgitation: long-term outcome and prognostic implications with quantitative Doppler assessment. Circulation 2001;103(13):1759–64.

11. Bursi F, Enriquez-Sarano M, Nkomo VT, et al. Heart failure and death after myocardial infarction in the community: the emerging role of mitral regurgitation. Circulation 2005;111(3):295–301.

12. Lamas GA, Mitchell GF, Flaker GC, et al. Clinical significance of mitral regurgitation after acute myocardial infarction. Survival and ventricular enlargement investigators. Circulation 1997;96:827–33.

13. Agricola E, Oppizzi M, Pisani M, et al. Ischemic mitral regurgitation: mechanisms and echocardiographic classification. Eur J Echocardiogr 2008;9(2):207–21.

14. Watanabe N, Ogasawara Y, Yamaura Y, et al. Geometric differences of the mitral valve tenting between anterior and inferior myocardial infarction with significant ischemic mitral regurgitation: quantitation by novel software system with transthoracic real-time three-dimensional echocardiography. J Am Soc Echocardiogr 2006;19(1):71–5.

15. Nagasaki M, Nishimura S, Ohtaki E, et al. The echocardiographic determinants of functional mitral regurgitation differ in ischemic and non-ischemic cardiomyopathy. Int J Cardiol 2006;108(2):171–6.

16. Kwan J, Shiota T, Agler DA, et al. Real-time three-dimensional echocardiography study. Geometric differences of the mitral apparatus between ischemic and dilated cardiomyopathy with significant mitral regurgitation: real-time three-dimensional echocardiography study. Circulation 2003;107(8):1135–40.

17. Kron IL, LaPar DJ, Acker MA, et al. 2016 update to the American Association for Thoracic Surgery (AATS) consensus guidelines: ischemic mitral valve regurgitation. J Thorac Cardiovasc Surg 2017;153(5):e97–114.

18. Nishimura RA, Otto CM, Bonow RO, et al. 2017 AHA/ACC focused update of the 2014 AHA/ACC guideline for the management of patients with valvular heart disease: a report of the American College of Cardiology/American Heart Association Task Force on clinical practice guidelines. Circulation 2017;135(25):e1159–95.

19. Enriquez-Sarano M, Avierinos JF, Messika-Zeitoun D, et al. Quantitative determinants of the outcome of asymptomatic mitral regurgitation. N Engl J Med 2005;352:875–83.

20. Suri RM, Vanoverschelde JL, Grigioni F, et al. Association between early surgical intervention vs. watchful waiting and outcomes for mitral regurgitation due to flail mitral valve leaflets. JAMA 2013;310:609–16.

21. Mohty D, Orszulak TA, Schaff HV, et al. Very long-term survival and durability of mitral valve repair for mitral valve prolapse. Circulation 2001;104(12 Suppl 1):I1–7.

22. Enriquez-Sarano M, Schaff HV, Orszulak TA, et al. Valve repair improves the outcome of surgery for mitral regurgitation. A multivariate analysis. Circulation 1995;91(4):1022–8.

23. Vassileva CM, Mishkel G, McNeely C, et al. Long-term survival of patients undergoing mitral valve repair and replacement: a longitudinal analysis of Medicare fee-for-service beneficiaries. Circulation 2013;127:1870–6.

24. Suri RM, Schaff HV, Dearani JA, et al. Survival advantage and improved durability of mitral repair for leaflet prolapse subsets in the current era. Ann Thorac Surg 2006;82(3):819–26.

25. Jouan J, Berrebi A, Chauvaud S, et al. Mitral valve reconstruction in Barlow disease: long-term echographic results and implications for surgical management. J Thorac Cardiovasc Surg 2012;143(4 Suppl):S17–20.

26. David TE. Outcomes of mitral valve repair for mitral regurgitation due to degenerative disease. Semin Thorac Cardiovasc Surg 2007;19:116–20.

27. David TE, Burns RJ, Bacchus CM, et al. Mitral valve replacement for mitral regurgitation with and without preservation of chordae tendineae. J Thorac Cardiovasc Surg 1984;88:718–25.

28. Yun KL, Sintek CF, Miller C, et al. Randomized trial comparing partial versus complete chordal-sparing mitral valve replacement: effects on left ventricular volume and function. J. Thorac Cardiovasc Surg 2002;123:707–14.

29. Suri RM, Aviernos JF, Dearani JA, et al. Management of less-than-severe mitral regurgitation: should guidelines recommend earlier surgical intervention? Eur J Cardiothorac Surg 2011;40(2):496–502.

30. Velazquez EJ, Lee KL, Jones RH, et al, STICHES Investigators. Coronary-artery bypass surgery in patients with ischemic cardiomyopathy. N Engl J Med 2016;374(16):1511–20.

31. Michler RE, Rouleau JL, Al-Khalidi H, et al. Insights from the STICH trial: change in left ventricular size after coronary artery bypass grafting with and without surgical ventricular reconstruction. J Thorac Cardiovasc Surg 2013;146(5). https://doi.org/10.1016/j.jtcvs.2012.09.007.

32. Koene RJ, Kealhofer JV, Adabag S, et al. Effect of coronary artery bypass graft surgery on left ventricular systolic function. J Thorac Dis 2017;9(2):262–70.

33. Choi J, Daly RC, Lin G, et al. Impact of surgical ventricular reconstruction on sphericity index in patients with ischemic cardiomyopathy: follow-up from the STICH trial. Eur J Heart Fail 2015;17(4):453–63.

34. Bolling SF, Smolens IA, Pagani FD. Surgical alternatives for heart failure. J Heart Lung Transplant 2001;20:729–33.

35. Romano MA, Bolling SF. Update on mitral repair in dilated cardiomyopathy. J Card Surg 2004;19(5):396–400.

36. Spoor MT, Geltz A, Bolling SF. Flexible versus nonflexible mitral valve rings for congestive heart failure: differential durability of repair. Circulation 2006;114(1 Suppl):I67–71.

37. Kron IL, Hung J, Overbey JR, et al, CTSN Investigators. Predicting recurrent mitral regurgitation after mitral valve repair for severe ischemic mitral regurgitation. J Thorac Cardiovasc Surg 2015;149(3):752–761 e1.

38. Borger MA, Alam A, Murphy PM, et al. Chronic ischemic mitral regurgitation: repair, replace or rethink? Ann Thorac Surg 2006;81(3):1153–61.

39. Borger MA, Murphy PM, Alam A, et al. Initial results of the chordal-cutting operation for ischemic mitral regurgitation. J Thorac Cardiovasc Surg 2007;133:1483–92.

40. Maisano F, Caldarola A, Blasio A, et al. Midterm results of edge-to-edge mitral valve repair without annuloplasty. J Thorac Cardiovasc Surg 2003;126:1987–97.

41. De Bonis M, Lapenna E, La Canna G, et al. Mitral valve repair for functional mitral regurgitation in end-stage dilated cardiomyopathy: role of the "edge-to-edge" technique. Circulation 2005;112(9 Suppl):I402–8.

42. Kron IL, Green GR, Cope JT. Surgical relocation of the posterior papillary muscle in chronic ischemic mitral regurgitation. Ann Thorac Surg 2002;74:600–1.

43. Fattouch K, Castrovinci S, Murana G, et al. Papillary muscle relocation and mitral annuloplasty in ischemic mitral valve regurgitation: midterm results. J Thorac Cardiovasc Surg 2014;148(5):1947–50.

44. Goldstein D, Moskowitz AJ, Gelijns AC, et al, CTSN. Two-year outcomes of surgical treatment of severe ischemic mitral regurgitation. N Engl J Med 2016;374(4):344–53.

45. Magne J, Girerd N, Sénéchal M, et al. Mitral repair versus replacement for ischemic mitral regurgitation: comparison of short-term and long-term survival. Circulation 2009;120(11 Suppl):S104–11.

46. Lorusso R, Gelsomino S, Vizzardi E, et al. Mitral valve repair or replacement for ischemic mitral regurgitation? The Italian Study on the Treatment of Ischemic Mitral Regurgitation (ISTIMIR). J Thorac Cardiovasc Surg 2013;145:128–39 [discussion: 137–8].

47. Vahanian A, Alfieri O, Andreotti F, et al. Guidelines on the management of valvular heart disease (version 2012). Eur Heart J 2012;33:2451–96.

48. Acker MA, Parides MK, Perrault LP, et al, CTSN. Mitral-valve repair versus replacement for severe ischemic mitral regurgitation. N Engl J Med 2014;370(1):23–32.

49. Maltais S, Schaff HV, Daly RC, et al. Mitral regurgitation surgery in patients with ischemic cardiomyopathy and ischemic mitral regurgitation: factors that influence survival. J Thorac Cardiovasc Surg 2011;142(5):995–1001.

50. Bolling SF, Li S, O'Brien SM, et al. Predictors of mitral valve repair: clinical and surgeon factors. Ann Thorac Surg 2010;90(6):1904–11 [discussion: 1912].

51. Chikwe J, Toyoda N, Anyanwu AC, et al. Relation of mitral valve surgery volume to repair rate, durability, and survival. J Am Coll Cardiol 2017. https://doi.org/10.1016/j.jacc.2017.02.026.

52. Smith PK, Puskas JD, Ascheim DD, et al, Cardiothoracic Surgical Trials Network Investigators. Surgical treatment of moderate ischemic mitral regurgitation. N Engl J Med 2014;371(23):2178–88.

53. Michler RE, Smith PK, Parides MK, et al, CTSN. Two-year outcomes of surgical treatment of moderate ischemic mitral regurgitation. N Engl J Med 2016;374(20):1932–41.

54. Maltais S, Tchantchaleishvili V, Schaff HV, et al. Management of severe ischemic cardiomyopathy: left ventricular assist device as destination therapy versus conventional bypass and mitral valve surgery. J Thorac Cardiovasc Surg 2014;147(4):1246–50.

55. Ngaage DL, Schaff HV. Mitral valve surgery in non-ischemic cardiomyopathy. J Cardiovasc Surg (Torino) 2004;45(5):477–86 [review].

56. Geidel S, Lass M, Krause K, et al. Early and late results of restrictive mitral valve annuloplasty in 121 patients with cardiomyopathy and chronic mitral regurgitation. Thorac Cardiovasc Surg 2008;56(5): 262–8.

57. Gummert JF, Rahmel A, Bucerius J, et al. Mitral valve repair in patients with end stage cardiomyopathy: who benefits? Eur J Cardiothorac Surg 2003;23(6): 1017–22.

58. Hueb AC, Jatene FB, Moreira LF, et al. Ventricular remodeling and mitral valve modifications in dilated cardiomyopathy: new insights from anatomic study. J Thorac Cardiovasc Surg 2002; 124(6):1216–24.

59. Acker MA, Jessup M, Bolling SF, et al. Mitral valve repair in heart failure: five-year follow-up from the mitral valve replacement stratum of the Acorn randomized trial. J Thorac Cardiovasc Surg 2011; 142(3):569–74.

60. Bapat V, Rajagopal V, Meduri C, et al, Intrepid Global Pilot Study Investigators. Early experience with new transcatheter mitral valve replacement. J Am Coll Cardiol 2017. https://doi.org/10.1016/j.jacc.2017.10.061.

61. Maisano F, Alfieri O, Banai S, et al. The future of transcatheter mitral valve interventions: competitive or complementary role of repair vs. replacement? Eur Heart J 2015;36(26):1651–9.

62. Mauri L, Foster E, Glower DD, et al, EVEREST II Investigators. 4-year results of a randomized controlled trial of percutaneous repair versus surgery for mitral regurgitation. J Am Coll Cardiol 2013;62(4):317–28.

63. clinicaltrials.gov. Available at: https://clinicaltrials.gov/ct2/show/NCT01626079?term=COAPT&rank=1. Accessed November 3, 2017.

64. Dillon J, Yakub MA, Kong PK, et al. Comparative long-term results of mitral valve repair in adults with chronic rheumatic disease and degenerative disease: is repair for "burnt-out" rheumatic disease still inferior to repair for degenerative disease in the current era? J Thorac Cardiovasc Surg 2015;149(3):771–7 [discussion: 777–9].

Current Status of Inotropes in Heart Failure

Mahazarin Ginwalla, MD, MS*, David S. Tofovic, MD

KEYWORDS

- Inotropes • Heart failure • Cardiogenic • Shock • Palliative care • Milrinone • Dobutamine
- Dopamine

KEY POINTS

- In the contemporary era, inotrope use has increased and indications have broadened. Survival with chronic inotrope use has also improved compared with the previous era.
- Inotropes are indicated in acute decompensated heart failure or cardiogenic shock with evidence of hypoperfusion; in cardiogenic shock after myocardial infarction; as a bridge to other therapies, including mechanical circulatory support or cardiac transplantation; to improve renal perfusion in cardiorenal syndrome; in right ventricular heart failure; and as palliative inotrope therapy in end-stage heart failure.
- Selection of an inotropic agent is dictated predominantly by the clinical scenario and the desired physiologic effects. Milrinone and dobutamine are the most commonly used inotropes. Dopamine and digoxin are also useful adjuncts. Newer agents, including levosimendan, omecamtiv mecarbil, and istaroxamine, are being evaluated.
- Inotrope therapy has been noted to alleviate symptoms, improve quality of life, decrease hospitalizations, and reduce length of stay in end-stage heart failure. It has also been shown to be cost-effective as a palliative option.

HISTORY OF INOTROPES

Although the first mentions of edema and dyspnea can be found in Greek and Roman texts from antiquity, the modern age of the study of heart failure began in the twentieth century when advances in hemodynamic study and later heart catheterization allowed for newfound insight into cardiovascular function.[1,2] Effective treatment, however, lagged with early focus directed toward the discovery of improved diuretics.

Digitalis, or digoxin, was the first inotrope to be successfully implemented in the treatment of heart failure.[3] William Withering postulated its usefulness more than 200 years ago when giving herbal remedies containing the foxglove plant,[3] with digoxin being isolated from it as the active metabolite in the 1930s.[4]

Meanwhile, at the University College in London, England, George Oliver and Edward Albert Shäfer began studying the effects of the suprarenal gland, first witnessing the direct actions of catecholamines.[5,6] The Japanese chemist Jokichi Takamine isolated epinephrine in pure crystal form in 1901.[5,7] Over the next 60 years, the various other catecholamines and hundreds of sympathomimetic substances were discovered and purified. Our knowledge of their mechanisms of action was elucidated with the first uses of this group in heart failure and cardiogenic shock (CS) occurring in the 1960s to 1970s.[8]

Disclosure: The authors have nothing to disclose.
Division of Cardiovascular Medicine, Harrington Heart & Vascular Institute, University Hospitals Cleveland Medical Center, Cleveland, OH, USA
* Corresponding author. Division of Cardiovascular Medicine, Harrington Heart & Vascular Institute, University Hospitals Cleveland Medical Center, 11100 Euclid Avenue, Mailstop LKS 5038, Cleveland, OH 44106.
E-mail address: Mahazarin.Ginwalla@UHhospitals.org

Heart Failure Clin 14 (2018) 601–616
https://doi.org/10.1016/j.hfc.2018.06.010
1551-7136/18/© 2018 Elsevier Inc. All rights reserved.

Beginning toward the end of this period, the next big breakthroughs arrived. With the catecholamine pathway elucidated, phosphodiesterase inhibitors became a novel treatment by altering downstream targets in this conduit.[9] More recently, sarcoplasmic reticulum calcium ATPase isoform 2a (SERCA2a) stimulators, myosin/actin cross-bridge enhancers, and calcium sensitizers have come to show significant promise.

FROM THEN TO NOW: CURRENT INDICATIONS FOR INOTROPES

In the contemporary era, inotrope use has increased and indications have broadened. Survival with chronic inotrope use has also improved compared with the previous era before the early 2000s. Current guidelines suggest their utilization in CS or in hypotension/hypoperfusion due to heart failure (**Box 1**).[10,11] Their usefulness extends to after a myocardial infarction (MI); perioperatively during cardiac surgery; as a bridge to advanced therapies, including transplantation; and as chronic palliative inotrope therapy in end-stage heart failure (**Box 2**). Selection of an inotropic agent in advanced heart failure is dictated predominantly by clinical scenario and the desired physiologic effects.[12] The major indications of inotropes are reviewed next.

Acute Decompensated Heart Failure/ Cardiogenic Shock

Inotropic therapy may be beneficial in patients with severely depressed cardiac output, systemic hypoperfusion, and end-organ dysfunction. Milrinone and dobutamine are the commonly used inotropes for patients with acutely decompensated heart failure. Several studies show improvement in heart failure symptoms with the use of dobutamine and milrinone at continuous infusion doses; however, there is associated increased mortality and it should be used only if evidence of hypoperfusion.[12,13]

The OPTIME (Outcomes of a Prospective Trial of Intravenous Milrinone for Exacerbations of Chronic Heart Failure) study of short-term milrinone use in patients with acute decompensated heart failure without CS suggested a more favorable response in patients with nonischemic cardiomyopathy compared with ischemic cardiomyopathy on subgroup analysis.[14] Overall, milrinone use did not show a benefit in days spent hospitalized for cardiovascular cause, short-term to midterm mortality, nor a composite of death or readmission and was associated with increased rates of atrial arrhythmias and sustained hypotension requiring intervention.[14] These results

---

Box 1
Current guidelines regarding oral and intravenous inotrope use in heart failure

American College of Cardiology Foundation/ American Heart Association 2013

- Acute CS to maintain end-organ perfusion until definitive therapy or resolution of acute cause (*class I, level C*)
- Stage D heart failure refractory to standard therapy as a bridge to ventricular assist devices or transplantation (*class IIa, level B*)
- Patients with stage D heart failure refractory to standard therapy who are not candidates for ventricular assist devices or transplantation as a palliative measure (*class IIa, level B*)
- Documented severe systolic heart failure presenting with low blood pressure and worsened cardiac output as a short-term therapy to maintain end-organ perfusion (*class IIa, level B*)
- Low-dose dopamine infusion to loop diuretics in the decompensated heart to preserve renal function and improve diuresis (*class IIb, level B*)
- Digoxin in reduced left ventricular ejection fraction and persistent heart failure symptoms despite optimal medical therapy (*class IIa, level B*)

European Society of Cardiologists 2016

- Acute heart failure complicated by hypotension (SBP <85 mm Hg), hypoperfusion, and/ or shock (*class IIb, level C*)
- Levosimendan or phosphodiesterase inhibitor in patients with hypotension, hypoperfusion, or shock thought to be due to over beta-blockade (*class IIa, level C*)
- Digoxin in concomitant NYHA class IV and atrial fibrillation with rapid ventricular rate in patients who are digoxin naive (*class IIa, level B*)
- Digoxin in concomitant NYHA class I to III and atrial fibrillation with inadequate response, intolerance, or contraindication to beta-blockers (*class IIa, level B*)
- Digoxin in reduced left ventricular ejection fraction and persistent heart failure symptoms despite ACE-I (or ARB), beta-blockers, and mineralocorticoid receptor agonist (*class IIb, level B*)

Abbreviations: ACE-I, angiotensin-converting enzyme inhibitor; ARB, angiotensin-receptor blocker; NYHA, New York Heart Association; SBP, systolic blood pressure.

Box 2
Indications for inotrope use
Acute decompensated heart failure or CS
Chronic heart failure as a bridge to other therapies
Right ventricular heart failure
Improve renal perfusion in cardiorenal syndrome
After cardiac surgery for hemodynamic support
Palliative home inotrope therapy

indicate that routine use of intravenous milrinone is not indicated in patients hospitalized with acute heart failure.

Levosimendan was studied in acute decompensated heart failure in REVIVE II (Randomized Evaluation of Intravenous Levosimendan Efficacy) and showed increased incidence of hypotension and cardiac arrhythmias.[15] The largest levosimendan trial, SURVIVE (Survival of Patients With Acute Heart Failure in Need of Intravenous Inotropic Support), randomized 1327 patients with acute decompensated heart failure and systolic blood pressure (SBP) greater than 85 mm Hg to short-term levosimendan versus dobutamine.[16] Levosimendan failed to improve the primary outcome of all-cause mortality at 180 days and was associated with increased incidence of atrial fibrillation, headache, and hypokalemia.[16]

Thus, inotropes may be used with close monitoring in patients with documented severe systolic heart failure presenting with low cardiac output as a short-term therapy to maintain end-organ perfusion, while optimizing oral heart failure therapy, or as a bridge to advanced therapies.

Chronic Heart Failure as Bridge to Other Therapies

The limited availability of donor organs creates a need for more effective management of heart disease when bridging patients to cardiac transplant. Inotropic therapy is becoming more commonly used in the long-term to maintain baseline function, whereby it has been shown to be effective in patients with refractory end-stage heart failure as a bridge to cardiac transplantation or left ventricular assist device (LVAD) implantation. In one study, both milrinone (84.8%) and dobutamine (15.2%) were used as a bridge to transplant/LVAD.[17] Median survival was 9 months with an actuarial 1-year survival of 47.6% and 2-year survival of 38.4%. Of the

60 patients placed on inotropes as a bridge to transplant/LVAD, 55 were successfully maintained on inotropes until transplant/LVAD.[17]

A separate study found that 46 of 60 patients studied were successfully bridged to transplant with milrinone, but 14 required LVAD because of clinical deterioration. Mean waiting times were significantly shorter in the transplant group (59.5 vs 112.0 days) for patients receiving milrinone who did not require an LVAD.[18] This study suggests that chronic intravenous milrinone provides an adequate strategy as a bridge to transplant if the waiting time is short (<100 days), whereas an elective ventricular assist device implantation may be a safer strategy for patients expected to wait longer.

Fixed pulmonary hypertension is a contraindication to cardiac transplantation in patients with advanced heart failure, and inotropes may help reduce pulmonary vascular resistance (PVR). A query of the United Network for Organ Sharing (UNOS) registry for all adult patients listed for primary heart transplantation with evidence of pulmonary hypertension noted similar rates of PVR reduction, rates of PVR normalization, and waitlist mortality between inotrope and LVAD therapy.[19] This finding suggests that inotropes may be used in patients with advanced heart failure with elevated PVR as an effective strategy to achieve normalization of PVR before cardiac transplantation.[19]

Cardiogenic Shock After Acute Myocardial Infarction

Inotropes may be used as an adjunctive/supportive therapy in patients with acute CS after acute MI (AMI). The American College of Cardiology Foundation/American Heart Association's current ST-segment elevation MI (STEMI) guidelines recommend individualized support with inotropes guided by invasive hemodynamic monitoring but do not specify a preferred agent.[20] However, they note that use of dopamine may be associated with excess hazard,[21] whereas the German-Austrian S3 CS guidelines state that its use is contraindicated.[22] In contrast to this, the European Society of Cardiology's (ESC) 2012 STEMI guidelines make a IIa recommendation for the use of dopamine in patients with STEMI with hypotension and hypoperfusion.[23]

Dobutamine carries a IIa recommendation in the ESC 2012 STEMI guidelines[23] and is deemed the drug of choice in the German-Austrian S3 guidelines for inotropic support in AMI complicated by CS.[22] Although it has previously been the inotrope of choice in this scenario, little prospective evidence exists and no compelling evidence demonstrates the superiority of dobutamine over another agent. Several investigators have suggested a hemodynamic benefit of combined dobutamine and dopamine to improve hemodynamics and limit side effects,[24,25] yet the source commonly cited for this practice is from a study of 8 patients,[26] limiting the evidence for its utility.

In contrast to dobutamine, milrinone is associated with less tachycardia and does not increase myocardial oxygen consumption,[27] which could provide a theoretic benefit.[28] Systemic inflammatory response syndrome (SIRS) leading to lower systemic vascular resistance (SVR) can be seen in patients with CS following AMI.[29] Introduction of milrinone, known to have significant arterial vasodilatory effects, could be problematic in such individuals. No large scale randomized, controlled trials have been performed to assess the utility of milrinone for use in CS complicating AMI. A meta-analysis of 4 small studies suggests that treatment with milrinone may be safe and effective for the treatment of CS following AMI.[30]

Levosimendan was also assessed in patients with left ventricular failure following AMI in 2 small trials showing clear benefit[31,32] and one noting a significant decrease in both short and midterm survival with its use.[33] Nonetheless, the ESC's 2012 STEMI guidelines give levosimendan a IIb recommendation, citing particular usefulness in patients on chronic beta-blocker therapy.[23]

A recent Cochrane review of randomized controlled trials in patients with AMI complicated by CS concluded that at present there are no robust and convincing data to support a distinct superior inotropic or vasodilator drug to reduce mortality.[34] Therefore, pharmacologic support with inotropic agents for CS complicating AMI should be individualized and used as an adjunct to prompt revascularization with or without concomitant temporary mechanical support.

Right-Sided Heart Failure

Right ventricular (RV) dysfunction may occur in isolation or in combination with left heart dysfunction. Few clinical studies have evaluated inotropes in the setting of primary RV failure. Therefore, the choice of inotropic agent is guided by pharmacologic properties and patient characteristics.

At low doses, dobutamine improves RV-pulmonary artery coupling via reduced PVR and increased RV contractility.[35] It has been successfully used for RV failure in the setting of AMI,[36] pulmonary arterial hypertension,[37] and pulmonary

hypertension in the setting of liver transplantation.[38] Milrinone may also be used in RV failure to augment RV performance via increased contractility. Milrinone decreases PVR more than dobutamine[39] and is, thus, typically considered the inotrope of choice in RV failure due to high pulmonary afterload.[40,41] However, its propensity to decrease SVR and induce hypotension limits its use, often requiring the addition of a vasopressor. Dopamine may also be used in RV failure to help with congestive hepatopathy or renal disease via splanchnic vasodilation.[37] Experimental data suggest levosimendan improves RV-pulmonary artery coupling more effectively than dobutamine.[42] In patients with left ventricular dysfunction and pulmonary hypertension, levosimendan causes similar reductions in PVR and mean pulmonary artery pressure as milrinone but comparatively causes more tachycardia and pressor requiring hypotension.[43]

Improve Renal Perfusion in Cardiorenal Syndrome

Literature documenting improved outcomes with inotropic therapy in acute cardiorenal syndrome is lacking. Nonetheless, inotropic agents, including dopamine, dobutamine, and milrinone, are commonly used in this setting. Although logical inotropic agent choices should be guided by patient and drug characteristics, previous research suggests that agent choice is also affected by individual and institutional preferences.[44]

Of note, dopamine was evaluated in the ROSE AHF trial (Renal Optimization Strategies Evaluation in Acute Heart Failure), which noted no difference between low-dose dopamine, low-dose nesiritide, and placebo in diuresis or preservation of renal function in patients with decompensated heart failure and renal dysfunction[45] However, the study found that there may be differential responses to dopamine in patients with reduced versus preserved ejection fraction (EF). Compared with placebo, dopamine was associated with higher urine output and improved clinical outcomes in heart failure with reduced EF and worse clinical outcomes in heart failure with preserved EF. Moreover, the trial only enrolled individuals with an SBP of greater than 90 mm Hg.[45] Therefore, dopamine may still play a role in patients with heart failure with SBPs of less than 90 mm Hg, and its use should be individualized.

Post Cardiac Surgery for Hemodynamic Support

Inotropes are commonly used to treat myocardial dysfunction, which is the major complication after coronary artery bypass graft (CABG) and valve surgeries. Several trials have evaluated milrinone in patients with low ventricular EF undergoing CABG surgery, but results have been inconclusive. A recent meta-analysis determined that perioperative continuous infusion of milrinone is effective in lowering the incidence of myocardial ischemia and MI after CABG, but it was unable to improve morbidity and mortality or decrease the duration of intensive care unit stay.[46] Some studies found that it increased the incidence of postoperative atrial arrhythmias. However, the sample size was small.[46]

Prophylactic renal-dosed dopamine administration after CABG was prospectively assessed in 41 patients.[47] The dopamine group was found to have lower creatinine and earlier mobilization compared with placebo. Larger studies are warranted to better determine the role of perioperative prophylactic renal-dosed dopamine.[47]

Recent evidence suggests that levosimendan enhances cardiac function after cardiopulmonary bypass in patients with both normal and reduced left ventricular function.[48] In addition to being used as postoperative rescue therapy for low cardiac output syndrome, preoperative levosimendan infusion in high-risk patients with poor cardiac function may reduce inotropic requirements, the need for mechanical support, the duration of intensive care stay, and postoperative mortality.[48] A comparison of the hemodynamic effects of milrinone, dobutamine, and levosimendan in 60 patients after cardiac valve surgeries showed levosimendan to be equally effective in increasing and maintaining adequate cardiac index (CI) as compared with dobutamine ($P>.05$) but better than milrinone.[49] Larger multicenter randomized trials in cardiac surgery are still needed to deduce its potential.

Palliative Home Inotrope Therapy

Long-term continuous intravenous inotropic support may be considered as palliative therapy for symptom control in select patients with advanced heart failure on optimal therapy who are not candidates for durable mechanical circulatory support or transplant.[10,50] Medicare coverage requires a right heart catheterization within 6 months before the initiation of home inotropic therapy, with documented evidence of poor hemodynamics before and favorable response after initiation of inotrope.[50] The median survival on chronic continuous inotropic therapy has improved in the recent era to 9 to 18 months as compared with 3 to 6 months previously. This improvement may be related to the higher use of guideline-based

heart failure therapy, including beta-blockers, and the presence of defibrillators.[50]

Suitable candidates must understand the goals of palliation and have adequate caregiver support. Given the arrhythmogenic potential of inotropic therapy, patient preference for ongoing implantable cardioverter-defibrillator (ICD) therapy must be discussed, as almost one-fifth of patients on home inotropes will receive an appropriate ICD shock if the device remains activated.[51] Other issues include infection risk due to chronic indwelling intravenous catheter, availability of caregiver assistance, dressing care, inotrope infusion bag changes, and quick access to community and hospice services. Unfortunately, financial coverage for continuous inotropes is often limited if patients transition to hospice care, necessitating discontinuation of the inotrope.

TYPES OF INOTROPES

There are 5 different classes of inotropes according to mechanism of action (**Table 1**). **Fig. 1** summarizes the mechanisms of inotrope action within cardiomyocytes.

Catecholamines

First discovered at the turn of the twentieth century, catecholamines mediate their effects through adrenergic (α_1, α_2, β_1, β_2) and dopaminergic (primary D_1, D_2) receptors. Each receptor type induces a different physiologic response: α_1 receptors increase systemic vascular resistance, β_1 and β_2 receptors heighten cardiac contractility, and D_1 and D_2 receptors produce splanchnic and renal vasodilation. In current practice, 2 catecholamines, dopamine and dobutamine, have been more commonly used.

Dopamine

Dopamine, the precursor to both epinephrine and norepinephrine, was initially discovered as a neurotransmitter in 1957.[52] Since then, laboratory studies have shown a unique dose-dependent mechanism of action due to its differing affinity for various receptors.[53] At low doses, dopamine primarily acts on D_1 and D_2 receptors, inducing localized vasodilation in the cerebral, coronary, splanchnic (or mesenteric), and renal vasculature. Intermediate doses increase cardiac contractility due to activation of β_2 receptors, with even higher doses increasing SVR via α_1 receptor stimulation.[53]

Given its ability to increase renal blood flow via D_1/D_2 receptors,[54] as well as independent natriuretic and diuretic effects, low-dose dopamine has been theorized to be renally protective.[55] In

Table 1
Inotrope pharmacology

	Inotrope Class	Predominant Mechanisms of Action	Half-Life	Excretion
Dobutamine	Catecholamine	Strong beta-adrenergic stimulator causes ↑↑cAMP levels→ actives L-type Ca channel → ↑↑ increase Ca intracellularly	2 min	Tissue metabolism to inactive metabolite
Dopamine	Catecholamine	D_1/D_2 stimulation at low dose, β and α adrenergic stimulator at higher doses; ↑↑cAMP levels→ actives L-type Ca channel → ↑↑Ca intracellularly	2 min	Tissue metabolism to inactive metabolite
Milrinone	PDE inhibitor	PDE inhibitor, prevents cAMP breakdown, which active L-type Ca channels→ ↑↑ increase Ca intracellularly	2.3 h	Renal excretion
Digoxin	Na-K pump inhibitor	Inhibits Na/K antiporter→ ↑↑ increase Ca intracellularly	36–48 h	85% renal excretion
Istaroxime	Na-K pump inhibitor and SERCA2a stimulator	Inhibits Na/K antiporter→ ↑↑ increase Ca intracellularly stimulates SERCA2 on the sarcoplasmic reticulum, improves Ca management, ↑↑ lusitropy	<1 h	Systemic conversion to less active metabolite
Levosimendan	Calcium sensitizer	Sensitizes troponin C to Ca++, improving myosin/actin interaction	~ 1 h for substrate 70–80 h for active metabolite	Renal and gastrointestinal excretion
Omecamtiv mecarbil	Myosin/actin cross-bridge enhancer	Interacts with ATPase on myosin, improving myosin/actin interaction	18.5 h	Renal and gastrointestinal excretion

Abbreviations: Ca, calcium; cAMP, cyclic adenosine monophosphate; K, potassium; Na, sodium; PDE, phosphodiesterase.

one study, renal ultrasounds were compared in patients with chronic heart failure who were given dopamine.[56] Both an increase in cardiac output and in renal perfusion was noted with dopamine administration. However, the increase in perfusion was out of proportion to the level expected to be induced by the increase in cardiac output alone, suggesting a direct effect of dopamine on the renal vasculature.[56]

Previously, a large meta-analysis comparing placebo with low-dose dopamine noted no difference in mortality and need for renal replacement therapy between the two groups.[57] More recently, the aforementioned ROSE AHF trial demonstrated no enhancement in diuresis or improvement in renal function with the addition of either medication compared with placebo.[58] When these trial data were included in a 2016 meta-analysis of 5

other randomized controlled trials and a retrospective study, low-dose dopamine improved renal function and diuresis but did not alter readmission rates or mortality.[59] The addition of low-dose dopamine to oral furosemide has similarly produced no difference in length of stay, all-cause hospitalizations, or mortality; but the dopamine group had a more stable renal and electrolyte profile.[60] Similar results were previously seen with oral furosemide doses used in treatment of refractory cases of decompensated heart failure and with intravenous diuretics in those with renal insufficiency.[61,62] Hence, this potential renoprotective effect of dopamine remains controversial, with a recommendation to consider it in patients with decompensated heart failure and renal dysfunction, a group already at risk of inadequate diuresis, further kidney injury, and mortality.[63–67]

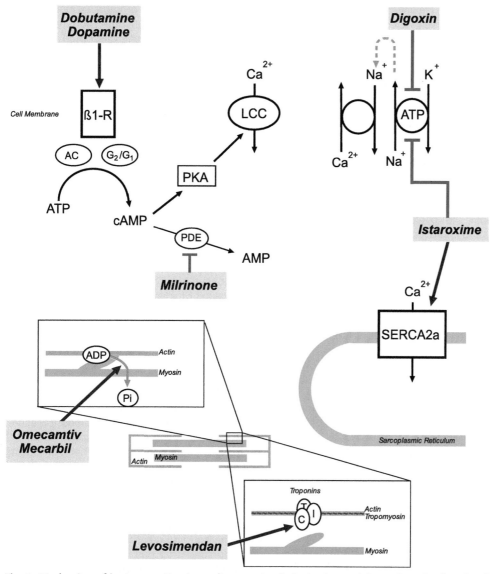

Fig. 1. Mechanism of inotrope action in cardiomyocytes. Dobutamine and dopamine stimulate β_1 adrenergic receptors, activating an adenylate cyclase that increases intracellular cyclic adenosine monophosphate (cAMP). cAMP activates protein kinase A (PKA), which stimulates L-type calcium (Ca) channels (LCC) to increase intracellular Ca levels. Milrinone inhibits the action of phosphodiesterase (PDE), the enzyme that breaks down cAMP into AMP. Digoxin and istaroxime both inhibit a cellular membrane sodium (Na)-potassium (K) ATPase. This inhibition decreases the Na gradient across the myocyte membrane, inhibiting a Na-Ca antiporter and maintaining higher intracellular levels of Ca. Istaroxime also stimulates a sarcoplasmic reticulum Ca ATPase, improving cardiomyocyte relaxation. Levosimendan sensitizes troponin-C on actin to Ca. Omecamtiv mecarbil acts on an ATPase located on myosin to improve actin-myosin crosslinking.

Dobutamine

Dobutamine, a sympathomimetic amine first developed in 1975, acts primarily via β_1 receptors to increase cardiac contractility and, to a lesser degree, heart rate.[68,69] Through α_1 and β_2 receptor activation, it also produces peripheral vasodilation at lower concentrations and vasoconstriction at higher concentrations.[68] Particular care

is warranted during its administration, given its proarrhythmogenic profile.[70] Uncommonly, eosinophilia[71,72] and fever have also been reported with dobutamine use.[73,74]

Given at low doses for a short duration, dobutamine has been shown to provide symptomatic relief in advanced decompensated heart failure, with the effects lasting weeks to months after discontinuation.[75–78] However, this benefit was not readily reproducible in intermittent ambulatory infusions with dobutamine.[79,80] Moreover, its use has been suggested to increase mortality due to arrhythmias,[81] particularly with long-term continuous infusion.[70,82,83] It also demonstrates development of tolerance.[84]

Phosphodiesterase Inhibitors

Phosphodiesterase inhibitors work downstream of adrenergic receptors within cardiomyocytes and vascular smooth muscle to inhibit breakdown of cyclic adenosine monophosphate (cAMP). Within the heart, this increases both calcium entry and removal, with the overall effect of increased contractility and improved lusitropy. In the periphery, increased levels of cAMP predominantly increase calcium expulsion from vascular smooth muscle and cause vasodilation. The most commonplace phosphodiesterase inhibitor currently used is milrinone.

Milrinone

First discovered in the late 1970s,[85] milrinone is a potent systemic vasodilator and weak inotrope.[86] Unlike dobutamine, it produces little change in heart rate or cardiac oxygen consumption.[27,86] It decreases pulmonary artery pressures, broadening its potential utility into patients with co-occurring pulmonary hypertension or RV failure.[27,39] Given that milrinone bypasses ß-adrenergic receptors to exert its affects, it may produce a stronger response in patients on beta-blockers and induce less tolerance compared with the catecholaminergic inotropes.[86] With its strong vasodilator response and long half-life, caution must be taken with its administration in individuals with low filling pressures or low systemic vascular resistance as prolonged and severe hypotension can develop. Moreover, as it is renally excreted, milrinone is generally contraindicated in advanced kidney disease.[87]

Although available in an oral formulation, prolonged oral administration has been linked to increased mortality and is no longer used.[88] Short-term intravenous use has provided mixed results. In comparison with dobutamine, milrinone was shown to more greatly decrease pulmonary capillary wedge pressures in patients after an MI with acute heart failure.[89] Moreover, 2-day infusions of milrinone were shown to improve cardiovascular output, reduce systemic vascular resistance, and improve diuresis.[90] However, these results were not supported when short-course intravenous milrinone was added to standard heart failure therapy, whereby milrinone failed to decreased symptoms, reduce hospitalization lengths, or improve mortality, but did result in more hypotension and atrial arrhythmias.[14] Subset analysis noted increased mortality in ischemic cardiomyopathy but not in nonischemic patients.[91] A potential benefit from milrinone may also be derived in certain subgroups, such as in end-stage cardiac transthyretin-related cardiac amyloidoses (ATTR) amyloidosis. The authors reported the case of one of their patients with end-stage cardiac ATTR amyloidosis who received chronic home milrinone and enjoyed an acceptable quality of life for more than 2 years.[92]

Sodium-Potassium Pump Inhibitors

The first known sodium (Na)-potassium (K) pump inhibitor is the cardiac glycoside digoxin. Inhibition of this pump causes increased intracellular concentrations of Na. This increase, in turn, changes the workload of a Na/calcium channel, increasing intracellular calcium levels. As a result, cardiac contractility increases. More recently, a new drug in this class, istaroxime, has been discovered.

Digoxin

Current guidelines recommend the use of digoxin in heart failure with reduced EF with continued symptoms despite optimal medical therapy.[10] It exhibits little to no effect on blood pressure, heart rate, or myocardial oxygen demand.[93,94] There is also a neurohormonal benefit, producing reduced activation of cardiac sympathetic drive.[94,95] In concomitant heart failure and atrial fibrillation, digoxin has dual value by providing both inotropic support and rate control. It has shown utility in weaning from intravenous inotrope therapy and mechanical support, although no large-scale trial has yet been conducted to confirm this.[96] Its role in end-stage renal disease remains controversial.[97–100] Outside of this group, however, it is known to reduce heart failure admissions and episodes of clinical deterioration but with no discernible effect on mortality.[101–104] This finding was recently supported by an updated Cochrane review of 7896 participants from 13 separate studies.[102] More recently, a post hoc analysis of one of the largest studies to date provided support for its use in diabetic patients with heart failure whereby it similarly reduced heart failure hospitalizations without a reduction in mortality.[104]

Istaroxime

Similar to digoxin, istaroxime acts to block Na-K ATPase, resulting in increased intracellular Na levels.[105,106] Via a second mechanism of action, it also stimulates SERCA2a.[105,106] SERCA2a regulates intracellular cardiomyocyte calcium levels, influencing both inotropy and lusitropy.[107] Its downregulation has been noted in heart failure.[107]

Istaroxime was recently evaluated in a double-blind trial involving 120 patients with systolic heart failure.[106] Improvements in pulmonary wedge pressure, CI, and left ventricular end-diastolic pressure were noted with administration. Interestingly, istaroxime decreased heart rate and increased SBP, making it unique among inotropes. No effect was seen on neurohormone levels, renal function, or troponin levels.[106] Further trials are needed to deduce its safety in heart failure.

Calcium-Sensitizing Agents

Elevated intracellular calcium has been suggested to produce maladaptive changes and adverse events in the heart.[108] As both catecholamine and phosphodiester inhibitor inotropes increase calcium levels within cardiomyocytes, potential exists for poor outcomes with their chronic administration. In an effort to bypass these effects, agents aimed directly at improving the calcium-myosin relationship have been developed. Levosimendan has been approved for clinical use in Europe but not in the United States.

Levosimendan

Levosimendan acts within cardiomyocytes to sensitize troponin C to calcium. This sensitization improves myosin-actin interaction, thereby increasing both inotropy and lusitropy.[109] These effects are thought to occur without increased myocardial oxygen consumption,[110] with evidence of improved coronary perfusion.[111] Although the half-life of levosimendan is 1 hour, its metabolites demonstrated half-lives of 70 to 80 hours and peak serum concentrations at approximately 48 hours.[112] Because of its complex pharmacodynamics, the use of levosimendan is generally contraindicated in patients with significant liver injury or renal disease.

When added to standard therapy for heart failure, infusions of levosimendan provided subjective and objective symptomatic relief in hospitalized patients.[15] Although treatment reduced the hospital stay length, no difference in mortality was seen, although it was noted that the treatment group had more numerical deaths. Moreover, levosimendan was associated with more adverse cardiac events, including hypotension and arrhythmias, but with less cardiac failure.[15]

Similar benefit was seen in patients after MI randomized to levosimendan versus placebo, with increased survival extending to 180 days post-treatment.[33] This finding may be due to improved

left ventricular contractility after infarction, as was seen in a smaller study.[113] Improvement in LVEF with levosimendan in patients with CS complicating AMI was further supported by 2 recent meta-analyses, but only one reached statistical significance.[114,115]

The use of intermittent levosimendan was evaluated in 3 recent double blinded, placebo controlled trials: the Efficacy and safety of the pulsed infusions of levosimendan in outpatients with advanced heart failure study (LevoRep) study, Long-Term Intermittent Administration of Levosimendan in Patients With Advanced Heart Failure (LAICA) study, and Efficacy and safety of intermittent intravenous outpatient administration of levosimendan in patients with advanced heart failure (LION-HEART) study.[116–118] The results showed a nonsignificant trend toward fewer hospitalizations for heart failure.[116–118] Additionally, the LION-HEART study demonstrated a significantly higher rate of survival at 180 days in the levosimendan group.[118]

Two major trials have directly compared levosimendan to dobutamine. In a randomized double-blinded study involving 203 subjects, short-course levosimendan produced a greater improvement in hemodynamics, was associated with less arrhythmogenesis, and had less mortality compared with dobutamine.[119] Contrarily, in the largest trial to date involving 1327 patients, levosimendan and dobutamine showed no significant differences in mortality at 31 or 180 days after infusion; but levosimendan was associated with more hypotension, arrhythmia, and hypokalemia.[16]

Myosin/Actin Cross-Bridge Enhancers

A second class of drugs aimed at circumventing the cAMP-calcium pathway to increase inotropy is currently under investigation. These inotropic enhancers directly interact with either myosin or actin to produce more efficient cardiac sarcomere shortening.[120] To date, only one such molecule, omecamtiv mecarbil, is undergoing clinical evaluation in humans.[120,121]

Omecamtiv mecarbil

Omecamtiv mecarbil directly interacts with the S1 domain on an ATPase found exclusive in cardiac myosin.[122] By increasing ATP turnover, omecamtiv mecarbil increases the effective number of myosin-actin interactions at any time, thus, prolonging contraction.[122]

In individuals with normal ventricular function, omecamtiv mecarbil produced a dose-dependent increase in left ventricular EF (LVEF).[121] Dosing was limited by myocardial ischemia attributed to excessive prolongation of systolic ejection.[121] A phase-II trial evaluated omecamtiv mecarbil in 45 individuals with stable heart failure, showing improvements in LVEF, stroke volume, and left ventricular systolic and diastolic volumes with therapy.[123] Of note, 2 of the participants had cardiac ischemia at higher concentrations of the drug.[123] In a larger phase-II study named Chronic Oral Study of Myosin Activation to Increase Contractility in Heart Failure (COSMIC-HF), 448 patients with stable heart failure symptoms and LVEF of 40% or less were randomized to a fixed dose of omecamtiv mecarbil, a titrated dose of omecamtiv mecarbil, or placebo.[124] Both omecamtiv mecarbil treatment groups noted increases in systolic ejection time and stroke volume compared with placebo. NT-proBNP levels were also lower than in the placebo, with reductions persisting for 4 weeks after therapy discontinuation. Adverse events were similar across all groups.[124] In a separate trial, it produced a concentration-dependent increase in left ventricular systolic ejection time and decrease in end-systolic dimension.[125] Plasma troponin concentrations were higher in the treatment group, suggesting a potential ischemic effect.[125] An ongoing study, Registrational Study With Omecamtiv Mecarbil/AMG 423 to Treat Chronic Heart Failure With Reduced Ejection Fraction (GALACTIC-HF), is under way to evaluate the benefit of omecamtiv mecarbil in patients with heart failure and reduced ejection fraction.

COMPARISON OF DOBUTAMINE VERSUS MILRINONE AS INOTROPIC THERAPY

Selection of an inotrope agent is dictated predominantly by clinical scenario and the desired physiologic effects, with the choice falling largely between dobutamine and milrinone in the United States. Both milrinone and dobutamine remain options as either bridging or palliative therapy.[12,50] In comparison with dobutamine, milrinone therapy causes a greater decrease in mean pulmonary artery pressure, pulmonary capillary wedge pressure, and systemic vascular resistance compared with dobutamine in patients with advanced heart failure.[126] In CS complicating AMI, milrinone may be preferable because of a reduced effect on the heart rate and myocardial oxygen consumption. Because of its propensity to reduce PVR,[39] milrinone is often more suitable in right-sided heart failure due to pulmonary hypertension.[12,41] Caution should be taken with milrinone in individuals with severe renal dysfunction given its aforementioned longer half-life and renal clearance.[34]

Milrinone may provide a better safety profile compared with dobutamine in patients unable to be weaned off of inotropic therapy. Additionally, patients on milrinone can simultaneously remain on beta-blockers, which may help reduce the proarrhythmogenic risk.[127] Two recent studies indicate that milrinone may pose a lesser risk than dobutamine. A retrospective study using the Acute Decompensated Heart Failure National Registry concluded that patients with dobutamine have higher in-hospital mortality after adjustment for both covariates and propensity score compared with milrinone.[128] A 2017 retrospective cohort study sought to evaluate posthospitalization mortality risk after inotropic treatment of heart failure.[13] Overall, an 18% mortality rate in the dobutamine group and 12% mortality rate in the milrinone group were observed during the study period. Most of these deaths were attributable to cardiovascular causes. Although both groups had elevated weighted relative risks, dobutamine showed a disproportionately strong trend toward harm. Subset analysis showed a greater likelihood of death from worsening heart failure in the dobutamine group at all time periods studied.[13] **Table 2** summarizes the main points in the comparison of dobutamine with milrinone.

Overall, inotrope therapy using milrinone and dobutamine has been noted to alleviate symptoms, improve quality of life, decrease hospitalizations, and reduce length of stay in end-stage heart failure.[129,130] UNOS IB status patients placed on these drugs after in-hospital optimization of hemodynamics showed improved resting hemodynamics, renal function, functional capacity, and decreased hospitalizations.[131] Furthermore, it has been shown to be cost-effective as a palliative option.[130]

FINANCIAL CONSIDERATIONS FOR INOTROPE USE

Outpatient inotropic therapy may be considered cost saving after an average of 22 to 33 days after discharge,[131] with average home treatment totaling only 4.2% per day compared with daily inpatient averages.[132] A later study has reaffirmed these results, showing average cost savings per home-going patient estimated at more than $115,000.[133]

Among the two commonly used inotropes, dobutamine and milrinone, there is a significant difference in total treatment cost of $380 ±$533 (dobutamine) versus $16227 ±$1334 (milrinone) (P<.00001).[130] As of July 2017, the average wholesale prices as determined by the Centers for Medicare and Medicaid Services for dobutamine and milrinone are $15.03 (250 mL, 2 mg/mL) and $48.00 (50 mL, 50 mg/50 mL),

Table 2
Comparison of dobutamine and milrinone

	Dobutamine	Milrinone
Inotrope class	Catecholamine	PDE inhibitor
Mechanism of action	Strong ß-adrenergic Agonist → Activates G-coupled Protein → Increases cAMP → Activates L-type calcium channel → Increases intracellular calcium levels	Inhibits PDE → Prevents breakdown of cAMP → Activates L-type calcium channel → Increases intracellular calcium levels
Dosage	2–20 µg/kg/min	0.125–0.75 µg/kg/min
Intracellular calcium	↑	↑
Heart rate	↑↑	↔
Myocardial O$_2$ demand	↑↑	↔
Cardiac output	↑↑	↑
Pulmonary vascular resistance	↓	↓↓
Systemic vascular resistance	↔	↓↓
Cost	$	$$$
Side effects	Arrhythmogenic Tachyphylaxis Peripheral eosinophilia Eosinophilic myocarditis	Arrhythmogenic Hypotension
Utilization	Advanced heart failure or CS complicated by renal failure, vasoplegia, hypotension; beta-blocker–induced low CO	CS complicating AMI; right-sided heart failure complicating pulmonary hypertension

Abbreviations: CO, carbon monoxide; O$_2$, oxygen; PDE, phosphodiesterase.

respectively. Thus, average dosing costs of using either dobutamine or milrinone alone would range between $250 and $500 and $800 and $1400, respectively.[134] Cost may ultimately play a large role in inotrope selection, especially when services are being delivered through an agency hospice benefit that compensates per diem.[135]

SUMMARY

The modern-day usage of inotropes remains broad, including as a temporizing measure in CS, as a bridge to other therapies, or as a palliative measure. The risks and benefits of each medication should be considered. Their unique physiologic actions and potential side effects must be aligned with the clinical status of the individual patient. Digoxin remains as a safe and well-tolerated adjunct to standard heart-failure therapies, with the added benefit of rate control for atrial fibrillation. Ongoing studies are evaluating the potential applications of omecamtiv mecarbil, levosimendan, and istaroxime and may provide further armamentarium in the management of heart failure.

REFERENCES

1. Katz AM. The "modern" view of heart failure: how did we get here? Circ Heart Fail 2008;1(1):63–71.
2. Ferrari R, Balla C, Fucili A. Heart failure: an historical perspective. Eur Heart J Suppl 2016;18(suppl_G):G3–10.
3. Bean WB. An account of the foxglove and some of its medical uses: practical remarks on dropsy and other diseases. Arch Intern Med 1963;112(1):143–4.
4. Smith S. LXXII.-Digoxin, a new digitalis glucoside. J Chem Soc 1930;0:508–10.
5. Goldstein DS. Catecholamines 101. Clin Auton Res 2010;20(6):331–52.
6. Oliver G, Schäfer EA. The physiological effects of extracts of the suprarenal capsules. J Physiol 1895;18(3):230–76.
7. Yamashima T. Jokichi Takamine (1854-1922), the samurai chemist, and his work on adrenalin. J Med Biogr 2003;11(2):95–102.
8. Goldberg LI, Hsieh YY, Resnekov L. Newer catecholamines for treatment of heart failure and shock: an update on dopamine and a first look at dobutamine. Prog Cardiovasc Dis 1977;19(4):327–40.

9. Uretsky BF. Phosphodiesterase inhibitors in heart failure: an overview. In: Hosenpud JD, Greenberg BH, editors. Congestive heart failure: pathophysiology, diagnosis, and comprehensive approach to management. New York: Springer; 1994. p. 493–506.

10. Yancy CW, Jessup M, Bozkurt B, et al. 2013 ACCF/AHA guideline for the management of heart failure: a report of the American College of Cardiology Foundation/American Heart Association Task Force on Practice Guidelines. J Am Coll Cardiol 2013; 62(16):e147–239.

11. Ponikowski P, Voors AA, Anker SD, et al. 2016 ESC Guidelines for the diagnosis and treatment of acute and chronic heart failure: the Task Force for the diagnosis and treatment of acute and chronic heart failure of the European Society of Cardiology (ESC). Developed with the special contribution of the Heart Failure Association (HFA) of the ESC. Eur J Heart Fail 2016;18(8):891–975.

12. Ginwalla M, Bianco C. Inotropes in heart failure. Reference module in biomedical sciences. Elsevier; 2017.

13. King JB, Shah RU, Sainski-Nguyen A, et al. Effect of inpatient dobutamine versus milrinone on out-of-hospital mortality in patients with acute decompensated heart failure. Pharmacotherapy 2017; 37(6):662–72.

14. Cuffe MS, Califf RM, Adams KF Jr, et al. Short-term intravenous milrinone for acute exacerbation of chronic heart failure: a randomized controlled trial. JAMA 2002;287(12):1541–7.

15. Packer M, Colucci W, Fisher L, et al. Effect of levosimendan on the short-term clinical course of patients with acutely decompensated heart failure. JACC Heart Fail 2013;1(2):103–11.

16. Mebazaa A, Nieminen MS, Packer M, et al. Levosimendan vs dobutamine for patients with acute decompensated heart failure: the SURVIVE randomized trial. JAMA 2007;297(17):1883–91.

17. Hashim T, Sanam K, Revilla-Martinez M, et al. Clinical characteristics and outcomes of intravenous inotropic therapy in advanced heart failure. Circ Heart Fail 2015;8(5):880–6.

18. Assad-Kottner C, Chen D, Jahanyar J, et al. The use of continuous milrinone therapy as bridge to transplant is safe in patients with short waiting times. J Card Fail 2008;14(10):839–43.

19. Al-Kindi SG, Farhoud M, Zacharias M, et al. Left ventricular assist devices or inotropes for decreasing pulmonary vascular resistance in patients with pulmonary hypertension listed for heart transplantation. J Card Fail 2017;23(3): 209–15.

20. American College of Emergency Physicians, Society for Cardiovascular Angiography and Interventions, O'Gara PT, et al. 2013 ACCF/AHA guideline for the management of ST-elevation myocardial infarction: a report of the American College of Cardiology Foundation/American Heart Association Task Force on Practice Guidelines. J Am Coll Cardiol 2013;61(4):e78–140.

21. De Backer D, Biston P, Devriendt J, et al. Comparison of dopamine and norepinephrine in the treatment of shock. N Engl J Med 2010;362(9):779–89.

22. Werdan K, Russ M, Buerke M, et al. Cardiogenic shock due to myocardial infarction: diagnosis, monitoring and treatment: a German-Austrian S3 Guideline. Dtsch Arztebl Int 2012;109(19):343–51.

23. Task Force on the Management of ST-Segment Elevation Acute Myocardial Infarction of the European Society of Cardiology (ESC), Steg PG, James SK, et al. ESC guidelines for the management of acute myocardial infarction in patients presenting with ST-segment elevation. Eur Heart J 2012;33(20):2569–619.

24. Khalid L, Dhakam SH. A review of cardiogenic shock in acute myocardial infarction. Curr Cardiol Rev 2008;4(1):34–40.

25. Overgaard CB, Dzavik V. Inotropes and vasopressors: review of physiology and clinical use in cardiovascular disease. Circulation 2008;118(10): 1047–56.

26. Richard C, Ricome JL, Rimailho A, et al. Combined hemodynamic effects of dopamine and dobutamine in cardiogenic shock. Circulation 1983; 67(3):620–6.

27. Grose R, Strain J, Greenberg M, et al. Systemic and coronary effects of intravenous milrinone and dobutamine in congestive heart failure. J Am Coll Cardiol 1986;7(5):1107–13.

28. Opie LH. The mechanism of myocyte death in ischaemia. Eur Heart J 1993;14(Suppl G):31–3.

29. Kohsaka S, Menon V, Lowe AM, et al. Systemic inflammatory response syndrome after acute myocardial infarction complicated by cardiogenic shock. Arch Intern Med 2005;165(14):1643–50.

30. Tang X, Liu P, Li R, et al. Milrinone for the treatment of acute heart failure after acute myocardial infarction: a systematic review and meta-analysis. Basic Clin Pharmacol Toxicol 2015;117(3):186–94.

31. Samimi-Fard S, Garcia-Gonzalez MJ, Dominguez-Rodriguez A, et al. Effects of levosimendan versus dobutamine on long-term survival of patients with cardiogenic shock after primary coronary angioplasty. Int J Cardiol 2008;127(2):284–7.

32. Omerovic E, Ramunddal T, Albertsson P, et al. Levosimendan neither improves nor worsens mortality in patients with cardiogenic shock due to ST-elevation myocardial infarction. Vasc Health Risk Manag 2010;6:657–63.

33. Moiseyev VS, Poder P, Andrejevs N, et al. Safety and efficacy of a novel calcium sensitizer, levosimendan, in patients with left ventricular failure

due to an acute myocardial infarction. A randomized, placebo-controlled, double-blind study (RUSSLAN). Eur Heart J 2002;23(18):1422–32.

34. Unverzagt S, Wachsmuth L, Hirsch K, et al. Inotropic agents and vasodilator strategies for acute myocardial infarction complicated by cardiogenic shock or low cardiac output syndrome. Cochrane Database Syst Rev 2014;(1):CD009669.

35. Kerbaul F, Rondelet B, Motte S, et al. Effects of norepinephrine and dobutamine on pressure load-induced right ventricular failure. Crit Care Med 2004;32(4):1035–40.

36. Ferrario M, Poli A, Previtali M, et al. Hemodynamics of volume loading compared with dobutamine in severe right ventricular infarction. Am J Cardiol 1994;74(4):329–33.

37. Sztrymf B, Souza R, Bertoletti L, et al. Prognostic factors of acute heart failure in patients with pulmonary arterial hypertension. Eur Respir J 2010;35(6):1286–93.

38. Romson JL, Leung JM, Bellows WH, et al. Effects of dobutamine on hemodynamics and left ventricular performance after cardiopulmonary bypass in cardiac surgical patients. Anesthesiology 1999;91(5):1318–28.

39. Eichhorn EJ, Konstam MA, Weiland DS, et al. Differential effects of milrinone and dobutamine on right ventricular preload, afterload and systolic performance in congestive heart failure secondary to ischemic or idiopathic dilated cardiomyopathy. Am J Cardiol 1987;60(16):1329–33.

40. Price LC, Wort SJ, Finney SJ, et al. Pulmonary vascular and right ventricular dysfunction in adult critical care: current and emerging options for management: a systematic literature review. Crit Care 2010;14(5):R169.

41. Green EM, Givertz MM. Management of acute right ventricular failure in the intensive care unit. Curr Heart Fail Rep 2012;9(3):228–35.

42. Kerbaul F, Rondelet B, Demester JP, et al. Effects of levosimendan versus dobutamine on pressure load-induced right ventricular failure. Crit Care Med 2006;34(11):2814–9.

43. Mishra A, Kumar B, Dutta V, et al. Comparative effect of levosimendan and milrinone in cardiac surgery patients with pulmonary hypertension and left ventricular dysfunction. J Cardiothorac Vasc Anesth 2016;30(3):639–46.

44. Allen LA, Fonarow GC, Grau-Sepulveda MV, et al. Hospital variation in intravenous inotrope use for patients hospitalized with heart failure: insights from get with the guidelines. Circ Heart Fail 2014;7(2):251–60.

45. Wan SH, Stevens SR, Borlaug BA, et al. Differential response to low-dose dopamine or low-dose nesiritide in acute heart failure with reduced or preserved ejection fraction: results from the ROSE

AHF Trial (Renal Optimization Strategies Evaluation in Acute Heart Failure). Circ Heart Fail 2016;9(8) [pii:e002593].

46. You Z, Huang L, Cheng X, et al. Effect of milrinone on cardiac functions in patients undergoing coronary artery bypass graft: a meta-analysis of randomized clinical trials. Drug Des Devel Ther 2016;10:53–8.

47. Gatot I, Abramov D, Tsodikov V, et al. Should we give prophylactic renal-dose dopamine after coronary artery bypass surgery? J Card Surg 2004;19(2):128–33.

48. Shi WY, Li S, Collins N, et al. Peri-operative levosimendan in patients undergoing cardiac surgery: an overview of the evidence. Heart Lung Circ 2015;24(7):667–72.

49. Sunny, Yunus M, Karim HM, et al. Comparison of levosimendan, milrinone and dobutamine in treating low cardiac output syndrome following valve replacement surgeries with cardiopulmonary bypass. J Clin Diagn Res 2016;10(12):UC05–8.

50. Ginwalla M. Home inotropes and other palliative care. Heart Fail Clin 2016;12(3):437–48.

51. Acharya D, Sanam K, Revilla-Martinez M, et al. Infections, arrhythmias, and hospitalizations on home intravenous inotropic therapy. Am J Cardiol 2016;117(6):952–6.

52. Yeragani VK, Tancer M, Chokka P, et al. Arvid Carlsson, and the story of dopamine. Indian J Psychiatry 2010;52(1):87–8.

53. Goldberg LI. Cardiovascular and renal actions of dopamine: potential clinical applications. Pharmacol Rev 1972;24(1):1–29.

54. Maskin CS, Ocken S, Chadwick B, et al. Comparative systemic and renal effects of dopamine and angiotensin-converting enzyme inhibition with enalaprilat in patients with heart failure. Circulation 1985;72(4):846–52.

55. Denton MD, Chertow GM, Brady HR. "Renal-dose" dopamine for the treatment of acute renal failure: scientific rationale, experimental studies and clinical trials. Kidney Int 1996;50(1):4–14.

56. Elkayam U, Ng TM, Hatamizadeh P, et al. Renal vasodilatory action of dopamine in patients with heart failure: magnitude of effect and site of action. Circulation 2008;117(2):200–5.

57. Friedrich JO, Adhikari N, Herridge MS, et al. Metaanalysis: low-dose dopamine increases urine output but does not prevent renal dysfunction or death. Ann Intern Med 2005;142(7):510–24.

58. Chen HH, Anstrom KJ, Givertz MM, et al. Low-dose dopamine or low-dose nesiritide in acute heart failure with renal dysfunction: the ROSE acute heart failure randomized trial. JAMA 2013;310(23):2533–43.

59. Xing F, Hu X, Jiang J, et al. A meta-analysis of low-dose dopamine in heart failure. Int J Cardiol 2016;222:1003–11.

60. Giamouzis G, Butler J, Starling RC, et al. Impact of dopamine infusion on renal function in hospitalized heart failure patients: results of the Dopamine in Acute Decompensated Heart Failure (DAD-HF) Trial. J Card Fail 2010;16(12):922–30.

61. Cotter G, Weissgarten J, Metzkor E, et al. Increased toxicity of high-dose furosemide versus low-dose dopamine in the treatment of refractory congestive heart failure. Clin Pharmacol Ther 1997;62(2):187–93.

62. Varriale P, Mossavi A. The benefit of low-dose dopamine during vigorous diuresis for congestive heart failure associated with renal insufficiency: does it protect renal function? Clin Cardiol 1997; 20(7):627–30.

63. Ronco C, McCullough P, Anker SD, et al. Cardio-renal syndromes: report from the consensus conference of the acute dialysis quality initiative. Eur Heart J 2010;31(6):703–11.

64. Hillege HL, Girbes AR, de Kam PJ, et al. Renal function, neurohormonal activation, and survival in patients with chronic heart failure. Circulation 2000;102(2):203–10.

65. Heywood JT, Fonarow GC, Costanzo MR, et al. High prevalence of renal dysfunction and its impact on outcome in 118,465 patients hospitalized with acute decompensated heart failure: a report from the ADHERE database. J Card Fail 2007;13(6):422–30.

66. Brandimarte F, Vaduganathan M, Mureddu GF, et al. Prognostic implications of renal dysfunction in patients hospitalized with heart failure: data from the last decade of clinical investigations. Heart Fail Rev 2013;18(2):167–76.

67. Smith GL, Lichtman JH, Bracken MB, et al. Renal impairment and outcomes in heart failure: systematic review and meta-analysis. J Am Coll Cardiol 2006;47(10):1987–96.

68. Ruffolo RR Jr. The pharmacology of dobutamine. Am J Med Sci 1987;294(4):244–8.

69. Tuttle RR, Mills J. Dobutamine: development of a new catecholamine to selectively increase cardiac contractility. Circ Res 1975;36(1):185–96.

70. Burger AJ, Horton DP, LeJemtel T, et al. Effect of nesiritide (B-type natriuretic peptide) and dobutamine on ventricular arrhythmias in the treatment of patients with acutely decompensated congestive heart failure: the PRECEDENT study. Am Heart J 2002;144(6):1102–8.

71. El-Sayed OM, Abdelfattah RR, Barcelona R, et al. Dobutamine-induced eosinophilia. Am J Cardiol 2004;93(8):1078–9.

72. Spear GS. Eosinophilic explant carditis with eosinophilia: ?Hypersensitivity to dobutamine infusion. J Heart Lung Transplant 1995;14(4):755–60.

73. Chapman SA, Stephan T, Lake KD, et al. Fever induced by dobutamine infusion. Am J Cardiol 1994;74(5):517.

74. Lee CC, Luthringer DJ, Czer LS. Dobutamine-induced fever and isolated eosinophilic myocarditis in a 66-year-old male awaiting heart transplantation: a case report. Transplant Proc 2014;46(7):2464–6.

75. Liang CS, Sherman LG, Doherty JU, et al. Sustained improvement of cardiac function in patients with congestive heart failure after short-term infusion of dobutamine. Circulation 1984; 69(1):113–9.

76. Unverferth DV, Magorien RD, Lewis RP, et al. Long-term benefit of dobutamine in patients with congestive cardiomyopathy. Am Heart J 1980;100(5): 622–30.

77. Leier CV, Webel J, Bush CA. The cardiovascular effects of the continuous infusion of dobutamine in patients with severe cardiac failure. Circulation 1977;56(3):468–72.

78. Patel MB, Kaplan IV, Patni RN, et al. Sustained improvement in flow-mediated vasodilation after short-term administration of dobutamine in patients with severe congestive heart failure. Circulation 1999;99(1):60–4.

79. Oliva F, Latini R, Politi A, et al. Intermittent 6-month low-dose dobutamine infusion in severe heart failure: DICE multicenter trial. Am Heart J 1999; 138(2 Pt 1):247–53.

80. Krell MJ, Kline EM, Bates ER, et al. Intermittent, ambulatory dobutamine infusions in patients with severe congestive heart failure. Am Heart J 1986; 112(4):787–91.

81. Elkayam U, Tasissa G, Binanay C, et al. Use and impact of inotropes and vasodilator therapy in hospitalized patients with severe heart failure. Am Heart J 2007;153(1):98–104.

82. Stevenson LW. Inotropic therapy for heart failure. N Engl J Med 1998;339(25):1848–50.

83. O'Connor CM, Gattis WA, Uretsky BF, et al. Continuous intravenous dobutamine is associated with an increased risk of death in patients with advanced heart failure: insights from the Flolan International Randomized Survival Trial (FIRST). Am Heart J 1999;138(1 Pt 1):78–86.

84. Unverferth DA, Blanford M, Kates RE, et al. Tolerance to dobutamine after a 72 hour continuous infusion. Am J Med 1980;69(2):262–6.

85. Farah AE, Alousi AA. New cardiotonic agents: a search for digitalis substitute. Life Sci 1978; 22(13–15):1139–47.

86. Shipley JB, Tolman D, Hastillo A, et al. Milrinone: basic and clinical pharmacology and acute and chronic management. Am J Med Sci 1996;311(6): 286–91.

87. Cox ZL, Calcutt MW, Morrison TB, et al. Elevation of plasma milrinone concentrations in stage D heart failure associated with renal dysfunction. J Cardiovasc Pharmacol Ther 2013;18(5):433–8.

88. Packer M, Carver JR, Rodeheffer RJ, et al. Effect of oral milrinone on mortality in severe chronic heart failure. The PROMISE Study Research Group. N Engl J Med 1991;325(21):1468–75.

89. Karlsberg RP, DeWood MA, DeMaria AN, et al. Comparative efficacy of short-term intravenous infusions of milrinone and dobutamine in acute congestive heart failure following acute myocardial infarction. Milrinone-Dobutamine Study Group. Clin Cardiol 1996;19(1):21–30.

90. Anderson JL, Baim DS, Fein SA, et al. Efficacy and safety of sustained (48 hour) intravenous infusions of milrinone in patients with severe congestive heart failure: a multicenter study. J Am Coll Cardiol 1987;9(4):711–22.

91. Felker GM, Benza RL, Chandler AB, et al. Heart failure etiology and response to milrinone in decompensated heart failure: results from the OPTIME-CHF study. J Am Coll Cardiol 2003; 41(6):997–1003.

92. Panhwar MS, Al-Kindi S, Oliveira GH, et al. Successful use of palliative inotrope therapy in end-stage cardiac ATTR amyloidosis. Amyloid 2017; 24(4):217–8.

93. Gheorghiade M, St Clair J, St Clair C, et al. Hemodynamic effects of intravenous digoxin in patients with severe heart failure initially treated with diuretics and vasodilators. J Am Coll Cardiol 1987; 9(4):849–57.

94. Gheorghiade M, van Veldhuisen DJ, Colucci WS. Contemporary use of digoxin in the management of cardiovascular disorders. Circulation 2006; 113(21):2556–64.

95. Newton GE, Tong JH, Schofield AM, et al. Digoxin reduces cardiac sympathetic activity in severe congestive heart failure. J Am Coll Cardiol 1996; 28(1):155–61.

96. Naqvi S, Ahmed I, Siddiqi R, et al. Digoxin as a rescue drug in intra aortic balloon pump and inotrope dependent patients. J Ayub Med Coll Abbottabad 2010;22(2):8–12.

97. Thiemann DR. Digitalis and hemodialysis is a bad combination. J Am Soc Nephrol 2010;21(9): 1418–20.

98. Chan KE, Lazarus JM, Hakim RM. Digoxin associates with mortality in ESRD. J Am Soc Nephrol 2010;21(9):1550–9.

99. Abdo AS, Basu A, Geraci SA. Managing chronic heart failure patient in chronic kidney disease. Am J Med 2011;124(1):26–8.

100. Segall L, Nistor I, Covic A. Heart failure in patients with chronic kidney disease: a systematic integrative review. Biomed Res Int 2014;2014: 937398.

101. Jaeschke R, Oxman AD, Guyatt GH. To what extent do congestive heart failure patients in sinus rhythm benefit from digoxin therapy? A systematic overview and meta-analysis. Am J Med 1990;88(3): 279–86.

102. Hood WB Jr, Dans AL, Guyatt GH, et al. Digitalis for treatment of heart failure in patients in sinus rhythm. Cochrane Database Syst Rev 2014;(4): CD002901.

103. Digitalis Investigation Group. The effect of digoxin on mortality and morbidity in patients with heart failure. N Engl J Med 1997;336(8):525–33.

104. Abdul-Rahim AH, MacIsaac RL, Jhund PS, et al. Efficacy and safety of digoxin in patients with heart failure and reduced ejection fraction according to diabetes status: an analysis of the Digitalis Investigation Group (DIG) trial. Int J Cardiol 2016;209: 310–6.

105. Shah SJ, Blair JE, Filippatos GS, et al. Effects of istaroxime on diastolic stiffness in acute heart failure syndromes: results from the hemodynamic, echocardiographic, and neurohormonal effects of istaroxime, a novel intravenous inotropic and lusitropic agent: a randomized controlled trial in patients hospitalized with Heart Failure (HORIZON-HF) trial. Am Heart J 2009;157(6):1035–41.

106. Gheorghiade M, Blair JE, Filippatos GS, et al. Hemodynamic, echocardiographic, and neurohormonal effects of istaroxime, a novel intravenous inotropic and lusitropic agent: a randomized controlled trial in patients hospitalized with heart failure. J Am Coll Cardiol 2008; 51(23):2276–85.

107. Gianni D, Chan J, Gwathmey JK, et al. SERCA2a in heart failure: role and therapeutic prospects. J Bioenerg Biomembr 2005;37(6):375–80.

108. Fearnley CJ, Roderick HL, Bootman MD. Calcium signaling in cardiac myocytes. Cold Spring Harb Perspect Biol 2011;3(11):a004242.

109. Givertz MM, Andreou C, Conrad CH, et al. Direct myocardial effects of levosimendan in humans with left ventricular dysfunction: alteration of force-frequency and relaxation-frequency relationships. Circulation 2007;115(10):1218–24.

110. Ukkonen H, Saraste M, Akkila J, et al. Myocardial efficiency during levosimendan infusion in congestive heart failure. Clin Pharmacol Ther 2000;68(5): 522–31.

111. Michaels AD, McKeown B, Kostal M, et al. Effects of intravenous levosimendan on human coronary vasomotor regulation, left ventricular wall stress, and myocardial oxygen uptake. Circulation 2005; 111(12):1504–9.

112. Sundberg S, Antila S, Scheinin H, et al. Integrated pharmacokinetics and pharmacodynamics of the novel calcium sensitizer levosimendan as assessed by systolic time intervals. Int J Clin Pharmacol Ther 1998;36(12):629–35.

113. Husebye T, Eritsland J, Muller C, et al. Levosimendan in acute heart failure following primary

percutaneous coronary intervention-treated acute ST-elevation myocardial infarction. Results from the LEAF trial: a randomized, placebo-controlled study. Eur J Heart Fail 2013;15(5):565–72.

114. Fang M, Cao H, Wang Z. Levosimendan in patients with cardiogenic shock complicating myocardial infarction: a meta-analysis. Med Intensiva 2017 [pii:S0210-5691(17)30283-8]. [Epub ahead of print].

115. Shang G, Yang X, Song D, et al. Effects of levosimendan on patients with heart failure complicating acute coronary syndrome: a meta-analysis of randomized controlled trials. Am J Cardiovasc Drugs 2017;17(6):453–63.

116. Altenberger J, Parissis JT, Costard-Jaeckle A, et al. Efficacy and safety of the pulsed infusions of levosimendan in outpatients with advanced heart failure (LevoRep) study: a multicentre randomized trial. Eur J Heart Fail 2014;16(8):898–906.

117. García-González MJ. Efficacy and security of intermittent repeated levosimendan administration in patients with advanced heart failure: a randomized, double-blind, placebo controlled multicenter trial: LAICA study. Paper presented at: The European Society of Cardiology–Heart Failure Association Congress. Florence, Italy, May 21, 2016.

118. Comin Colet J. Multicenter, double blind, randomized, placebo controlled trial evaluating the efficacy and safety of intermittent levosimendan in outpatients with advanced chronic heart failure: the LION Heart study. Paper presented at: The European Society of Cardiology–Heart Failure Association Congress. Seville, Spain, May 24, 2015.

119. Follath F, Cleland JG, Just H, et al. Efficacy and safety of intravenous levosimendan compared with dobutamine in severe low-output heart failure (the LIDO study): a randomised double-blind trial. Lancet 2002;360(9328):196–202.

120. Teerlink JR. A novel approach to improve cardiac performance: cardiac myosin activators. Heart Fail Rev 2009;14(4):289–98.

121. Teerlink JR, Clarke CP, Saikali KG, et al. Dose-dependent augmentation of cardiac systolic function with the selective cardiac myosin activator, omecamtiv mecarbil: a first-in-man study. Lancet 2011;378(9792):667–75.

122. Malik FI, Hartman JJ, Elias KA, et al. Cardiac myosin activation: a potential therapeutic approach for systolic heart failure. Science 2011;331(6023):1439–43.

123. Cleland JG, Teerlink JR, Senior R, et al. The effects of the cardiac myosin activator, omecamtiv mecarbil, on cardiac function in systolic heart failure: a double-blind, placebo-controlled, crossover, dose-ranging phase 2 trial. Lancet 2011;378(9792):676–83.

124. Teerlink JR, Felker GM, McMurray JJ, et al. Chronic Oral Study of Myosin Activation to Increase Contractility in Heart Failure (COSMIC-HF): a phase 2, pharmacokinetic, randomised, placebo-controlled trial. Lancet 2016;388(10062):2895–903.

125. Teerlink JR, Felker GM, McMurray JJV, et al. Acute treatment with omecamtiv mecarbil to increase contractility in acute heart failure: the ATOMIC-AHF Study. J Am Coll Cardiol 2016;67(12):1444–55.

126. Yamani MH, Haji SA, Starling RC, et al. Comparison of dobutamine-based and milrinone-based therapy for advanced decompensated congestive heart failure: hemodynamic efficacy, clinical outcome, and economic impact. Am Heart J 2001;142(6):998–1002.

127. Jimenez J, Jara J, Bednar B, et al. Long-term (>8 weeks) home inotropic therapy as destination therapy in patients with advanced heart failure or as bridge to heart transplantation. Int J Cardiol 2005;99(1):47–50.

128. Abraham WT, Adams KF, Fonarow GC, et al. In-hospital mortality in patients with acute decompensated heart failure requiring intravenous vasoactive medications: an analysis from the Acute Decompensated Heart Failure National Registry (ADHERE). J Am Coll Cardiol 2005;46(1):57–64.

129. Harjai KJ, Mehra MR, Ventura HO, et al. Home inotropic therapy in advanced heart failure: cost analysis and clinical outcomes. Chest 1997;112(5):1298–303.

130. Hauptman PJ, Mikolajczak P, George A, et al. Chronic inotropic therapy in end-stage heart failure. Am Heart J 2006;152(6):1096.e1-8.

131. Upadya S, Lee FA, Saldarriaga C, et al. Home continuous positive inotropic infusion as a bridge to cardiac transplantation in patients with end-stage heart failure. J Heart Lung Transplant 2004;23(4):466–72.

132. Brozena SC, Twomey C, Goldberg LR, et al. A prospective study of continuous intravenous milrinone therapy for status IB patients awaiting heart transplant at home. J Heart Lung Transplant 2004;23(9):1082–6.

133. Lang CC, Hankins S, Hauff H, et al. Morbidity and mortality of UNOS status 1B cardiac transplant candidates at home. J Heart Lung Transplant 2003;22(4):419–26.

134. Aranda JM Jr, Schofield RS, Pauly DF, et al. Comparison of dobutamine versus milrinone therapy in hospitalized patients awaiting cardiac transplantation: a prospective, randomized trial. Am Heart J 2003;145(2):324–9.

135. Malotte K, Saguros A, Groninger H. Continuous cardiac inotropes in patients with end-stage heart failure: an evolving experience. J Pain Symptom Manage 2018;55(1):159–63.

Palliative Therapy in Heart Failure

Christopher M. Hritz, MD

KEYWORDS

- Palliative care • Heart failure • Prognostication • Symptom management • Referral

KEY POINTS

- Palliative care is a multidisciplinary approach to patient care with the aim to improve quality of life alongside disease-directed management.
- Recent studies suggest that palliative care consultation improves quality of life and symptom burden for both patients and families.
- Challenges remain in providing quality end-of-life care in patients with heart failure, especially when patients have undergone left-ventricular assist device implantation.

INTRODUCTION

Heart failure in most cases is a chronic, ultimately terminal illness accompanied by increased symptom burden throughout the progression of the disease. Palliation, meaning to treat symptoms without curing, is a virtual necessity in the management of heart failure and is often provided by multiple clinicians including cardiologists as well as palliative medicine specialists. The American Academy of Hospice and Palliative Medicine defines palliative care as "[focusing] on improving a patient's quality of life by managing pain and other distressing symptoms of a serious illness. Palliative care should be provided along with other medical treatments."[1] Along with symptom management, a palliative care team provides support for various aspects of caring for someone with a serious illness. It is becoming apparent that palliative care can provide significant improvements in patients with heart failure, both throughout disease management and at end of life. Palliative care can also provide much needed support for patients undergoing invasive, life-altering treatment modalities often required in end-stage heart failure.

THE PALLIATIVE CARE ASSESSMENT AND DOMAINS

To adequately care for patients suffering from life-limiting illnesses, 8 domains have been identified as essential for quality care. These domains include "structure and process of care," "physical aspects of care," "psychological and psychiatric aspects of care," "social aspects of care," "spiritual, religious, and existential aspects of care," "cultural aspects of care," "care of the patient at end of life," and "ethical and legal aspects of care." A dedicated palliative care team is often multidisciplinary to better address these domains as they expand beyond medical issues. Examples of information or opportunities elicited through exploring these domains includes identifying unmanaged symptoms, recognizing grief, evaluating family support, exploring living situations, striving for respectful communication in the setting of different cultures, educating families about the dying process, and ensuring a bereavement plan is in place. Because these domains are broad, an interdisciplinary team is required and often includes physicians, nurses, social workers, chaplains, rehabilitative experts, and psychiatrists.[2]

Disclosure Statement: The author has nothing to disclose.
Division of Palliative Medicine, Department of Internal Medicine, The Ohio State University Wexner Medical Center, McCampbell Hall, 5th Floor, 1581 Dodd Drive, Columbus, OH 43210, USA
E-mail address: christopher.hritz@osumc.edu

Heart Failure Clin 14 (2018) 617–624
https://doi.org/10.1016/j.hfc.2018.06.011
1551-7136/18/© 2018 Elsevier Inc. All rights reserved.

Social workers and chaplains can contribute significantly to the effectiveness of support and management of patient and family issues falling under the later domains. A comparable focus on domains including "medical," "mind and emotion," and "social environment" along with goals-of-care discussion has been recently suggested for geriatric patients suffering from heart failure. These domains are analogous to the palliative domains of "structure and process of care," "physical aspects of care," "psychological and psychiatric aspects of care," and "social aspects of care."[3]

REFERRAL/UTILIZATION

Although access to subspecialty palliative care has expanded over the past 2 decades, it remains a limited resource. There is approximately 1 palliative care specialist per 1200 patients with life-limiting illnesses. In the United States access varies depending on geographic location and size of hospital system, with the south lacking somewhat in palliative care support relative to the rest of the United States. Hospitals smaller than 50 beds are much less likely to have palliative care support, with only 29% having palliative care teams in 2015. Around 90% of larger hospitals with more than 300 beds have palliative care support, although this can vary depending on region.[4] These statistics show that although palliative care support has grown, many practice settings still lack a palliative care team and the importance of exploring support options available in a patient's current clinical setting.

Unfortunately palliative care training during cardiology fellowship is currently limited despite nearly all cardiologists recognizing its importance.[5] Although palliative care continues to grow as a subspecialty, the immense need will require the delivery of primary palliative care by nonpalliative specialists as an essential part of providing excellent care to patients with heart failure, underscoring the need to develop more robust palliative care training for cardiology fellows. The primary palliative care assessment should include a physical and psychological symptom assessment, identification of social or spiritual concerns, exploring understanding of illness, prognosis and treatment options, identifying goals of care, and exploring safe care following discharge.[6]

Subspecialty palliative care may be sought in the setting of complex symptom management or difficulties in defining goals of care. Given the limited subspecialty palliative care resources and prognostic uncertainty associated with heart failure, timing of palliative care consultation is challenging. Prognostic models may be beneficial in identifying heart failure patients with palliative care needs. Events associated with heart failure, such as a change in baseline New York Heart Association (NYHA) class to IV, implantable cardioverter defibrillator (ICD) discharge, a resuscitation event, or frequent hospital readmissions, may also trigger palliative care consultation.[7] Recently, the PAL-HF trial compared patients with heart failure who received cardiologist-driven usual care with patients who received usual care along with palliative care intervention over a period of 6 months. The study population included currently hospitalized patients with a previous hospitalization in the last year and the Evaluation Study of Congestive Heart Failure and Pulmonary Artery Catheterization Effectiveness (ESCAPE) risk score of greater than or equal to 4. Patients on chronic inotropes, at least 3 heart failure hospitalizations in the past year, or patients with an ESCAPE risk greater than 4 regardless of recent hospitalization were also included.[8] The palliative care intervention involved assessment and management of multiple quality-of-life domains by a palliative care–trained nurse practitioner, a board-certified hospice and palliative medicine physician, and a counselor. The usual care + palliative care arm of the study exhibited improved quality of life and spiritual well-being along with decreased anxiety and depression.[9] This supports integration of palliative care throughout a patient's heart failure trajectory rather than relying on the previously mentioned event triggers.[10]

Although most common in the inpatient setting, palliative care intervention is likely beneficial in the outpatient setting as well. Currently the most common patient population addressed in outpatient palliative care clinics is patients with cancer, although patients with heart failure do currently receive outpatient palliative care in some practices.[11] Exploration of outpatient palliative care over the past few years has suggested a possible benefit in symptom reduction, depression, and quality of life in patients with heart failure.[12] The ENABLE CHF-PC pilot has shown promise in the outpatient setting for patients with NYHA Class III and IV heart failure. This study provided outpatient palliative care consultation, weekly sessions with a nurse, and monthly sessions focusing on an educational guidebook. In this pilot, patients receiving intervention experienced improved quality of life, symptom burden, and mental health, as well as improved caregiver quality of life and mental health.[13]

Hospice care is a subset of palliative care for patients thought to have a prognosis of 6 months or less and who choose to focus only on comfort

Table 1	
Symptom prevalence in heart failure	
Shortness of breath	60%–88%
Pain	63%–80%
Fatigue	69%–82%
Depression	9%–60%
Anxiety	49%
Insomnia	36%–48%
Constipation	32%–48%
Nausea	17%–48%
Decreased Appetite	21%–41%
Delirium	18%–32%

Data from Rutledge T, Reis VA, Linke SE, et al. Depression in heart failure a meta-analytic review of prevalence, intervention effects, and associations with clinical outcomes. J Am Coll Cardiol 2006;48(8):1527–37; and Solano JP, Gomes B, Higginson IJ. A comparison of symptom prevalence in far advanced cancer, AIDS, heart disease, chronic obstructive pulmonary disease and renal disease. J Pain Symptom Manage 2006;31(1):58–69.

care. It is generally provided in the home. Medicare does not cover room and board under the hospice benefit, which may limit patients who require prolonged continuous care.[14] Hospice can be an extremely beneficial service and support for the patient with end-stage heart failure who wishes to forgo further hospitalizations and focus on comfort. Hospice will often continue many heart failure–directed therapies such as diuretics and, in certain circumstances inotropes, because these are essential to providing the best quality of life for patients with end-stage heart failure. Hospice care in the United States also provides support to the patient's family both during care and after death.

SYMPTOM MANAGEMENT

Heart failure often carries a significant symptom burden similar to other terminal illnesses. **Table 1** provides a list of common symptoms patients with heart failure may encounter. Often these symptoms will subside following optimization of disease-directed heart failure therapies such as angiotensin-converting enzyme inhibitors, diuretics, vasodilators, inotropes, and surgical interventions such as mechanical circulatory support or transplantation. Despite optimal management, symptoms may become refractory to heart failure therapies. Refractory symptoms can be improved by combining optimal management along with palliative care interventions and are important to address throughout the disease trajectory.

Shortness of Breath

Shortness of breath is a hallmark symptom of heart failure. Beyond heart failure management aimed at reducing pulmonary congestion, stimulation of the trigeminal nerve via oxygen supplementation or simply providing a fan to blow over a patient's face can be effective in providing dyspnea relief.[15] Movement of air through the nares provides relief regardless of oxygenation status, supporting the fan-to-face technique in the setting of adequate oxygenation. In the setting of comfort-focused care where comfort takes priority over oxygenation, fans are ideal because oxygen delivery devices may cause unnecessary discomfort.[16] Shortness of breath refractory to management of heart failure and trigeminal nerve stimulation can be alleviated through the use of opioid medications. Opioids are thought to reduce dyspnea through acting on both central and peripheral opioids receptors as well as decreasing respiratory drive.[17] Low doses of opioids have been shown to be effective in managing shortness of breath when compared with common analgesic doses.[18] Historically there have been concerns of significant respiratory depression from opioid administration, although this should not be a concern when dosed appropriately. A study showing no difference in time to death with increased opioid usage following palliative extubation demonstrates that this concern is unfounded.[19] In addition, a recent evaluation of opioid use in hospitalized patients with heart failure showed little difference in 30-day readmission rates or 90-day mortality when compared with similar patients who were not prescribed opioids.[20] This further supports that opioid management can be a safe and effective modality when indicated in refractory heart failure symptoms.

Pain

Although pain is a very common symptom experienced by patients with heart failure, it is often underrecognized in heart failure.[21] Pain in heart failure can have multiple causes including an ischemic or neuropathic nature as well as edematous pain commonly found in the lower extremities or abdomen. In addition, comorbid pain conditions such as osteoarthritis are often present, raising challenges because nonsteroidal antiinflammatory drugs (NSAIDs), a critical medication in osteoarthritis management, should be avoided in the heart failure population. NSAIDs can produce undesirable effects in this population such as increase in fluid retention and renal impairment.[22] Acetaminophen may be considered a first-line analgesic in patients with heart failure, although limited in patients at risk for liver dysfunction or other co-morbid hepatic impairments. Right heart failure and associated venous congestion can lead to decreased hepatic and renal function; therefore, clinicians should avoid NSAIDs and acetaminophen in this population.[23] Given the pharmacologic pain management limitations in heart failure, it is sometimes necessary to use opioid medications for pain management in this clinical scenario. As stated earlier, opioid use seems to have little effect on hospitalization and mortality, although general issues with opioids such as side effects, dependence, and diversion are still present and must be monitored.

Special considerations must be made in the patient with heart failure requiring opioid medications. Bowel, renal, and hepatic function must be closely followed in patients with refractory heart failure symptoms requiring opioid management. Patients with heart failure are at risk for constipation due to fluid shifts and potential for decreased ambulation. This risk is furthered with opioid medications and commonly requires titration of stimulant laxatives such as senna.

Careful opioid selection is needed in settings of hepatic or renal insufficiency. Morphine is renally excreted and should be avoided in renal dysfunction. Codeine is a prodrug of morphine and should be avoided in renal dysfunction as well. Oxycodone undergoes hepatic metabolism, requiring careful dosing or avoidance in hepatic insufficiency.[24] In addition, oxycodone is often provided in a combination pill with acetaminophen, which limits titration of dosage and should be used with caution in hepatic insufficiency to avoid exceeding the recommended dosage in the setting of hepatic disease. If dosed appropriately, all opioids should be comparably effective in both pain and shortness of breath management, allowing the clinician to choose the best opioid in the setting of organ dysfunction.

Fatigue

Adequate management of fatigue involves identifying and managing comorbid conditions such as anemia, hypothyroidism, depression, and sleep disorders. Aerobic exercise training in combination with medical therapy used in patients with heart failure has shown to improve scores on the Kansas City Cardiomyopathy Questionnaire. There was also significant improvement in each subgroup of the questionnaire including physical limitations and symptoms, which contain questions about fatigue and shortness of breath.[25] An additional strategy includes the concept of energy conservation. This has been applied to palliative

care patients suffering from fatigue-causing terminal illnesses. It involves planning activities around observed times of heightened fatigue and prioritizing activities to allow engagement during these periods of lessened fatigue.[26] Prolonged rest should be avoided because it will lead to worsened deconditioning.

Depression

Depression in advanced illness such as heart failure can be difficult to identify because many depressive symptoms such as decreased appetite, fatigue, and changes in sleep are shared with heart failure.[27] Furthermore, it is evident that depression is underrecognized in heart failure.[28] Screening tools that do not assess somatic symptoms such as the Hospital Anxiety and Depression Scale or simply asking "are you depressed?" have been shown to be effective depression screening tools in the palliative care setting.[29] Intuitively, as a patient's NYHA functional class worsens, the incidence of depression increases, with a prevalence exceeding 40% in class IV. Depression has been linked to increased mortality and health care utilization making adequate management an integral part of heart failure care.[28]

As with depression in the general population, cognitive behavioral therapy (CBT) can effectively improve depression scores. Alhough effective in managing depression, CBT has not been shown to affect mortality or the incidence of hospital readmissions in patients with heart failure.[30] Aerobic exercise has also been shown to improve depressive symptoms in heart failure.[31]

Should nonpharmacologic interventions fail, selective serotonin reuptake inhibitors (SSRIs) may be considered. The SSRI sertraline has been evaluated and shown to be a safe modality when used in relatively low doses in heart failure.[32] Tricyclic antidepressants (TCAs) may be considered as an alternative, although they carry the risk of QT prolongation. TCAs also have undesirable side effects such as dry mouth and orthostatic hypotension, which may already be present and bothersome in a patient with advanced heart failure.[33]

Stimulants such as methylphenidate may be considered as well, though with caution due to increased risk for arrhythmias. Stimulants normally provide symptom relief in as little as 2 days.[34] Given the increased cardiac risk, stimulants should be limited to clinical scenarios where rapid improvement of symptoms is needed, such as end-of-life care.

COMMUNICATION

Communication is paramount to adequately addressing the "structure and process" and "ethical and legal" domains of care. Robust communication will ensure patient preferences are followed regardless of a patient's condition. It can also explore a patient's understanding of their disease state and prognosis as well as their desired physical environment.

Advanced care planning is a process that explores the adult patient's values, goals, and preferences for future medical care. It often involves identifying a surrogate decision maker to assume the decision-making role, should the patient lose their medical decision-making capacity. This surrogate should be included in advanced care planning conversations when possible, along with the patient and their health care providers. Advanced care planning can be explored at any stage of health, should be revisited as needed due to change in health status, and should be documented for future reference.[35] Advanced care planning can be extremely helpful when exploring goals of care in the event of a change in clinical status because it can lay the framework for medical decisions before a health crisis. The periodic exploration of values, goals, and preferences is especially valuable in heart failure because patients are at high risk of losing medical decision-making capacity due to various medical complications. This includes neurologic sequela following cardiac arrest, complications from advanced cardiac therapies, or delirium from decreased cardiac output. Suggested documentation for a goals-of-care conversation[36]:

1. Assessment of Medical Knowledge.
2. Prognostic Awareness.
3. Goals of Care—including minimal acceptable mental and physical status as well as location of care.
4. Psychosocial concerns.

While exploring overall values through advanced care planning, specific issues should be addressed in the patient with heart failure. It has been found that initiation of prognostic discussions by physicians at the time of diagnosis is preferred by patients.[37] Prognostic information is a useful foundation when exploring goals of care. Resuscitation preferences are also important to explore, as it has been seen that historically these preferences are outdated or unnoticed if elicited at all.[38] Should a patient decide to forgo resuscitation, the presence or absence of an ICD should be confirmed. If present, discussion regarding the risks and benefits of the ICD is warranted because it has been shown that many clinicians fail to discuss this before death.[39] Pacemakers do not reverse terminal events and are likely to only contribute to a patient's comfort. In most cases pacing should be continued, although discontinuation is ethically permissible in rare cases such as prolonged suffering.[40]

PROGNOSTICATION

Prognostication in heart failure is challenging because the clinical course contains multiple episodes of exacerbation and incomplete recovery. Although 5-year mortality following the onset of heart failure approaches 50%, this can vary significantly.[41] Clinical decline in the form of decreased functional status, increased NYHA class, cachexia, and depression signal a worsening prognosis.[42] Clinical signs are currently the prognostic basis for hospice eligibility.

There are a multitude of scoring models that may act as alternative method to determining prognosis. The Seattle Heart Failure Model is a widely used prognostic tool and uses a combination of laboratory values, vital signs, medication requirements, and NYHA class to predict 1-, 2-, and 3-year survival rates. The population used to develop the model was in the outpatient setting with a reduced ejection fraction, possibly limiting its value in the inpatient setting or in patients with a preserved ejection fraction.[43] Another prognostic tool, ESCAPE risk models, aims to predict mortality at the time of discharge using a combination of laboratory and vitals data along with medication requirements, hospital events, and physical ability to create a risk score.[44]

Although many tools exist to assist with prognostication in heart failure, prognostication is almost always imprecise regardless of terminal illness. Prognostic uncertainty has been noted as a source of distress in patients with cancer.[45] This is likely true in patients with heart failure as well and prognostic uncertainty should be addressed as part of an overall goals-of-care discussion.

MECHANICAL CIRCULATORY SUPPORT, TRANSPLANTATION, AND PALLIATIVE CARE

The increased utilization of mechanical circulatory support in the management of end-stage heart failure has provided increased opportunities to reverse the symptoms of heart failure at the expense of greater risk for prolonged unacceptable outcomes and increased complexity in understanding patient preferences for care.

The presence of a palliative care specialist is required by the Centers for Medicare & Medicaid

Services to be part of the multidisciplinary team managing destination therapy left ventricular assist devices (DT-LVADs).[46] Although recognized as crucial aspect of mechanical circulatory support, the extent of palliative care involvement depends on the institution. This can vary from only end-of-life care to active involvement in LVAD selection preparation.[47] When involved before LVAD implementation, a palliative care specialist may incorporate a type of advanced care planning geared toward patients with an LVAD referred to as preparedness planning.[48] The risks associated with LVADs threaten acceptable quality of life in recipients, and therefore, it is imperative to explore the "minimal acceptable outcome" with both patient and the surrogate decision maker. This approach should also be considered for bridge to transplant patients with LVAD because potential risks are similar and the trajectory may ultimately end up as destination therapy due to a change in transplant candidacy. A similar process can be applied to biventricular and temporary mechanical circulatory support, given the similar risk profile and possible outcomes. A potential barrier to preparedness planning before temporary support is the often emergent nature of its initiation.

The role of palliative care in heart transplantation is still being explored. As end-stage heart failure is always present before transplantation as well as the likelihood of mechanical circulatory support is also very likely prior transplant, there are certainly opportunities for palliative care involvement. Data also suggest that there is a role for palliative care in managing pretransplant quality of life and anxiety related to the uncertainty of transplant candidacy as well as posttransplant symptom burden.[49]

Optimal end-of-life care in patients with LVADs is an evolving process. Unfortunately, many patients with an LVAD die in the hospital. At Mayo Clinic in Rochester, Minnesota, 78% of patients with an LVAD died in the hospital between 2007 and 2014. It was also noted that 60% of patients deactivated before death and only 6% of deactivations were at home.[50] Multiple factors likely contribute to the high number of in-hospital deaths in patients with an LVAD. It can be challenging to find hospice agencies that will accept patients with an LVAD because technical knowledge is required to deactivate the LVAD and it is a relatively uncommon clinical situation that hospice providers may not be comfortable with. Another contributing factor is patients with LVADs may also decline quickly during hospitalization before the decision to seek comfort care and transportation home may be medically unfeasible or not desired by the patient or family.

It is generally accepted that deactivation of LVAD support following patient request is ethical similar to other life-sustaining treatments.[51] An optimal symptom management plan addressing shortness of breath, pain, and anxiety must be in place before deactivation because circulation may cease rapidly following deactivation making further dosing difficult.

SUMMARY

Heart failure, although manageable, remains a terminal illness with high incidence of symptom burden. Palliative assessment and management is essential for high-quality heart failure care. Subspecialty palliative care is proving to be beneficial in multiple heart failure patient populations and is an integral part of the mechanical circulatory support team. As we strive to improve the care of heart failure patients, we must continue to explore the optimal timing, location, and overall benefits of palliative care integration into heart failure management.

REFERENCES

1. AAHPM and the Specialty of Hospice and Palliative Medicine. Available at: http://aahpm.org/about/about. Accessed November 23, 2017.
2. Clinical practice guidelines for quality palliative care. Pittsburgh (PA): National Consensus Project for Quality Palliative Care; 2013. Available at: https://www.nationalcoalitionhpc.org/ncp-guidelines-2013/. Accessed August 1, 2018.
3. Gorodeski EZ, Goyal P, Hummel SL, et al. Domain management approach to heart failure in the geriatric patient: present and future. J Am Coll Cardiol 2018;71(17):1921–36.
4. Dumanovsky T, Augustin R, Rogers M, et al. The growth of palliative care in U.S. hospitals: a status report. J Palliat Med 2016;19(1):8–15.
5. Crousillat DR, Keeley BR, Buss MK, et al. Palliative care education in cardiology. J Am Coll Cardiol 2018;71(12):1391–4.
6. Weissman DE, Meier DE. Identifying patients in need of a palliative care assessment in the hospital setting: a consensus report from the Center to Advance Palliative Care. J Palliat Med 2011;14(1):17–23.
7. Lemond L, Allen LA. Palliative care and hospice in advanced heart failure. Prog Cardiovasc Dis 2011;54(2):168–78.
8. Mentz RJ, Tulsky JA, Granger BB, et al. The palliative care in heart failure trial: rationale and design. Am Heart J 2014;168(5):645–51.e1.
9. Rogers JG, Patel CB, Mentz RJ, et al. Palliative care in heart failure: the PAL-HF randomized,

controlled clinical trial. J Am Coll Cardiol 2017; 70(3):331–41.

10. Kavalieratos D, Gelfman LP, Tycon LE, et al. Palliative care in heart failure: rationale, evidence, and future priorities. J Am Coll Cardiol 2017;70(15): 1919–30.

11. Smith AK, Thai JN, Bakitas MA, et al. The diverse landscape of palliative care clinics. J Palliat Med 2013;16(6):661–8.

12. Evangelista LS, Lombardo D, Malik S, et al. Examining the effects of an outpatient palliative care consultation on symptom burden, depression, and quality of life in patients with symptomatic heart failure. J Card Fail 2012;18(12):894–9.

13. Bakitas M, Dionne-Odom JN, Pamboukian SV, et al. Engaging patients and families to create a feasible clinical trial integrating palliative and heart failure care: results of the ENABLE CHF-PC pilot clinical trial. BMC Palliat Care 2017;16(1):45.

14. Your Medicare Coverage. Available at: https://www.medicare.gov/coverage/hospice-and-respite-care.html. Accessed November 23, 2017.

15. Schwartzstein RM, Lahive K, Pope A, et al. Cold facial stimulation reduces breathlessness induced in normal subjects. Am Rev Respir Dis 1987; 136(1):58–61.

16. Liss HP, Grant BJ. The effect of nasal flow on breathlessness in patients with chronic obstructive pulmonary disease. Am Rev Respir Dis 1988; 137(6):1285–8.

17. Mahler DA. Opioids for refractory dyspnea. Expert Rev Respir Med 2013;7(2):123–34 [quiz: 135].

18. Johnson MJ, McDonagh TA, Harkness A, et al. Morphine for the relief of breathlessness in patients with chronic heart failure–a pilot study. Eur J Heart Fail 2002;4(6):753–6.

19. Chan JD, Treece PD, Engelberg RA, et al. Narcotic and benzodiazepine use after withdrawal of life support: association with time to death? Chest 2004; 126(1):286–93.

20. Dawson NL, Roth V, Hodge DO, et al. Opioid use in patients with congestive heart failure. Pain Med 2018;19(3):485–90.

21. Setoguchi S, Glynn RJ, Stedman M, et al. Hospice, opiates, and acute care service use among the elderly before death from heart failure or cancer. Am Heart J 2010;160(1):139–44.

22. Heerdink ER, Leufkens HG, Herings RM, et al. NSAIDs associated with increased risk of congestive heart failure in elderly patients taking diuretics. Arch Intern Med 1998;158(10):1108–12.

23. Konstam MA, Kiernan MS, Bernstein D, et al. Evaluation and management of right-sided heart failure: a scientific statement from the american heart association. Circulation 2018;137(20):e578–622.

24. Smith HS. Opioid metabolism. Mayo Clin Proc 2009; 84(7):613–24.

25. Flynn KE, Piña IL, Whellan DJ, et al. Effects of exercise training on health status in patients with chronic heart failure: HF-ACTION randomized controlled trial. JAMA 2009;301(14):1451–9.

26. Radbruch L, Strasser F, Elsner F, et al. Fatigue in palliative care patients – an EAPC approach. Palliat Med 2008;22(1):13–32.

27. Goodlin SJ. Sadness in heart failure: what is a clinician to do? J Am Coll Cardiol 2010;56(9):700–1.

28. Rutledge T, Reis VA, Linke SE, et al. Depression in heart failure a meta-analytic review of prevalence, intervention effects, and associations with clinical outcomes. J Am Coll Cardiol 2006;48(8): 1527–37.

29. Lloyd-Williams M, Spiller J, Ward J. Which depression screening tools should be used in palliative care? Palliat Med 2003;17(1):40–3.

30. Jeyanantham K, Kotecha D, Thanki D, et al. Effects of cognitive behavioural therapy for depression in heart failure patients: a systematic review and meta-analysis. Heart Fail Rev 2017;22(6):731–41.

31. Blumenthal JA, Babyak MA, O'Connor C, et al. Effects of exercise training on depressive symptoms in patients with chronic heart failure: the HF-ACTION randomized trial. JAMA 2012;308(5): 465–74.

32. O'Connor CM, Jiang W, Kuchibhatla M, et al. Safety and efficacy of sertraline for depression in patients with heart failure: results of the SADHART-CHF (sertraline against depression and heart disease in chronic heart failure) trial. J Am Coll Cardiol 2010; 56(9):692–9.

33. Teply RM, Packard KA, White ND, et al. Treatment of depression in patients with concomitant cardiac disease. Prog Cardiovasc Dis 2016;58(5):514–28.

34. Woods SW, Tesar GE, Murray GB, et al. Psychostimulant treatment of depressive disorders secondary to medical illness. J Clin Psychiatry 1986;47(1):12–5.

35. Sudore RL, Lum HD, You JJ, et al. Defining advance care planning for adults: a consensus definition from a multidisciplinary delphi panel. J Pain Symptom Manage 2017;53(5):821–32.e1.

36. Barrett T. Cardiac palliative medicine. Curr Heart Fail Rep 2017;14(5):428–33.

37. Caldwell PH, Arthur HM, Demers C. Preferences of patients with heart failure for prognosis communication. Can J Cardiol 2007;23(10):791–6.

38. Krumholz HM, Phillips RS, Hamel MB, et al. Resuscitation preferences among patients with severe congestive heart failure: results from the SUPPORT project. Study to understand prognoses and preferences for outcomes and risks of treatments. Circulation 1998;98(7):648–55.

39. Goldstein NE, Lampert R, Bradley E, et al. Management of implantable cardioverter defibrillators in end-of-life care. Ann Intern Med 2004;141(11): 835–8.

40. Mueller PS, Hook CC, Hayes DL. Ethical analysis of withdrawal of pacemaker or implantable cardioverter-defibrillator support at the end of life. Mayo Clin Proc 2003;78(8):959–63.

41. Levy D, Kenchaiah S, Larson MG, et al. Long-term trends in the incidence of and survival with heart failure. N Engl J Med 2002;347(18):1397–402.

42. Stuart B. Palliative care and hospice in advanced heart failure. J Palliat Med 2007;10(1):210–28.

43. Levy WC, Mozaffarian D, Linker DT, et al. The Seattle Heart Failure Model: prediction of survival in heart failure. Circulation 2006;113(11):1424–33.

44. O'Connor CM, Hasselblad V, Mehta RH, et al. Triage after hospitalization with advanced heart failure: the ESCAPE (evaluation study of congestive heart failure and pulmonary artery catheterization effectiveness) risk model and discharge score. J Am Coll Cardiol 2010;55(9):872–8.

45. Gramling R, Stanek S, Han PKJ, et al. Distress due to prognostic uncertainty in palliative care: frequency, distribution, and outcomes among hospitalized patients with advanced cancer. J Palliat Med 2018;21(3):315–21.

46. Jacques M, Louis, Syrek Jensen J, et al. Decision memo for ventricular assist devices for bridge-to-transplant and destination therapy (CAG-00432R). 2013. Available at: https://www.cms.gov/medicare-coverage-database/details/nca-decision-memo.aspx?NCAId=268. Accessed November 24, 2017.

47. Wordingham SE, McIlvennan CK, Fendler TJ, et al. Palliative care clinicians caring for patients before and after continuous flow-left ventricular assist device. J Pain Symptom Manage 2017; 54(4):601–8.

48. Swetz KM, Kamal AH, Matlock DD, et al. Preparedness planning before mechanical circulatory support: a "how-to" guide for palliative medicine clinicians. J Pain Symptom Manage 2014;47(5): 926–35.e6.

49. Bayoumi E, Sheikh F, Groninger H. Palliative care in cardiac transplantation: an evolving model. Heart Fail Rev 2017;22(5):605–10.

50. Dunlay SM, Strand JJ, Wordingham SE, et al. Dying with a left ventricular assist device as destination therapy. Circ Heart Fail 2016;9(10) [pii: e003096].

51. Mueller PS, Swetz KM, Freeman MR, et al. Ethical analysis of withdrawing ventricular assist device support. Mayo Clin Proc 2010;85(9):791–7.

Interventional Heart Failure and Hemodynamic Monitoring

Umair Ahmad, MD[a], Scott M. Lilly, MD, PhD[a,b],*

KEYWORDS

- Heart failure • Hemodynamic monitoring • Implantable devices • Intervention

KEY POINTS

- Device-based therapies for heart failure have several advantages; they may reduce polypharmacy and attenuate the consequences of medical nonadherence.
- Although new, the interventional heart failure discipline is based on previous examples of successful device-based heart failure therapies, including cardiac resynchronization therapy and devices for invasive hemodynamic monitoring.
- The potential spectrum of interventional heart failure devices is broad and may include temporary mechanical left ventricular support devices (eg, intra-aortic balloon pump, extracorporeal membrane oxygenation), and transcatheter-based therapies for valvular heart disease.

INTERVENTIONAL HEART FAILURE

Device-based therapies for heart failure (HF) have several advantages, they may reduce polypharmacy and attenuate the consequences of medical nonadherence.[1] Although new, the interventional HF discipline is based on previous examples of successful device-based HF therapies, including cardiac resynchronization therapy and devices for invasive hemodynamic monitoring (eg, CardioMEMS HF System, St. Jude Medical, St. Paul, MN). The potential spectrum of interventional HF devices is indeed broad, and may include temporary mechanical left ventricular (LV) support devices (eg, intra-aortic balloon pump, Impella, TandemHeart extracorporeal membrane oxygenation) and transcatheter-based therapies for valvular heart disease.[1] However, the focus next is on novel, nonvalvular, and percutaneously implantable devices for the management of HF.

INTERATRIAL SHUNT DEVICES

HF with preserved ejection fraction accounts for approximately 50% of HF admissions. Unfortunately, effective pharmacologic treatment strategies remain elusive.[2] The clinical manifestation of HF with preserved ejection fraction is exertional breathlessness often caused by an abnormal increase left atrial pressure (LAP) leading to increased pulmonary venous pressure. Although diuretic therapy is commonly used to reduce LAP, side effects and diuretic resistance are common, and the effectiveness of diuretics on long-term outcomes is difficult to establish.[3] Mechanical devices intended to reduce LAP have been developed, and operate by creating an interatrial shunt.[3] Three such devices are currently being investigated and early clinical experience has been promising.[4,5]

Disclosure: The authors have nothing to disclose.
[a] Department of Cardiology, Ohio State University Wexner Medical Center, 473 West 12th Avenue, Suite 200, Columbus, OH 43210-1252, USA; [b] Interventional Cardiology, 473 West 12th Avenue, Suite 200, Columbus, OH 43210, USA
* Corresponding author. Interventional Cardiology, 473 West 12th Avenue, Suite 200, Columbus, OH 43210.
E-mail address: Scott.Lilly@osumc.edu

Heart Failure Clin 14 (2018) 625–634
https://doi.org/10.1016/j.hfc.2018.06.007
1551-7136/18/© 2018 Elsevier Inc. All rights reserved.

V-Wave Device

The V-Wave device (V-Wave Ltd, Or Akiva, Israel) is a trileaflet porcine tissue valve housed in a hourglass-shaped nickel titanium frame (**Fig. 1**).[6] This device is a unidirectional (valve) left-to-right shunt device that is implanted via 14F catheter femoral venous approach under fluoroscopic and echocardiographic guidance. After transseptal puncture ideally through the center of the fossa ovalis, the waist of the hourglass (5-mm diameter) is placed across the fossa, securing the device in place.[4] The device allows blood to flow from the left to right only, and requires a pressure difference of greater than or equal to 5 mm Hg. Following device placement, patients have been provided anticoagulation (warfarin or direct-acting oral anticoagulant) for 3 months in addition to low-dose aspirin indefinitely.[4] The use of this unidirectional left-to-right interatrial shunt device was reported in a patient with New York Heart Association (NYHA) functional class III HF and an LV ejection fraction of less than 35%. Implantation was associated with a pulmonary artery (PA) to systemic (ascending aorta) blood flow ratio (Qp/Qs) of 1.17, improvement in the NYHA functional class, quality of life score, and exercise capacity at 3 months.[4] Following device implantation there was also an observed decrease in LV volumes and pulmonary capillary wedge pressures (PCWP; 23–17 mm Hg at 3 months; $P = .035$).

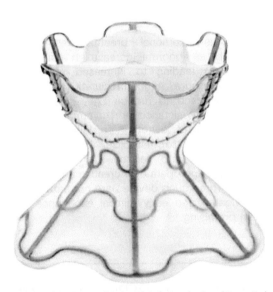

Fig. 1. The V-Wave interatrial shunt device. (*From* Del Trigo M, Bergeron S, Bernier M, et al. Unidirectional left-to-right interatrial shunting for treatment of patients with heart failure with reduced ejection fraction: a safety and proof-of-principle cohort study. Lancet 2016;387:1290–7; with permission.)

These findings are consistent with those reported in a pilot study of 10 patients, and the large animal preclinical studies that preceded human utilization.[6]

InterAtrial Shunt Device System

The InterAtrial Shunt Device (IASD) system (Corvia Medical Inc, Tewkesbury, MA) consists of a nitinol device (outer diameter 19 mm) inserted percutaneously via a 16F catheter venous approach into the interatrial septum to produce a permanent 8-mm atrial septal communication (**Fig. 2**). Unlike the V-Wave device this does not incorporate a biologic tissue. REDUCE LAP-HF (REDUCe Elevated Left Atrial Pressure in Patients with Heart Failure) was a phase I, open-label nonrandomized trial that evaluated the safety and performance of this device.[5,7] Within this trial 68 patients were enrolled with an average ejection fraction of 57% and mean PCWP at rest of 17 mm Hg. The coprimary end points of the study were reduction of PCWP at rest and exercise along with evidence of left-to-right shunt on echocardiography.[5] IASD placement was successful in 66 of 68 patients (97%). All patients received dual antiplatelet therapy with aspirin and clopidogrel post-procedure. There were no major adverse events and there was no need for cardiac surgical intervention for device-related complications. After 6 months, IASD system implantation demonstrated a reduced rest or exercise mean PCWP in 71% of patients (n = 42).[5] The follow-up to the REDUCE LAP-HF trial subsequently recruited additional patients that were randomized (n = 44) to device placement versus a sham procedure (REDUCE LAP-HF I).[8] Distribution of results was just presented at the American Heart Association Scientific Sessions in 2017 and simultaneously published in *Circulation*.[8–10] Results showed that at 1 month, the interatrial shunt device resulted in a greater reduction in PCWP pressure versus the sham procedure ($P = .028$ accounting for all stages of exercise). In addition, peak PCWP decreased by 3.5 ± 6.4 mm Hg in the interatrial shunt device group versus 0.5 ± 5.0 mm Hg in the sham procedure group ($P = .14$).[8]

A larger scale trial (REDUCE LAP-HF II) has initiated recruitment with the enrollment goal of 380 patients and completion date of July 2024 (NCT03088033).

Atrial Flow Regulator

The Atrial flow regulator (Occlutech International AB, Helsingborg, Sweden), is a self-expandable double-disc wire mesh device constructed from nitinol and braided into two flat discs connected

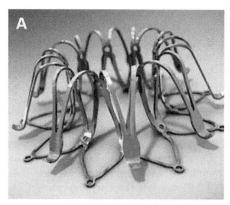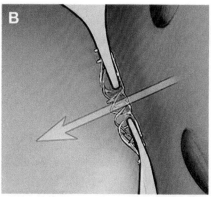

Fig. 2. (A) IASD system. (B) An illustration of the final position of the device in the interatrial septum. The flow goes from the left to the right atrium. The flow occurs according to pressure gradient (it is not unidirectional like V-Wave). ([A] *Courtesy of* Corvia Medical, Tewkesbury, MA; with permission; and [B] *From* Hasenfuß G, Hayward C, Burkhoff D, et al. A transcatheter intracardiac shunt device for heart failure with preserved ejection fraction (REDUCE LAP-HF): a multicentre, open-label, single-arm, phase 1 trial. Lancet 2016;387(10025):1300; with permission.)

by a waist of 1 to 2 mm with a central fenestration that permits bidirectional flow (**Fig. 3**). The device is available with central fenestration sizes of 6, 8, or 10 mm. A delivery catheter system is used via percutaneous 10F to 12F catheter venous approach. The device was first used in a person with severe irreversible pulmonary arterial hypertension to permit right atrial decompression.[11] However, its efficacy in HF patients is being explored in the upcoming Pilot Study to Assess Safety and Efficacy of a Novel Atrial Flow Regulator (AFR) in Heart Failure Patients (PRELIEVE trial).[12]

VENTRICULAR REMODELING

Ischemic heart disease is one of the principal causes of HF with reduced ejection fraction. Remodeling postinfarction is associated with

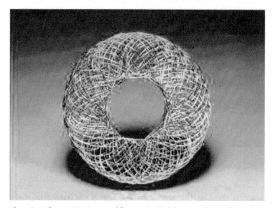

Fig. 3. The AFR is a self-expandable double-disc wire mesh device. (*Courtesy of* Occlutech International AB, Helsingborg, Sweden; with permission.)

increase ventricular volumes and poorer outcomes, particularly among those with anterior or anteroapical infarcts. Current interventions aim to interrupt and/or reverse the remodeling process by medical and cardiac resynchronization-based therapies. Historically surgical techniques have been used to restore LV dimensions and spatial differences in wall stress, although the largest clinical trial of this technique (Surgical Treatment for Ischemic Heart Failure; STITCH) failed to establish a benefit with respect to composite death and rehospitalization for cardiac causes.[13] With this and operative risks in mind, transcatheter approaches for ventricular reconstruction have been developed.

Parachute

An LV partitioning device known as Parachute (CardioKinetix, Inc, Menlo Park, CA) is composed of a self-expanding nitinol frame with a conical shape and 16 struts that serve to anchor the device at the ventricular apex. This device is deployed percutaneously in retrograde fashion via the femoral artery, and placing the delivery sheath in the LV apex, then "unsheathing" the device in patients with an existing anteroapical aneurysm (**Fig. 4**). The aim is to exclude infarcted and akinetic or dyskinetic regions, partly restore the internal LV geometry, and reduce LV volume and wall stress. Early clinical results were favorable among patients with LV ejection fraction less than 35%, NYHA functional class III or greater symptoms, and a prior infarction in the left anterior descending artery territory with associated anteroapical aneurysm.[14] However, the randomized PARACHUTE IV trial was terminated early and

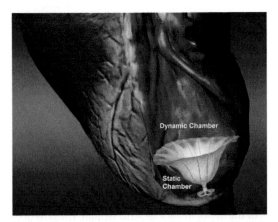

Fig. 4. The ventricular partitioning device is positioned in the aneurysmal apex. (*Adapted from* Mazzaferri EL, Gradinac S, Sagic D, et al. Percutaneous left ventricular partitioning in patients with chronic heart failure and a prior anterior myocardial infarction: results of the PercutAneous Ventricular RestorAtion in Chronic Heart failUre PaTiEnts Trial. Am Heart J 2012;163(5); with permission.)

the company had closed.[15] Whether or not this device, or a similar one has merit awaits additional development and clinical trials.

Revivent

The Revivent-TC System (Bioventrix, Inc, San Ramon, CA) implants an internal and external anchor into scarred and akinetic LV myocardium. Each anchor is composed of a small titanium bar covered by polyester cloth (**Fig. 5**). This procedure is performed with a hybrid approach by an interventional cardiologist and cardiothoracic surgeon. It is a "beating-heart" procedure (ie, cardiopulmonary bypass not necessary). Surgical procedure is performed via a minithoracotomy; the scarred LV segments are exposed; and a curved needle is inserted through the LV free wall, across the

interventricular septum where its tip is captured via a 14F jugular venous catheter. Once this connection is created, a fastening anchor is introduced over the wire via the right internal jugular vein and placed on the right ventricular (RV) side of the septum. The external anchor is then introduced and positioned via the minithoracotomy to plicate the scarred myocardium and restore the LV to a more conical shape. Initial data from the original Revivent device revealed a reduction in LV volume, increase of LV ejection fraction, and an increase in 6-minute-walk test.[16] The BRAVE-TC (BioVentrix Registry Assessment of Ventricular Enhancement for the Revivent TC) trial is currently recruiting up to 100 subjects, with anticipated 5-year follow-up to assess the safety of this device.[17] The ALIVE (American Less Invasive Ventricular Enhancement) trial is randomized 2:1 device to control, aims to enroll 120 patients with primary end point analysis (LV volume reduction, NYHA functional class, ejection fraction, quality of life, 6-minute-walk test, and rehospitalization) at 12-months; this trial began enrollment in October 2017.[18]

INJECTABLE BIOMATERIAL THERAPIES

Injectable acellular biomaterials have recently been investigated and shown early promise with respect to tissue regeneration and functional improvements in patients with HF with reduced ejection fraction. One such biomaterial is Algisyl (LoneStar Heart, Inc, Irvine, CA). This gel, derived from marine algae, is injected directly into specific areas of the LV myocardium. As the hydrogel thickens it reduces regional wall tension of the LV, with the intent of interrupting progressive LV remodeling.[19] The danger of progressive LV remodeling is that as HF progresses this leads to LV dilatation, thereby increasing wall stress and worsening clinical symptoms of HF.[20] In the AUGMENT-HF trial, patients with advanced

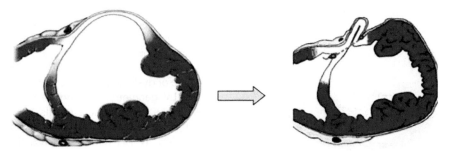

Fig. 5. The Revivent TC system, which includes an internal anchor that is delivered percutaneously into the right ventricle and an external anchor that is positioned surgically. (*From* Zaouter C, Cornolle C, Labrousse L, et al. Perioperative management of a patient undergoing a novel mini-invasive percutaneous transcatheter left ventricular reconstruction procedure. J Clin Anesth 2016;32:203–7; with permission.)

chronic HF were randomized (1:1) to alginate-hydrogel (n = 40) in plus standard medical therapy or standard medical therapy alone (control; n = 38). The primary end point of this trial was assessing for a change in peak oxygen consumption (V_{O_2}) from baseline to 6 months.[20] Improvement in peak V_{O_2} was seen starting from a mean baseline of 12.2 ± 1.8 mL/kg/min to an improved peak V_{O_2} with an additional 1.2 ± 1.24 mL/kg/min (P = .014). One-year follow-up results from the AUGMENT-HF trial also demonstrated further improvement in peak V_{O_2} in the Algisyl treatment arm when compared with the control treatment; at 12 months the mean treatment effect was an increase of 2.10 mL/kg/min (P≤.001).[21]

Although still investigational, the local delivery of compounds that can interrupt or arrest remodeling processes that occur in the context of myocardial injury represent exciting new frontiers in catheter-based HF therapies.

DURABLE PERCUTANEOUS CIRCULATORY SUPPORT
Aortix Device

Device company Procyrion, Inc (Houston, TX) has developed a catheter-deployed circulatory support assist device intended for ambulatory use in chronic HF patients. This device anchored into the descending thoracic aorta with self-expanding struts harnesses fluid entrainment to increase downstream total velocity and aortic flow (**Fig. 6**). The potential benefits include reduction of cardiac afterload, reduction of myocardial work and filling pressures, and increase in renal perfusion.[22] In a short-term animal study the device was implanted safely starting from access, strut fixation, and pump operation.[22] The device

is not intended for full mechanical circulatory support and currently only designed for partial support (2–3 L/min). Earlier this year Procyrion announced that they have partnered with Millar, Inc (Houston, TX) to use transcutaneous energy transfer technology to transfer energy from a coil mounted outside the body across the intact skin to a coil implanted inside the body, thereby eliminating the need for an indwelling power driveline.[23]

HEART FAILURE MONITORING

The diagnosis of acute decompensated HF is a clinical one, based on history, clinical findings, and corroborated at times with laboratory results. Traditional approaches to prevent recurrent hospitalization, such as monitoring weight gain and symptoms or even serologic markers, are unreliable and are often not adequately predictive.[24,25] Right heart catheterization is not routinely used for the management of patients with acute decompensated HF because of concerns about invasiveness, cost, and risk of complications and perhaps appropriate interpretation.[26,27] Although invaluable in some clinical settings, the right heart catheterization is indeed only a snapshot in time and cannot provide chronic hemodynamic data that may be most useful to titrate medical therapy, and prevent or reduce rehospitalizations. Devices and strategies for remote longitudinal hemodynamic and other surrogate assessments in the outpatient setting have been developed.[28]

IMPLANTABLE HEMODYNAMIC MONITORS

Many devices have been developed over the past decade to remotely monitor intracardiac and pulmonary arterial pressures. Collectively, these

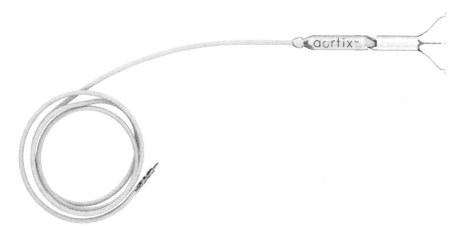

Fig. 6. Novel fully implantable percutaneous partial circulatory support device, which can provide 2–3 L/min. (*Courtesy of* Procyrion, Inc, Houston, TX; with permission.)

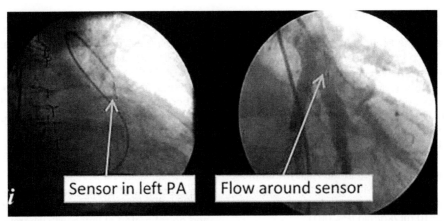

Fig. 7. Pulmonary angiography at the time of CardioMEMS implantation. (*Adapted from* Sandhu AT, Heidenreich PA. Heart failure management with ambulatory pulmonary artery pressure monitoring. Trends Cardiovasc Med 2018;28(3):212–9; with permission.)

devices are known as implantable hemodynamic monitors (IHMs).[28]

Right Ventricular Pressure Monitoring

The technology of IHMs can be traced back to the Chronicle Offers Management to Patients with Advanced Signs and Symptoms of Heart Failure (COMPASS-HF) trial.[29] In this trial patients who met an indication for implantable cardioverter-defibrillator and/or pacemaker were implanted with an RV lead that had the ability to continuously monitor RV systolic and diastolic pressures. This trial randomized 274 NYHA functional class III and IV patients with HF to standard outpatient management versus standard care plus guided information received from the RV sensor. In the active arm of the trial there was a nonsignificant 21% reduction ($P = .33$) in HF hospitalizations and emergency or urgent care visits requiring intravenous therapy.[29] At the end of the trial, the primary end point (HF event reduction) was not met, perhaps because of patients in the guided-therapy group not being managed to specific hemodynamic goals.[30] The RV sensor technologically was eventually discontinued because of several technical limitations that included generator battery depletion, which somewhat reflected the demands of continuous RV pressure.[29,30]

Pulmonary Artery Pressure Monitoring

Newer sensors developed in the form of micro-electric and nanoelectric mechanical systems have led to novel and more widely accepted application of IHMs.[31] The CardioMEMS (Abbott, Abbott Park, IL) system is the first and currently sole remote hemodynamic monitoring system approved by the US Food and Drug

Administration.[32] This system is comprised of three distinct parts. The first part is a specialized delivery system with of a transvenous over-the-wire catheter, designed to deploy the implantable sensor into a branch of the PA tree during right heart catheterization.[33] The ideal placement of the PA pressure (PAP) sensor is within an inferior and lateral branch of the left PA assuming a diameter of 7 to 15 mm. The rationale for this location is that as opposed to right-sided PA branches, left-sided branches tend to course in a posterior orientation such that interrogation of the sensor is more effective.[33,34] After identifying a segmental branch of the left PA by using selective pulmonary angiography, the sensor is deployed by withdrawing a tether release wire that unfolds the nitinol wire loops of the sensor and lodging the unit into the a branch of the left PA (**Figs. 7 and 8**A).[34] The second component is the leadless PAP sensor that is implanted permanently into the branch of the PA. The sensor does not require batteries and never needs to be replaced. It contains a pressure-sensitive capacitor that is encased in a silicone capsule with a nitinol wire loop attached to each end (**Fig. 8**B).[34] The third component is an external antenna wand that is placed against the patient's supine body or enclosed in a pillow (see **Fig. 8**B).[33,34] This antenna provides power to the sensor based on the microelectromechanical principles of resonance whereby this external antenna wand emits radiofrequency energy causing varying degrees of oscillations in the sensor depending on the surrounding pressure. The resonant frequency information is then converted to a pressure waveform. The data collected include PA systolic pressures, PA diastolic pressures, mean PA pressures, and heart rate.[33] These data are then transmitted wirelessly to a secure Web site accessible

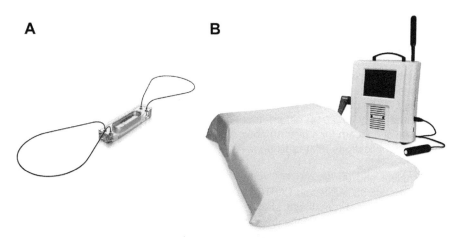

Fig. 8. CardioMEMS measurement system. (*A*) The MEMS-based sensor. (*B*) An antenna embedded in a pillow simultaneously powers and interrogates the sensor using radiofrequency. (*Adapted from* Abraham WT. The role of implantable hemodynamic monitors to manage heart failure. Heart Fail Clin 2015;11(2):183–9; with permission.)

to authorized health care providers who can evaluate and make treatment decisions.[33]

The CardioMEMS Heart Sensor Allows Monitoring of Pressure to Improve Outcomes in NYHA Class III Heart Failure Patients (CHAMPION) study evaluated this technology in ambulatory patients.[33] In CHAMPION, 550 patients with NYHA functional class III symptoms (regardless of LV systolic function) all underwent the implant of a PA sensor. Patients were subsequently randomized to a treatment arm (270 patients) or a control group (280 patients).[33] Health care professionals had access to the PA pressures of the patients in the treatment group only, allowing medications to be adjusted based on the generated data. The control group received traditional HF management using signs, symptoms, and clinical assessments. Unlike previous studies that used IHMs, specific pressure goals and treatment algorithms were dictated.[33] The goal for PA systolic pressures was 15 to 35 mm Hg, PA diastolic pressure goal of 8 to 20 mm Hg, and mean PA goal of 10 to 25 mm Hg. The foundation of these recommendations was derived from published data using RV pressure monitors.[35] In CHAMPION, if pressures were found to be elevated, then the treatment algorithm included intensifying diuretics, initiating or increasing long-acting nitrates, and/or continued education of dietary salt and fluid restrictions. At the end of 6 months the primary efficacy end point was met with a 28% relative risk reduction for HF hospitalizations in the treatment arm (*P* = .0002).[33]

Left Atrial Pressure Monitoring

A device that enables direct measurement of the LAP has been developed and consists of a transducer lead that is secured to the interatrial septum and coupled to a subcutaneous antenna coil. It is implanted via transvenous access and transseptal puncture of the interatrial septum. The tip of the sensor lead is oriented in the left atrium, which then provides LAP, temperature, and an intracardiac electrogram.[36] Similar to early heart rhythm management devices, LAP monitors (HeartPOD, Abbott Laboratories, Abbott Park, IL) can transmit data through radiofrequency wireless transmissions by direct interrogation of the coil antenna using a handheld patient advisory module (PAM).[36–38] High-fidelity LAP waveforms are captured and stored in the PAM and also available for a health care professional to review through a secure Web site. The use of this technology initially demonstrated reduction in HF events in the Hemodynamically Guided Home Self-Therapy in Severe Heart Failure Patients (HOMEOSTASIS) trial.[38] This early phase trial looked at the feasibility, safety, accuracy, and reliability of LAP monitoring using a novel self-management protocol via the PAM, analogous to diabetic self-management using glucometers in the ambulatory setting. In HOMEOSTASIS, 40 patients with NYHA functional class III or IV HF were implanted with a LAP monitor. There was an initial 3-month observation period where patients and clinicians were blinded to readings of LAP measurements, after which individualized therapy instructions based on reading was initiated. The pressure-guided and patient self-management treatment strategy was associated with reduced rate of HF hospitalizations, lower mean LAP (decreased from 17.6 mm Hg in the first 3 months to 14.8 mm Hg), increased LV ejection fraction, and improved NYHA functional class.[37]

The encouraging results from the HOMEOSTA-SIS study formed the basis for the Left Atrial Pressure Monitoring to Optimize Heart Failure Therapy Study (LAPTOP-HF), which was designed to determine the safety and clinical effectiveness of a physician-directed, patient self-management therapeutic strategy.[38] The pivotal trial for this device was terminated early in 2014 before trial completion because of concern for a high number of implant-related complications related to transseptal catheterization.[39,40]

Although incomplete and underpowered, data gathered from the HOMEOSTASIS and LAPTOP-HF studies are informative. From these studies one can hope for a future where patients can adjust medications guided by hemodynamic data.[39]

Future Roles for Implantable Hemodynamic Monitors

In the future there could be a role for IHMs in the risk stratification of patients requiring advanced HF therapies.[40] Data from the CHAMPION trial found that the treatment group progressed faster to LV assist device therapy and had a shorter time to heart transplantation.[41] PAP sensors in patients with LV assist devices can also longitudinally be followed for volume retention and possible development of pump thrombosis. Theoretically a rise in PAP may correlate with a concomitant rise in lactate dehydrogenase levels, which can be an early marker for pump thrombosis.[42] PAP sensors may also provide a novel way to measure PA pressures in those a total artificial heart whose PA pressures are unable to be measured because of obvious technical limitations of the total artificial heart implant. This technology is being used to remotely monitor patients with pulmonary hypertension, which can allow for recognition of optimal pulmonary hypertension medication dosing and decreasing the procedural risk of repeat right heart catheterizations.[43] CardioMEMS was also recently implanted in a patient with congenital heart disease that exhibited a single ventricle with Fontan anatomy, with which the goal of implantation was to further understand Fontan hemodynamics and guide treatment strategies in these patients.[44]

REFERENCES

1. Shah SJ. Interventional heart failure: a new field. EuroIntervention 2016;12(Suppl X):X85–8.
2. Li J, Becher PM, Blankenberg S, et al. Current treatment of heart failure with preserved ejection fraction: should we add life to the remaining years or add years to the remaining life? Cardiol Res Pract 2013;2013:1–9.
3. Cuthbert JJ, Pellicori P, Clark AL. Interatrial shunt devices for heart failure with normal ejection fraction: a technology update. Med Devices (Auckl) 2017;10:123–32.
4. Amat-Santos IJ, Bergeron S, Bernier M, et al. Left atrial decompression through unidirectional left-to-right interatrial shunt for the treatment of left heart failure: first-in-man experience with the V-Wave device. EuroIntervention 2015;10(9):1127–31.
5. Søndergaard L, Reddy V, Kaye D, et al. Transcatheter treatment of heart failure with preserved or mildly reduced ejection fraction using a novel interatrial implant to lower left atrial pressure. Eur J Heart Fail 2014;16(7):796–801.
6. Del Trigo MD, Bergeron S, Bernier M, et al. Unidirectional left-to-right interatrial shunting for treatment of patients with heart failure with reduced ejection fraction: a safety and proof-of-principle cohort study. Lancet 2016;387(10025):1290–7.
7. Malek F, Neuzil P, Gustafsson F, et al. Clinical outcome of transcatheter treatment of heart failure with preserved or mildly reduced ejection fraction using a novel implant. Int J Cardiol 2015;187:227–8.
8. Feldman T, Mauri L, Kahwash R, et al. A transcatheter interatrial shunt device for the treatment of heart failure with preserved ejection fraction (REDUCE LAP-HF I): a phase 2, randomized, sham-controlled trial. Circulation 2017;137(4):364–75.
9. Hasenfuß G, Hayward C, Burkhoff D, et al. A transcatheter intracardiac shunt device for heart failure with preserved ejection fraction (REDUCE LAP-HF): a multicentre, open-label, single-arm, phase 1 trial. Lancet 2016;387(10025):1298–304.
10. Feldman T, Komtebedde J, Burkhoff D, et al. Transcatheter interatrial shunt device for the treatment of heart failure: rationale and design of the randomized trial to REDUCE elevated left atrial pressure in heart failure (REDUCE LAP-HF I). Circ Heart Fail 2016;9(7) [pii:e003025].
11. Rajeshkumar R, Pavithran S, Sivakumar K, et al. Atrial septostomy with a predefined diameter using a novel Occlutech atrial flow regulator improves symptoms and cardiac index in patients with severe pulmonary arterial hypertension. Catheter Cardiovasc Interv 2017;90(7):1145–53.
12. The Prelieve Trial - Pilot Study to Assess Safety and Efficacy of a Novel Atrial Flow Regulator (AFR) in Heart Failure Patients. Available at: https://clinicaltrials.gov/ct2/show/NCT03030274. Accessed October 11, 2017.
13. Jones RH, Velazquez EJ, Michler RE, et al. Coronary bypass surgery with or without surgical ventricular reconstruction. N Engl J Med 2009;360(17):1705–17.
14. Mazzaferri EL, Gradinac S, Sagic D, et al. Percutaneous left ventricular partitioning in patients with chronic heart failure and a prior anterior myocardial

infarction: results of the PercutAneous Ventricular RestorAtion in Chronic Heart failUre PaTiEnts Trial. Am Heart J 2012;163(5):812–20.e1.

15. A Pivotal Trial to Establish the Efficacy and Long-term Safety of the Parachute Implant System - Full Text View. A Pivotal Trial to Establish the Efficacy and Long-term Safety of the Parachute Implant System - Full Text View - ClinicalTrials.gov. Available at: https://clinicaltrials.gov/ct2/show/NCT01614652. Accessed November 4, 2017.

16. Hernández-Enríquez, et al. New transcatheter treatment of the dilated ischaemic cardiomyopathy with Revivent system. Abstract presented at EuroPCR (Paris) France, May 6, 2016.

17. Observational study to collect data on health improvements after mini-invasive operation with Revivent TC device to reshape the heart and reduce its volume. ISRCTN - ISRCTN89757315: observational study to collect data on health improvements after mini-invasive operation with Revivent TC device to reshape the heart and reduce its volume. Available at: http://www.isrctn.com/ISRCTN89757315/. Accessed November 17, 2017.

18. First Patient Enrolled in U.S. Arm of ALIVE Pivotal Heart Failure Trial. DAIC. 2017. Available at: https://www.dicardiology.com/content/first-patient-enrolled-us-arm-alive-pivotal-heart-failure-trial. Accessed December 23, 2017.

19. Yu J, Christman KL, Chin E, et al. Restoration of left ventricular geometry and improvement of left ventricular function in a rodent model of chronic ischemic cardiomyopathy. J Thorac Cardiovasc Surg 2009;137(1):180–7.

20. Anker SD, Coats AJ, Cristian G, et al. A prospective comparison of alginate-hydrogel with standard medical therapy to determine impact on functional capacity and clinical outcomes in patients with advanced heart failure (AUGMENT-HF trial). Eur Heart J 2015;36(34):2297–309.

21. Mann DL, Lee RJ, Coats AJ, et al. One-year follow-up results from AUGMENT-HF: a multicentre randomized controlled clinical trial of the efficacy of left ventricular augmentation with Algisyl in the treatment of heart failure. Eur J Heart Fail 2015; 18(3):314–25.

22. Shabari FR, George J, Cuchiara MP, et al. Improved hemodynamics with a novel miniaturized intra-aortic axial flow pump in a porcine model of acute left ventricular dysfunction. ASAIO J 2013;59(3):240–5.

23. Micro Heart Pump Developer, Procyrion, to Test Transcutaneous Energy Transfer Technology from Millar. RSS. Available at: http://www.procyrion.com/news/micro-heart-pump-developer-procyrion-to-test-transcutaneous-energy-transfer-technology-from-millar. Accessed October 1, 2017.

24. Lewin J, Ledwidge M, O'Loughlin C, et al. Clinical deterioration in established heart failure: what is the value of BNP and weight gain in aiding diagnosis? Eur J Heart Fail 2005;7:953–7.

25. Stevenson LW, Perloff JK. The limited reliability of physical signs for estimating hemodynamics in chronic heart failure. JAMA 1989;261:884–8.

26. Binanay C, Califf RM, Hasselblad V, et al. Evaluation study of congestive heart failure and pulmonary artery catheterization effectiveness: the ESCAPE trial. JAMA 2005;294:1625–33.

27. Yancy CW, Jessup M, Bozkurt B, et al. 2013 ACCF/AHA guideline for the management of heart failure: a report of the American College of Cardiology Foundation/American Heart Association Task Force on Practice Guidelines. J Am Coll Cardiol 2013;62: e147–239.

28. Abraham WT. The role of implantable hemodynamic monitors to manage heart failure. Heart Fail Clin 2015;11(2):183–9.

29. Bourge RC, Abraham WT, Adamson PB, et al, the COMPASS-HF group. Randomized controlled trial of an implantable continuous hemodynamic monitor in patients with advanced heart failure: the COMPASS-HF study. J Am Coll Cardiol 2008;51: 1073–9.

30. Emani S. Remote monitoring to reduce heart failure readmissions. Curr Heart Fail Rep 2017; 14(1):40–7.

31. Sousa C, Leite S, Lagido R, et al. Telemonitoring in heart failure: a state-of-the-art review. Rev Port Cardiol 2014;33:229–39.

32. U.S. Food and Drug Administration FDA Executive Summary—Addendum. Presented December 8, 2011, at Gaithersburg MD. Available at: http://www.fda.gov/downloads/AdvisoryCommittees/CommitteesMeetingMaterials/MedicalDevices/MedicalDevicesAdvisoryCommittee/CirculatorySystemDevicesPanel/UCM282272.pdf. Accessed March 5, 2017.

33. Abraham WT, Adamson PB, Bourge RC, et al, CHAMPION Trial Study Group. Wireless pulmonary artery haemodynamic monitoring in chronic heart failure: a randomised controlled trial. Lancet 2011; 377:658–66.

34. Shavelle D, Jermyn R. The CardioMEMS heart failure sensor: a procedural guide for implanting physicians. J Invasive Cardiol 2016;28(7):273.

35. Stevenson LW, Zile M, Bennett TD, et al. Chronic ambulatory intracardiac pressures and future heart failure events. Circ Heart Fail 2010;3(5): 580–7.

36. Troughton RW, Ritzema J, Eigler NL, et al. Direct left atrial pressure monitoring in severe heart failure: long-term sensor performance. J Cardiovasc Transl Res 2011;4:3–13.

37. Ritzema J, Troughton R, Melton I, et al, the Hemodynamically Guided Home Self-Therapy in Severe Heart Failure Patients Study Group. Physician-directed patient self-management of left atrial

pressure in advanced chronic heart failure. Circulation 2010;121:1086–95.

38. Maurer MS, Adamson PB, Costanzo MR, et al. Rationale and design of the left atrial pressure monitoring to optimize heart failure therapy study (LAPTOP-HF). J Card Fail 2015;21:479–88.

39. Abraham WT, editor. Hemodynamic monitoring in advanced heart failure: results from the LAPTOP-HF trial. HFSA 20th Annual Scientific Meeting. Orlando (FL), September 18, 2016.

40. Mabote T, Wong K, Cleland JG. The utility of novel non-invasive technologies for remote hemodynamic monitoring in chronic heart failure. Expert Rev Cardiovasc Ther 2014;12:923–8.

41. Feldman D, Naka Y, Cabuay B, et al. A wireless hemodynamic pressure sensor before and after ventricular assist device placement: a sub-study of the CHAMPION trial. J Heart Lung Transplant 2011;30(Suppl 4):S86.

42. Lampert BC, Emani S. Remote hemodynamic monitoring for ambulatory left ventricular assist device patients. J Thorac Dis 2015;7(12):2165–71.

43. Raina A, Abraham WT, Adamson PB, et al. Limitations of right heart catheterization in the diagnosis and risk stratification of patients with pulmonary hypertension related to left heart disease: insights from a wireless pulmonary artery pressure monitoring system. J Heart Lung Transplant 2015;34:438–47.

44. Bradley EA, Berman D, Daniels CJ. First implantable hemodynamic monitoring device placement in single ventricle fontan anatomy. Catheter Cardiovasc Interv 2016;88(2):248–52.

Management of Sleep Apnea in Heart Failure

Ali Vazir, MBBS, PhD, FESC, FRCP[a,b,]*, Varun Sundaram, MD, FRCP[a,b,c]

KEYWORDS

- Sleep apnea • Heart failure • Adaptive servo-ventilation • CPAP

KEY POINTS

- Sleep apnea is common in patients with heart failure (HF), and is characterized by 2 phenotypes, central (CSA) and obstructive sleep apnea (OSA), and is associated with poor outcome.
- Patients with HF and sleep apnea do not usually report excessive daytime hypersomnolence, suggesting the need for screening.
- Registry data and small randomized controlled trials suggest that treatment of OSA in patients with HF with continuous positive airway pressure is beneficial; however, data from large randomized controlled studies are lacking.
- CSA is associated with severity of HF and improving the underlying HF may alleviate CSA.
- A recent randomized controlled trial of adaptive servo-ventilation (ASV) in patients with HF and CSA, despite ASV effectively alleviating CSA, ASV was associated with increased cardiovascular mortality.

INTRODUCTION

The prevalence of sleep-disordered breathing (SDB) in the general population is 2% to 4%,[1] in contrast SDB is much more common in patients with heart failure (HF), with the prevalence ranging between 50% and 75%.[2,3] The presence of SDB in patients with HF appears to be associated with increased risk of cardiovascular morbidity and mortality.[4] In this review, we describe the types, pathophysiology, and consequences of SDB and discuss ways in which SDB can be diagnosed. We also lay emphasis on the recent randomized controlled trials that have had a major impact on how SDB is managed and highlight the complex relationship between SDB and outcomes.

TYPES OF SLEEP-DISORDERED BREATHING AND PATHOPHYSIOLOGY

The predominant type of SDB in patients with HF is central sleep apnea (CSA), and is reported to occur in 45% to 55% of patients with HF,[2,3] with similar prevalence rates between the 2 main phenotypes of HF, reduced or preserved ejection fraction (ie, HFrEF or HFpEF).[5,6] The prevalence of SDB in decompensated HF may be higher.[7]

The presence of CSA is characterized by abnormal regulation of breathing within the respiratory centers located in the brainstem. The hallmark of CSA is the reduced or complete lack of efferent activity to respiratory pump muscles leading to periods of 10 or more seconds in which

Disclosure Statement: Dr A. Vazir has received an unrestricted grant from Boston Scientific and a travel grant from ResMED UK. Dr V. Sundaram has nothing to disclose.
[a] Department of Cardiology, Royal Brompton Hospital, Royal Brompton and Harefield NHS Foundation Trust, Sydney Street, London SW3 6NP, UK; [b] Royal Brompton Hospital, National Heart and Lung Institute, Imperial College London, Dovehouse Street, London SW3 6LR, UK; [c] Case Western Reserve University School of Medicine, 2109 Adelbert Rd, Cleveland, Ohio 44106, USA
* Corresponding author. Royal Brompton and Harefield NHS Foundation Trust, Sydney Street, London SW3 6NP, UK.
E-mail address: A.vazir@imperial.ac.uk

1551-7136/18/© 2018 Elsevier Inc. All rights reserved.

heartfailure.theclinics.com

there is significantly reduced (hypopnea) or complete cessation (apnea) of respiratory effort (**Fig. 1**). Thus, during a central apnea there is reduced or absent chest wall and abdominal movement and airflow, which is associated with a dip in oxygen saturation and a rise in arterial carbon dioxide ($Paco_2$) and terminated by an arousal, which is characterized with a rise in heart rate and blood pressure. Cheyne-Stokes respiration (CSR) is another type of SDB, which is similar to CSA, but is characterized by crescendo-decrescendo oscillation of tidal volume, with intervals of hyperventilation separated by periods of hypopnea and apnea. A major feature of CSR is that the cycle length of the crescendo-decrescendo breathing pattern is characteristically prolonged compared with CSA and appears to correlate with circulation time. CSR also may be detected in patients who are awake at rest or during exercise in patients with severe and advanced HF.[8,9]

The pathophysiology of CSA and CSR is complex and not completely understood. The changes in $Paco_2$ levels appear to play an important role in the pathophysiology of CSA.

The central chemoreceptors can detect changes in levels of $Paco_2$, such that a rise in $Paco_2$ leads to increased respiratory effort. By contrast, a fall in $Paco_2$ will lead to reduced respiratory effort. Central apnea will result when $Paco_2$ falls below the apneic threshold: the point at which respiratory effort is no longer triggered. Patients with HF characteristically have $Paco_2$ close to the lower limit of normal or may have hypocapnia in response to stimulation of the pulmonary stretch receptors (J-receptors), which are sensitive to pulmonary congestion.[10] Furthermore, patients with HF have increased hypercapnic ventilatory response, also termed enhanced chemosensitivity to $Paco_2$.[11]

Thus, in patients with HF, the fluctuations in the level of $Paco_2$ below and above the apneic threshold may switch the breathing on and off, and result in periods of central apnea/hypopnea and hyperventilation. The presence of circulatory delay, leading to a time lag between changes in arterial CO_2 and O_2 in the lung and their detection in the central chemoreceptors in the brainstem, may lengthen the apnea/hypopnea cycle.[12]

Obstructive sleep apnea (OSA) is also more frequently observed in patients with HF compared with the general population, with reported prevalence of 10% to 15%.[2,3] OSA remains the commonest form of SDB in the general population. The pathophysiology of OSA is characterized by the collapse of the pharyngeal airway. The latter may be either complete or partial, leading to an obstructive apnea or hypopnea, respectively. Obstructive apnea may occur because of loss of pharyngeal dilator muscle tone during sleep. The tendency of pharyngeal collapse is increased with obesity, large neck size, and retrognathia, and in patients with HF the presence of pharyngeal edema due to rostral fluid shift during sleep.[13] An obstructive apnea is characterized by the absence of airflow, with continued but paradoxic chest wall

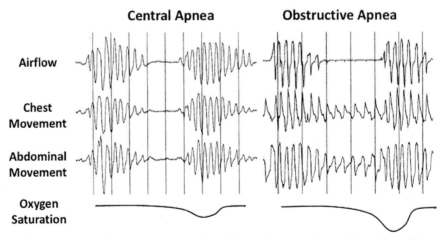

Fig. 1. Example of central and obstructive apnea with evidence of oxygen desaturation. Central apnea is characterized by absence of airflow of more than 10 seconds and lack of chest and abdominal movement, with associated oxygen desaturation, followed by period of hyperpnea (faster and deeper chest and abdominal movement) leading to increased airflow and rise in oxygen saturation level. Obstructive apnea is characterized by absence of airflow, but continued and paradoxic chest and abdominal movement, associated with a more marked oxygen desaturation compared with a central apnea, followed by hyperpnea with faster and deeper chest and abdominal movement and a rise in oxygen saturation.

and abdominal movement, in association with an arterial oxygen desaturation (see **Fig. 1**).

CLINICAL FEATURES OF SLEEP-DISORDERED BREATHING

One of the main clinical features of SDB in the general population is fatigue and daytime hypersomnolence. Contrary to this, patients with HF appear not to report excessive daytime sleepiness despite objective evidence that they may be sleepy.[14,15] Metrics of daytime somnolence that record subjective sleepiness, such as the Epworth sleepiness score (ESS), are normal in most patients with HF. Even patients with OSA and HF also have low ESS scores[16]; thus, raising the proposition that screening methods are required to detect SDB in patients with HF. Furthermore, patients who have HF regularly report nonspecific symptoms, such as fatigue and lethargy, that also may be linked to the underlying HF or as side effects of some of the medication, such as beta-blockers. A feature of SDB that also appears to be more frequent compared with patients with HF without SDB is paroxysmal nocturnal dyspnea (PND).[17] Often patients may be waking up immediately after having an apnea, during the hyperpnea phase and arousal, mimicking some of the features of PND.

Other symptoms that also may be reported in patients with SDB, with a degree of variation between individuals, are morning headaches, poor-quality sleep, frequently waking up from sleep, and low mood and depression. It is also very valuable to ask the bed partners of patients whether or not they have witnessed an apnea.

In large registry of patients with HFrEF and SDB, the presence of SDB was associated with obesity, male sex, atrial fibrillation, age, and poorer left ventricular systolic function.[18] Risk factors for CSA in patients with HF are age older than 60 years, male sex, atrial fibrillation, and presence of hypocapnia while awake.[19]

DIAGNOSING SLEEP-DISORDERED BREATHING

An apnea is defined as a reduction in airflow ≥90% of pre-event baseline for ≥10 seconds and a hypopnea is defined as a reduction in airflow ≥30% from baseline for ≥10 seconds, with a fall in oxygen saturation of ≥3% or detection of an arousal from sleep.[20] The diagnosis of SDB is made when at least more than 5 apnea/hypopnea events per hour of sleep (apnea-hypopnea index [AHI]) are detected. Thus, an AHI of less than 5 events per hour can usually occur in healthy individuals.

The severity of SDB is arbitrarily categorized as mild SDB, defined as an AHI of 5 to 15 per hour, moderate SDB as an AHI of 15 to 30 per hour, and severe SDB as an AHI of more than 30 per hour. Furthermore, SDB is arbitrarily categorized into 2 main phenotypes, CSA and OSA, when more than 50% of events are central or obstructive, respectively.

The gold standard test for the diagnosis of SDB is the use of nocturnal polysomnography (NPSG), which involves monitoring electroencephalography, electro-oculography, and electromyography to determine wakefulness and sleep. Monitoring of the electrocardiograph, respiratory parameters (oronasal airflow/pressure, abdominal and chest movements), and pulse oximetry are performed. The AHI is determined from oronasal airflow/pressure, and the abdominal and chest movement component of the NPSG. The latter may be set up in hospitals or in the home. However, NPSG is expensive and time-consuming.

The commonest type of test used for diagnosing SDB is polygraphy (PG). These devices monitor oronasal airflow/pressure, chest and abdominal movement, and pulse oximetry. PG devices may be used in hospitals or at home and offer the advantages of being easier and cheaper to use than NPSG. They are accepted as an alternative to standard NPSG in patients with a high pretest probability for SDB,[21] with a sensitivity and specificity of 90% to 100% when compared with NPSG.[22,23]

Overnight pulse oximetry when used alone may be a useful screening tool, with a sensitivity of 93% and specificity of 73% in detecting moderate to severe SDB (AHI of >15 events per hour) compared with NPSG when more than 12.5 desaturations of ≥3% occur per hour.[24] A disadvantage of pulse oximetry alone is that it cannot differentiate between the 2 main phenotypes of SDB.

Other methods of screening for SDB in patients with HF that remain under investigation include pacemaker algorithms that follow changes in thoracic impedance and minute ventilation that may be able to detect apnea and hypopneas. In one such study, the sensitivity and specificity of the pacemaker algorithm in detecting moderate to severe SDB was 89% and 85%, respectively.[25]

RATIONALE FOR TREATING SLEEP-DISORDERED BREATHING

Data suggest that there is a link between SDB and HF, such that the Sleep Heart Health Study showed that OSA is independently associated with incident HF.[26] Furthermore, data from the

Wisconsin Sleep Cohort Study showed that after adjusting for age, sex, smoking, and body mass index, there was an increased incidence of coronary heart disease or HF in the general population over 24 years of follow-up, with a hazard ratio of 2.6 (1.1–6.1) for severe SDB (AHI >30/h) relative to an AHI of 0 per hour.[27]

In patients with established HF, the presence of CSA or OSA are independently associated with increased mortality and morbidity.[4,28] The presence of CSA in patients with acute decompensated HF is usually severe (ie, AHI >30/h),[7] and these patients are at higher risk of readmission and mortality.[29] Optimizing HF syndrome with medical therapy (such as decongestion or disease-modifying medications) or cardiac resynchronization therapy may reduce AHI in patients with CSA or CSR.[30]

The pathophysiological consequences of SDB that have been linked with HF include increased sympathetic nervous system activation, increased negative intrathoracic pressure swings, intermittent hypoxia and hypercapnia, and increased arousal from sleep with associated sleep fragmentation and deprivation. Furthermore, metabolic and endothelial dysfunction[31,32] have also been reported, together with increased systemic inflammation characterized by elevated levels of interleukin-6 and high-sensitivity C-reactive protein.[33,34]

Patients with SDB have evidence of higher level of urinary catecholamines and higher sympathetic nervous system (SNS) activity within muscle. Activation of SNS is also linked with inflammatory cytokines.[35]

During an apnea or hypopnea, the repetitive inspiratory effort may lead to large swings of negative intrathoracic pressure. These negative swings in intrathoracic pressure may be as much as −50 mm Hg with obstructive apneas, but tend to be much lower during central apneas. The consequences of the negative intrathoracic pressure are an increased left ventricular (LV) afterload, increased LV transmural pressure, and increased right ventricular venous return leading to movement of the interventricular septum into the LV,[36] with subsequent impaired LV relaxation, increased myocardial oxygen demand, and reduced cardiac output. The rise in left atrial (LA) pressure may subsequently lead to adverse remodeling of the LA, characterized by LA dilation and predisposing to the development of atrial arrhythmias, such as atrial fibrillation, the latter of which is associated with SDB.[37] Severe SDB is also associated with LV diastolic dysfunction independent of obesity, diabetes mellitus, and hypertension.[38]

TREATING SLEEP-DISORDERED BREATHING IN PATIENTS WITH HEART FAILURE

For all patients with SDB and HF, medical optimization is paramount, particularly in patients with CSA or CSR, in which optimization with disease-modifying drugs, decongestion with diuretics, cardiac resynchronization therapy, treatment with LV assist devices or cardiac transplantation all appear to reduce AHI, and, in some circumstances, abolish CSA completely.[30,39] Weight loss in the general population that has OSA appears to be effective therapy,[40] and for obese patients with HF may also be beneficial, but its evidence base in HF is lacking.

Lateral sleeping position has a major beneficial effect on the severity of SDB in patients with HF, particularly in patients with HF with OSA than those with CSA.[41] In light of these data, positional therapy, for example, using a wedged cushion, can discourage patients sleeping on their backs and encourage a lateral position. In patients with mild OSA in the general population, mandibular advancement splint may reduce AHI, particularly in individuals with retrognathia.

Mask-Based Positive Airway Pressure Therapies in Patients with Heart Failure and Obstructive Sleep Apnea

Treatment of OSA with continuous positive airway pressure therapy (CPAP) is well established. CPAP delivers constant and continuous pressure throughout both inspiration and expiration through a nasal or face mask. It reduces episodes of obstructive apnea, hypopneas, and associated arousals. It also reduces daytime somnolence and daytime blood pressure.[42–44] Observational data also suggest that the use of CPAP in the general population appears to be associated with lower number of events compared with patients with OSA who were untreated or those with poor compliance to CPAP.[45]

In a randomized study of 24 patients with chronic heart failure (CHF) with OSA, 12 patients randomized to 1 month of CPAP therapy (average use of therapy 6.2 hours per night) had a significant improvement in LV ejection fraction (LVEF) of 9% (from 25.8% ± 2.8 to 33.8% ± 2.4%). Daytime heart rate and blood pressure were also decreased after use of CPAP for 1 month.[46] The improvement was attributed to the reversal of the mechanical and hemodynamic effects of OSA. In contrast, the control group did not experience any improvement in any of these variables. In a similar randomized controlled study, Mansfield and colleagues[47] showed in 55 patients with CHF with OSA, that 3 months of CPAP therapy significantly improved LVEF by 5%, reduced sympathetic activity, and improved quality of life measures. CPAP over 3 months also resulted in improvements in LV modeling, pulmonary hypertension, and also right ventricular function.

Registry data suggest that the use of CPAP in patients with HF is associated with reduced rate of death, heart transplantation, or implant of a ventricular assist device.[48] Furthermore, this was also observed in a large US registry in which treatment with CPAP was associated with better 2-year survival rate than those who were not treated (hazard ratio 0.49; 95% confidence interval [CI] 0.29–0.84; $P = .009$).[49] Adequately powered randomized controlled studies assessing the impact of CPAP on cardiovascular outcomes in patients with HF and OSA have not been performed. The ADVENT-HF study (NCT01128816) is currently assessing the utility of adaptive servo-ventilation (ASV) in patients with HF and SDB, with either predominant OSA or CSA, and the results are expected in 2020. ASV is a form of positive-pressure ventilation with variable pressure algorithm that delivers back-up breaths and high pressures during apnea and lower pressure during hyperpnea, resulting in resolution of AHI to normal levels in most cases.

Mask-Based Positive Airway Pressure Therapies in Patients with Heart Failure and Central Sleep Apnea

The 2 main mask-based positive-pressure treatments that have been extensively studied in patients with HF and CSA are CPAP and ASV. ASV has been shown to treat CSA more effectively than CPAP. In small studies, both CPAP and ASV have shown a fall in AHI levels coinciding with improvement in surrogate markers of HF, such as biomarkers (eg, brain natriuretic peptide), exercise capacity, ejection fraction, and symptoms.[19,43,50] The CANPAP (Canadian Continuous Positive Airway Pressure for Patients with Central Sleep Apnea and Heart Failure) trial of 203 patients with HFrEF and CSA assessed the effectiveness of CPAP versus medical therapy on transplant-free survival.[51] CPAP was shown to reduce mean AHI level from 40 ± 16 events per hour to approximately 19 ± 16 events per hour, but it did not improve survival rates. A post hoc analysis of CANPAP showed that in those patients who had their CSA suppressed by CPAP, that is, the AHI level being suppressed to less than 15 events per hour, had a significantly better survival rate compared with those in whom CPAP did not suppress CSA effectively. Caution is required when interpreting these results, however, as the number of events in this

analysis was low: 5 in the CPAP-suppressed versus 13 in the CPAP-unsuppressed group.[52]

The SERVE-HF trial (Treatment of Sleep-disordered Breathing by Adaptive Servo-ventilation in Heart Failure Patients) study assessed the effectiveness of ASV versus optimal medical therapy on survival in 1325 patients with HFrEF and CSA.[53] The results of the trial were unexpected, and they demonstrated that ASV, despite effectively treating CSA (with a drop in mean AHI levels from 31.2 events per hour at baseline to 6.6 events per hour at 12 months), did not result in a benefit in the primary endpoint of the trial, a composite endpoint of time-to-event analysis of first event of death from any cause, life-saving cardiovascular intervention (cardiac transplantation, implantation of a ventricular assist device, resuscitation after sudden cardiac arrest, or appropriate life-saving shock) or unplanned hospitalization for worsening HF (54.1% in the ASV group vs 50.8% in the medical group; hazard ratio 1.13; 95% CI 0.97–1.31; $P = .10$). Furthermore, to everyone's surprise, ASV was associated with harm with increased all-cause mortality rate (hazard ratio 1.28; 95% CI 1.06–1.55; $P = .01$), predominantly due to an increased risk of cardiovascular death (hazard ratio 1.34; 95% CI 1.09–1.65; $P = .006$), driven mainly by sudden cardiac death as opposed to pump failure death. The explanations for these findings have included a possible direct toxic effect of positive airway pressure on patients with reduced LV function and a low pulmonary capillary wedge pressure; another explanation included the fact that the presence of CSA may actually be beneficial in patients with HF.[54] Currently, the use of ASV for the treatment of CSA in patients with HF is not recommended.

Following the SERVE-HF trial, the CAT-HF trial, which was a randomized trial of ASV in patients presenting with acute decompensated HF, has been terminated. However, the ADVENT-HF trial (NCT01128816), as described previously, is ongoing and may provide more data on efficacy and safety in patients with SDB and HF. Smaller studies of ASV in patients with HFpEF have also been undertaken with benefits in surrogate markers of HF, such as brain-type natriuretic peptide levels; however, there are no randomized controlled studies of ASV in the HFpEF population assessing outcomes.[55,56]

Non–mask-Based Therapies for Patients with Heart Failure and Sleep-Disordered Breathing

Oxygen therapy may reduce AHI and frequency of oxygen desaturation in patients with HF and

CSA[57]; however, the impact of oxygen on prognosis is unclear.

Phrenic nerve stimulation using an implantable unilateral transvenous neurostimulator has shown a significant reduction in the severity of CSA, with a drop in AHI from 50 ± 15 to 28 ± 18 events per hour, together with improved oxygenation (reduced frequency of oxygen desaturation of >4% from 46 ± 19 to 27 ± 18 per hour). A significant proportion of patients in this study had HF. A potential advantage of this approach is pacing the diaphragm works by sucking air into the lungs, which may be more physiologic than positive airway pressure treatments.[58]

In patients with HF and CSA, acetazolamide may reduce AHI and improve oxygen saturation levels.[59] This has subsequently led to the design of the HF-ACZ study (Predicting Successful Sleep Apnea Treatment With Acetazolamide in Heart Failure Patients, NCT01377987), which is currently under way.

Should We Be Treating Central Sleep Apnea or Cheyne-Stokes Respiration in Patients with Heart Failure?

The surprising results of the SERVE-HF study highlighted the need to reassess the way we interpret CSA or CSR, in that this abnormal pattern of breathing may in fact be favorable and beneficial in HF and perhaps treating it may not be constructive, as was argued by Naughton.[54] The cycles of apnea and hyperventilation may bring several benefits. For example, the presence of apnea may prevent respiratory muscle fatigue that may develop with continuous tachypnea in the context of pulmonary congestion. Alternating hyperventilation and hypoventilation may lead to increase in stroke volume and circulation in the presence of swings in intrathoracic pressure. Furthermore, reduced sympathetic and increased vagal activity may occur during the hyperventilation phase following an apnea, and the development of hypocapnia and respiratory alkalosis may aid cardiac function during hypoxemia by improving oxygen delivery (via Bohr and Haldane effects). In addition, hyperventilation leads to a larger end-tidal volume that may act as a reservoir of oxygen-counteracting hypoxemia in the context of pulmonary edema. Thus, correcting CSA may lead to the loss of these protective mechanisms and may also partly explain the increased cardiovascular mortality rates observed in the SERVE-HF study.

SUMMARY

SDB is common in patients with HF, with the predominant type being CSA as opposed to OSA.

Patients with HF and SDB commonly do not report subjective symptoms of daytime hypersomnolence, emphasizing the need for screening for SDB in this population. SDB in patients with HF is associated with a poor prognosis, and this has been the rationale for treating this condition. The focus of alleviating SDB should always begin by improving and optimizing the underlying HF syndrome. A recent randomized study assessing the efficacy of ASV on outcomes in patients with HF and CSA, despite effectively treating CSA, was associated with increased cardiovascular mortality, raising concerns that perhaps CSA may be a beneficial adaptive response in patients with HF, and whether it should be treated at all. Other forms of treatment that are being assessed for CSA in patients with HF include phrenic nerve stimulation and use of acetazolamide.

The treatment of OSA in patients with HF with CPAP appears to be beneficial, but evidence for this is limited to data from observational datasets and small randomized trials, and data from adequately powered outcome studies using this therapy in patients with HF patients and OSA are necessary. Furthermore, similar outcome trials are also needed to assess the efficacy and safety of treating SDB in patients with HF and preserved ejection fraction or those presenting with acute decompensated HF.

REFERENCES

1. Young T, Palta M, Dempsey J, et al. The occurrence of sleep-disordered breathing among middle-aged adults. N Engl J Med 1993;328(17):1230–5.
2. Vazir A, Hastings PC, Dayer M, et al. A high prevalence of sleep disordered breathing in men with mild symptomatic chronic heart failure due to left ventricular systolic dysfunction. Eur J Heart Fail 2007;9(3):243–50.
3. Oldenburg O, Lamp B, Faber L, et al. Sleep-disordered breathing in patients with symptomatic heart failure: a contemporary study of prevalence in and characteristics of 700 patients. Eur J Heart Fail 2007;9(3):251–7.
4. Javaheri S, Shukla R, Zeigler H, et al. Central sleep apnea, right ventricular dysfunction, and low diastolic blood pressure are predictors of mortality in systolic heart failure. J Am Coll Cardiol 2007; 49(20):2028–34.
5. Chan J, Sanderson J, Chan W, et al. Prevalence of sleep-disordered breathing in diastolic heart failure. Chest 1997;111(6):1488–93.
6. Sekizuka H, Osada N, Miyake F. Sleep disordered breathing in heart failure patients with reduced versus preserved ejection fraction. Heart Lung Circ 2013;22(2):104–9.

7. Padeletti M, Green P, Mooney AM, et al. Sleep disordered breathing in patients with acutely decompensated heart failure. Sleep Med 2009; 10(3):353–60.

8. Arzt M, Harth M, Luchner A, et al. Enhanced ventilatory response to exercise in patients with chronic heart failure and central sleep apnea. Circulation 2003;107(15):1998–2003.

9. Corra U, Giordano A, Bosimini E, et al. Oscillatory ventilation during exercise in patients with chronic heart failure: clinical correlates and prognostic implications. Chest 2002;121(5):1572–80.

10. Naughton MT, Bradley TD. Sleep apnea in congestive heart failure. Clin Chest Med 1998;19(1):99–113.

11. Javaheri S. A mechanism of central sleep apnea in patients with heart failure. N Engl J Med 1999; 341(13):949–54.

12. Hall MJ, Xie A, Rutherford R, et al. Cycle length of periodic breathing in patients with and without heart failure. Am J Respir Crit Care Med 1996;154(2 Pt 1): 376–81.

13. Yumino D, Redolfi S, Ruttanaumpawan P, et al. Nocturnal rostral fluid shift: a unifying concept for the pathogenesis of obstructive and central sleep apnea in men with heart failure. Circulation 2010; 121(14):1598–605.

14. Atalla A, Carlisle TW, Simonds AK, et al. Sleepiness and activity in heart failure patients with reduced ejection fraction and central sleep-disordered breathing. Sleep Med 2017;34:217–23.

15. Hastings PC, Vazir A, O'Driscoll DM, et al. Symptom burden of sleep-disordered breathing in mild-to-moderate congestive heart failure patients. Eur Respir J 2006;27(4):748–55.

16. Arzt M, Young T, Finn L, et al. Sleepiness and sleep in patients with both systolic heart failure and obstructive sleep apnea. Arch Intern Med 2006; 166(16):1716–22.

17. Vazir A, Dayer M, Hastings PC, et al. Can heart rate variation rule out sleep-disordered breathing in heart failure? Eur Respir J 2006;27(3):571–7.

18. Arzt M, Woehrle H, Oldenburg O, et al. Prevalence and predictors of sleep-disordered breathing in patients with stable chronic heart failure: the SchlaHF registry. JACC Heart Fail 2016;4(2): 116–25.

19. Sin DD, Fitzgerald F, Parker JD, et al. Risk factors for central and obstructive sleep apnea in 450 men and women with congestive heart failure. Am J Respir Crit Care Med 1999;160(4):1101–6.

20. Berry RB, Budhiraja R, Gottlieb DJ, et al. Rules for scoring respiratory events in sleep: update of the 2007 AASM manual for the scoring of sleep and associated events. deliberations of the sleep apnea definitions task force of the American Academy of Sleep Medicine. J Clin Sleep Med 2012; 8(5):597–619.

21. Chesson AL Jr, Ferber RA, Fry JM, et al. The indications for polysomnography and related procedures. Sleep 1997;20(6):423–87.

22. Pinna GD, Robbi E, Pizza F, et al. Can cardiorespiratory polygraphy replace portable polysomnography in the assessment of sleep-disordered breathing in heart failure patients? Sleep Breath 2014;18(3): 475–82.

23. Quintana-Gallego E, Villa-Gil M, Carmona-Bernal C, et al. Home respiratory polygraphy for diagnosis of sleep-disordered breathing in heart failure. Eur Respir J 2004;24(3):443–8.

24. Ward NR, Cowie MR, Rosen SD, et al. Utility of overnight pulse oximetry and heart rate variability analysis to screen for sleep-disordered breathing in chronic heart failure. Thorax 2012;67(11):1000–5.

25. Defaye P, de la Cruz I, Marti-Almor J, et al. A pacemaker transthoracic impedance sensor with an advanced algorithm to identify severe sleep apnea: the DREAM European study. Heart Rhythm 2014;11(5):842–8.

26. Shahar E, Whitney CW, Redline S, et al. Sleep-disordered breathing and cardiovascular disease: cross-sectional results of the sleep heart health study. Am J Respir Crit Care Med 2001;163(1):19–25.

27. Hla KM, Young T, Hagen EW, et al. Coronary heart disease incidence in sleep disordered breathing: the Wisconsin sleep cohort study. Sleep 2015; 38(5):677–84.

28. Wang H, Parker JD, Newton GE, et al. Influence of obstructive sleep apnea on mortality in patients with heart failure. J Am Coll Cardiol 2007;49(15): 1625–31.

29. Ohmura T, Iwama Y, Kasai T, et al. Impact of predischarge nocturnal pulse oximetry (sleep-disordered breathing) on postdischarge clinical outcomes in hospitalized patients with left ventricular systolic dysfunction after acute decompensated heart failure. Am J Cardiol 2014;113(4):697–700.

30. Oldenburg O, Faber L, Vogt J, et al. Influence of cardiac resynchronisation therapy on different types of sleep disordered breathing. Eur J Heart Fail 2007; 9(8):820–6.

31. Kato M, Roberts-Thomson P, Phillips BG, et al. Impairment of endothelium-dependent vasodilation of resistance vessels in patients with obstructive sleep apnea. Circulation 2000;102(21):2607–10.

32. Punjabi NM, Polotsky VY. Disorders of glucose metabolism in sleep apnea. J Appl Physiol (1985) 2005; 99(5):1998–2007.

33. Born J, Lange T, Hansen K, et al. Effects of sleep and circadian rhythm on human circulating immune cells. J Immunol 1997;158(9):4454–64.

34. Meier-Ewert HK, Ridker PM, Rifai N, et al. Effect of sleep loss on C-reactive protein, an inflammatory marker of cardiovascular risk. J Am Coll Cardiol 2004;43(4):678–83.

35. Somers VK, Dyken ME, Clary MP, et al. Sympathetic neural mechanisms in obstructive sleep apnea. J Clin Invest 1995;96(4):1897–904.

36. Malone S, Liu PP, Holloway R, et al. Obstructive sleep apnoea in patients with dilated cardiomyopathy: effects of continuous positive airway pressure. Lancet 1991;338(8781):1480–4.

37. Oliveira W, Campos O, Bezerra Lira-Filho E, et al. Left atrial volume and function in patients with obstructive sleep apnea assessed by real-time three-dimensional echocardiography. J Am Soc Echocardiogr 2008;21(12):1355–61.

38. Kim SH, Cho GY, Shin C, et al. Impact of obstructive sleep apnea on left ventricular diastolic function. Am J Cardiol 2008;101(11):1663–8.

39. Vazir A, Hastings PC, Morrell MJ, et al. Resolution of central sleep apnoea following implantation of a left ventricular assist device. Int J Cardiol 2010;138(3): 317–9.

40. Araghi MH, Chen YF, Jagielski A, et al. Effectiveness of lifestyle interventions on obstructive sleep apnea (OSA): systematic review and meta-analysis. Sleep 2013;36(10):1553–62, 1562A–E.

41. Pinna GD, Robbi E, La Rovere MT, et al. Differential impact of body position on the severity of disordered breathing in heart failure patients with obstructive vs. central sleep apnoea. Eur J Heart Fail 2015; 17(12):1302–9.

42. Engleman HM, Martin SE, Deary IJ, et al. Effect of continuous positive airway pressure treatment on daytime function in sleep apnoea/hypopnoea syndrome. Lancet 1994;343(8897):572–5.

43. Pepperell JC, Maskell NA, Jones DR, et al. A randomized controlled trial of adaptive ventilation for Cheyne-Stokes breathing in heart failure. Am J Respir Crit Care Med 2003;168(9):1109–14.

44. Pepperell JC, Ramdassingh-Dow S, Crosthwaite N, et al. Ambulatory blood pressure after therapeutic and subtherapeutic nasal continuous positive airway pressure for obstructive sleep apnoea: a randomised parallel trial. Lancet 2002;359(9302):204–10.

45. Marin JM, Carrizo SJ, Vicente E, et al. Long-term cardiovascular outcomes in men with obstructive sleep apnoea-hypopnoea with or without treatment with continuous positive airway pressure: an observational study. Lancet 2005;365(9464):1046–53.

46. Kaneko Y, Floras JS, Usui K, et al. Cardiovascular effects of continuous positive airway pressure in patients with heart failure and obstructive sleep apnea. N Engl J Med 2003;348(13):1233–41.

47. Mansfield DR, Gollogly NC, Kaye DM, et al. Controlled trial of continuous positive airway pressure in obstructive sleep apnea and heart failure. Am J Respir Crit Care Med 2004;169(3):361–6.

48. Damy T, Margarit L, Noroc A, et al. Prognostic impact of sleep-disordered breathing and its treatment with nocturnal ventilation for chronic heart failure. Eur J Heart Fail 2012;14(9):1009–19.

49. Javaheri S, Caref EB, Chen E, et al. Sleep apnea testing and outcomes in a large cohort of Medicare beneficiaries with newly diagnosed heart failure. Am J Respir Crit Care Med 2011;183(4): 539–46.

50. Tkacova R, Liu PP, Naughton MT, et al. Effect of continuous positive airway pressure on mitral regurgitant fraction and atrial natriuretic peptide in patients with heart failure. J Am Coll Cardiol 1997; 30(3):739–45.

51. Bradley TD, Logan AG, Kimoff RJ, et al. Continuous positive airway pressure for central sleep apnea and heart failure. N Engl J Med 2005;353(19):2025–33.

52. Arzt M, Floras JS, Logan AG, et al. Suppression of central sleep apnea by continuous positive airway pressure and transplant-free survival in heart failure: a post hoc analysis of the Canadian continuous positive airway pressure for patients with central sleep apnea and heart failure trial (CANPAP). Circulation 2007;115(25):3173–80.

53. Cowie MR, Woehrle H, Wegscheider K, et al. Adaptive servo-ventilation for central sleep apnea in systolic heart failure. N Engl J Med 2015; 373(12):1095–105.

54. Naughton MT. Cheyne-Stokes respiration: friend or foe? Thorax 2012;67(4):357–60.

55. Bitter T, Westerheide N, Faber L, et al. Adaptive servoventilation in diastolic heart failure and Cheyne-Stokes respiration. Eur Respir J 2010;36(2):385–92.

56. Yoshihisa A, Suzuki S, Yamaki T, et al. Impact of adaptive servo-ventilation on cardiovascular function and prognosis in heart failure patients with preserved left ventricular ejection fraction and sleep-disordered breathing. Eur J Heart Fail 2013;15(5): 543–50.

57. Nakao YM, Ueshima K, Yasuno S, et al. Effects of nocturnal oxygen therapy in patients with chronic heart failure and central sleep apnea: CHF-HOT study. Heart Vessels 2016;31(2):165–72.

58. Jagielski D, Ponikowski P, Augostini R, et al. Transvenous stimulation of the phrenic nerve for the treatment of central sleep apnoea: 12 months' experience with the remede((R)) system. Eur J Heart Fail 2016;18(11):1386–93.

59. Javaheri S, Sands SA, Edwards BA. Acetazolamide attenuates Hunter-Cheyne-Stokes breathing but augments the hypercapnic ventilatory response in patients with heart failure. Ann Am Thorac Soc 2014;11(1):80–6.

UNITED STATES POSTAL SERVICE ® Statement of Ownership, Management, and Circulation (All Periodicals Publications Except Requester Publications)

1. Publication Title	2. Publication Number	3. Filing Date
HEART FAILURE CLINICS	025 – 055	6/18/2018

4. Issue Frequency	5. Number of Issues Published Annually	6. Annual Subscription Price
JAN, APR, JUL, OCT	4	$252.00

7. Complete Mailing Address of Known Office of Publication (Not printer) (Street, city, county, state, and ZIP+4®)

ELSEVIER INC.
230 Park Avenue, Suite 800
New York, NY 10169

Contact Person
STEPHEN R. BUSHING

Telephone (Include area code)
215-239-3688

8. Complete Mailing Address of Headquarters or General Business Office of Publisher (Not printer)

ELSEVIER INC.
230 Park Avenue, Suite 800
New York, NY 10169

9. Full Names and Complete Mailing Addresses of Publisher, Editor, and Managing Editor (Do not leave blank)

Publisher (Name and complete mailing address)

TAYLOR E. BALL, ELSEVIER INC.
1600 JOHN F KENNEDY BLVD. SUITE 1800
PHILADELPHIA, PA 19103-2899

Editor (Name and complete mailing address)

STACY EASTMAN, ELSEVIER INC.
1600 JOHN F KENNEDY BLVD. SUITE 1800
PHILADELPHIA, PA 19103-2899

Managing Editor (Name and complete mailing address)

PATRICK MANLEY, ELSEVIER INC.
1600 JOHN F KENNEDY BLVD. SUITE 1800
PHILADELPHIA, PA 19103-2899

10. Owner (Do not leave blank. If the publication is owned by a corporation, give the name and address of the corporation immediately followed by the names and addresses of all stockholders owning or holding 1 percent or more of the total amount of stock. If not owned by a corporation, give the names and addresses of the individual owners. If owned by a partnership or other unincorporated firm, give its name and address as well as those of each individual owner. If the publication is published by a nonprofit organization, give its name and address.)

Full Name	Complete Mailing Address
WHOLLY OWNED SUBSIDIARY OF REED/ELSEVIER, US HOLDINGS	1600 JOHN F KENNEDY BLVD. SUITE 1800 PHILADELPHIA, PA 19103-2899

11. Known Bondholders, Mortgagees, and Other Security Holders Owning or Holding 1 Percent or More of Total Amount of Bonds, Mortgages, or Other Securities. If none, check box ▶ ☐ None

Full Name	Complete Mailing Address
N/A	

12. Tax Status (For completion by nonprofit organizations authorized to mail at nonprofit rates) (Check one)
The purpose, function, and nonprofit status of this organization and the exempt status for federal income tax purposes:
☒ Has Not Changed During Preceding 12 Months
☐ Has Changed During Preceding 12 Months (Publisher must submit explanation of change with this statement)

PS Form 3526, July 2014 [Page 1 of 4 (see instructions page 4)] PSN: 7530-01-000-9931 PRIVACY NOTICE: See our privacy policy on www.usps.com.

13. Publication Title		14. Issue Date for Circulation Data Below
HEART FAILURE CLINICS		JULY 2018

15. Extent and Nature of Circulation			Average No. Copies Each Issue During Preceding 12 Months	No. Copies of Single Issue Published Nearest to Filing Date
a. Total Number of Copies (Net press run)			55	91
b. Paid Circulation (By Mail and Outside the Mail)	(1)	Mailed Outside-County Paid Subscriptions Stated on PS Form 3541 (Include paid distribution above nominal rate, advertiser's proof copies, and exchange copies)	16	23
	(2)	Mailed In-County Paid Subscriptions Stated on PS Form 3541 (Include paid distribution above nominal rate, advertiser's proof copies, and exchange copies)	0	0
	(3)	Paid Distribution Outside the Mails Including Sales Through Dealers and Carriers, Street Vendors, Counter Sales, and Other Paid Distribution Outside USPS®	9	13
	(4)	Paid Distribution by Other Classes of Mail Through the USPS (e.g., First-Class Mail®)	0	0
c. Total Paid Distribution (Sum of 15b (1), (2), (3), and (4))		▶	25	36
d. Free or Nominal Rate Distribution (By Mail and Outside the Mail)	(1)	Free or Nominal Rate Outside-County Copies included on PS Form 3541	30	55
	(2)	Free or Nominal Rate In-County Copies Included on PS Form 3541	0	0
	(3)	Free or Nominal Rate Copies Mailed at Other Classes Through the USPS (e.g., First-Class Mail)	0	0
	(4)	Free or Nominal Rate Distribution Outside the Mail (Carriers or other means)	0	0
e. Total Free or Nominal Rate Distribution (Sum of 15d (1), (2), (3) and (4))		▶	30	55
f. Total Distribution (Sum of 15c and 15e)		▶	55	91
g. Copies not Distributed (See Instructions to Publishers #4 (page 43))		▶	0	0
h. Total (Sum of 15f and g)		▶	55	91
i. Percent Paid (15c divided by 15f times 100)		▶	54.55%	39.56%

* If you are claiming electronic copies, go to line 16 on page 3. If you are not claiming electronic copies, skip to line 17 on page 3.

16. Electronic Copy Circulation		Average No. Copies Each Issue During Preceding 12 Months	No. Copies of Single Issue Published Nearest to Filing Date
a. Paid Electronic Copies	▶	0	0
b. Total Paid Print Copies (Line 15c) + Paid Electronic Copies (Line 16a)	▶	30	36
c. Total Print Distribution (Line 15f) + Paid Electronic Copies (Line 16a)	▶	55	91
d. Percent Paid (Both Print & Electronic Copies) (16b divided by 16c × 100)	▶	54.55%	39.56%

☒ I certify that 50% of all my distributed copies (electronic and print) are paid above a nominal price.

17. Publication of Statement of Ownership

☒ If the publication is a general publication, publication of this statement is required. Will be printed in the OCTOBER 2018 issue of this publication. ☐ Publication not required.

18. Signature and Title of Editor, Publisher, Business Manager, or Owner

STEPHEN R. BUSHING – INVENTORY DISTRIBUTION CONTROL MANAGER

Stephen R. Bushing   Date 6/18/2018

I certify that all information furnished on this form is true and complete. I understand that anyone who furnishes false or misleading information on this form or who omits material or information requested on the form may be subject to criminal sanctions (including fines and imprisonment) and/or civil sanctions (including civil penalties).

PS Form 3526, July 2014 (Page 3 of 4)   PRIVACY NOTICE: See our privacy policy on www.usps.com

Moving?

Make sure your subscription moves with you!

To notify us of your new address, find your **Clinics Account Number** (located on your mailing label above your name), and contact customer service at:

Email: journalscustomerservice-usa@elsevier.com

800-654-2452 (subscribers in the U.S. & Canada)
314-447-8871 (subscribers outside of the U.S. & Canada)

Fax number: 314-447-8029

Elsevier Health Sciences Division
Subscription Customer Service
3251 Riverport Lane
Maryland Heights, MO 63043

*To ensure uninterrupted delivery of your subscription, please notify us at least 4 weeks in advance of move.